Autoimmune Diseases in Paediatric Gastroenterology

FALK SYMPOSIUM 127

Autoimmune Diseases in Paediatric Gastroenterology

Edited by

F. Hadziselimovic
Kindertagesklinik
Liestal
Switzerland

Proceedings of Falk Symposium 127 (IV International Falk Symposium on Paediatric Gastroenterology) held in Basel, Switzerland, November 8–9, 2001

KLUWER ACADEMIC PUBLISHERS
DORDRECHT / BOSTON / LONDON

Library of Congress Cataloging-in-Publication Data is available.

ISBN 0–7923–8778–3

Published by Kluwer Academic Publishers, BV
P.O. Box 17, 3300 AA Dordrecht, The Netherlands.

Sold and distributed in North, Central and South America
by Kluwer Academic Publishers,
101 Philip Drive, Norwell, MA 02061, USA.

In all other countries, sold and distributed
by Kluwer Academic Publishers, Distribution Center,
P.O. Box 322, 3300 AH Dordrecht, The Netherlands.

Printed on acid-free paper

Printed and bound in Great Britain by MPG Books, Bodmin, Cornwall.

Contents

List of Principal Contributors

O Alpan
Laboratory of Cell and Molecular Immunology
National Institutes of Health
Bldg 3, Room 1011
900 Rockville Pike
Bethesda, MD 20850
USA

H Bantel
Innere Medizin B
Klinikum der Universität
Albert-Schweitzer-Str. 33
D-48149 Münster
Germany

R Behrens
Pädiatrische Gastroenterologie und Endoskopie
Universitätsklinik und Poliklinik für Kinder und Jugendliche
Loschgestr. 15
D-91054 Erlangen
Germany

Dr DC Belli
Hôpital Cantonal
Pédiatric
Gastroentérologie pédiatrique
Rue Willy Donzé 6
CH-1205 Geneva
Switzerland

CP Braegger
Abt. Gastroenterologie und Ernährung
Universitäts-Kinderklinik
Steinwiesstr. 75
CH-8032 Zürich
Switzerland

M Burdelski
Pädiatrische Gastroenterologie
Universitätsklinkum Hamburg-Eppendorf
Martinistr. 52
D-20246 Hamburg
Germany

J-O Gebbers
Pathologisches Institut
Kantonspital Luzern
CH-6000 Luzern
Switzerland

N Hadzic
Department of Child Health
King's College Hospital
Denmark Hill
London, SE5 9RS
UK

F Hadziselimovic
Kindertagesklinik
Oristalstrasse 87a
CH-4410 Liestal
Switzerland

HK Harms
Dr von Haunersches Kinderspital
Lindwurmstr. 4
D-80337 München
Germany

DS Huff
Department of Pathology
Children's Hospital of Philadelphia
34th Street and Civic Center Boulevard
Philadelphia, PA 19104-4399
USA

A Lanzavecchia
Institute for Research
in Biomedicine
Via Vincenzo Vela 6
CH-6500 Bellinzona
Switzerland

C Le Coultre
Department of Paediatric Surgery
Children's Hospital
HUC 1211
CH-1211 Geneva 14
Switzerland

E Lebenthal
Department of Pediatrics
Mount Scopus Hadassah-Hebrew
University Medical Center
POB 24035
IL-91031 Jerusalem
Israel

U Leuschner
Innere Medizin II
Klinikum der Johann Wolfgang
Goethe-Universität Frankfurt
Theodor-Stern-Kai 7
D-60590 Frankfurt
Germany

A Levine
Pediatric Gastroenterology Service
Edith Wolfson Medical Center
POB 5
IL-58100 Holon
Israel

GR Lichtenstein
Gastroenterology Division
Department of Medicine
University of Pennsylvania
School of Medicine
3rd Floor Ravdin Building
3400 Spruce Street
Philadelphia, PA 19104-4283
USA

G Mieli-Vergani
Institute of Liver Studies
King's College Hospital
London
SE5 9RS
UK

PJ Milla
University of London
Institute of Child Health
30 Guilford Street
London, WC1N 1EH
UK

EL Renner
Abteilung Gastroenterologie
Departement für Innere Medizin
Universitätsspital Zürich
Rämistr. 100
CH-8091 Zürich
Switzerland

M Rössle
Bismarckallee 4
D-79098 Freiburg
Germany

E Seidman
Centre de Recherche, #5736
Hôpital Ste Justine
3175 Côte Ste Catherine Road
Montreal
QC H3T 1C5
Canada

WB Storch
Netztal 32
D-69469 Weinheim
Germany

D Vergani
University College London
Institute of Hepatology
69–75 Chenies Mews
London, WC1E 6HX
UK

AJ Wakefield
Academic Department of Medicine
Royal Free Hospital
School of Medicine
Rowland Hill Street
London, NW3 2PF
UK

Preface

The fourth International Falk Symposium on Paediatric Gastroenterology featured autoimmunity and its significance in paediatric gastroenterology. In all three previous meetings, we focused our attention on the role of the innate immune system in the aetiology of inflammatory bowel disease (IBD). It has become increasingly clear in recent years that the innate system has a much more important and fundamental role in host defence. The decision to initiate an immune response is one of the major roles of the innate system. Mutations within this system could transform it into becoming constitutively active, resulting in an inflammatory reaction and thus eliciting an autoimmune response.

Various autoimmune diseases have been associated with a deficiency of natural killer (NK) cells, important components of the innate immune system. Type 1 diabetes mellitus and scleroderma are but two of the various autoimmune diseases that have been associated with NK deficiency; and, more recently, both IBD and coeliac disease have been implicated.

Following an introduction to the basic phenomena of autoimmunity, the clinical aspects of autoimmune diseases are discussed. In particular, it was intended to present to clinicians the relevant current knowledge, the state of the art so to speak, on the diagnosis and treatment of the autoimmune diseases of the gastrointestinal tract in children.

This book is proffered primarily to paediatric and adult gastroenterologists, and to paediatricians and general practitioners dealing with children with autoimmune diseases of the gut and liver.

F.H.
Kindertagesklinik
Liestal, Switzerland
May 2002

Section I
Autoimmunity of the gastrointestinal tract

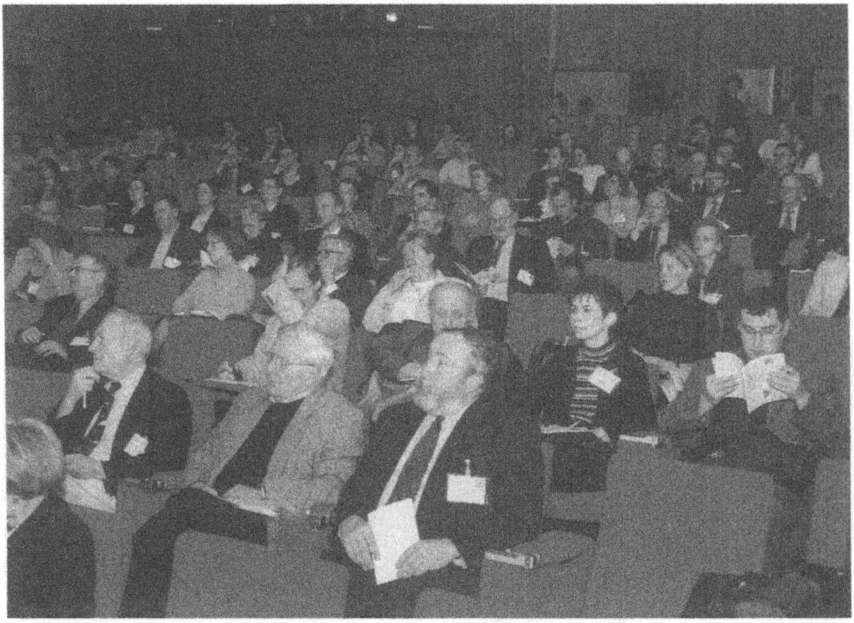

1
From antigen presentation to effector and memory T cells

A. LANZAVECCHIA

The relationship between T lymphocyte differentiation and migration has been studied in mouse and human systems. By stimulating mouse naïve T lymphocytes under defined *in-vitro* conditions, we found that T cells that receive a short antigenic stimulation in the absence of cytokines proliferate but remain *non-effectors* and retain the constitutive expression of the lymph node homing chemokine receptor CCR7. When transferred to syngeneic mice, these cells home to the T cell areas of lymph nodes and spleen and, in response to a secondary antigenic stimulation, proliferate and differentiate to effector cells. In contrast, T cells that receive a prolonged antigenic stimulation in the presence of IL-12 or IL-4 proliferate and differentiate to *effector cells* (type 1 or type 2) and lose CCR7 expression, while acquiring the capacity to home to inflamed peripheral tissues. Importantly, non-effector and effector T cells are present in the human memory pool as distinct populations of $CCR7^+$ '*central memory*' cells (devoid of immediate effector function) and $CCR7^-$ '*effector memory*' cells (endowed with type 1 or type 2 effector function). Memory T cells specific for recall antigens are present in both subsets even several years after priming. I will discuss how the strength of T cell stimulation and the stochastic interactions between antigen-presenting dendritic cells and T cells generate, in the primary immune response, both non-effector and effector cells within single T cell clones. I will also discuss how both cell types can be maintained for a lifetime as long-term memory cells in the absence of antigen.

References

1. Sallusto F, Lenig D, Forster R, Lipp M, Lanzavecchia A. Two subsets of memory T lymphocytes with distinct homing potentials and effector functions. Nature. 1999;401:708–12.
2. Lanzavecchia A, Sallusto F. Dynamics of T lymphocyte responses: intermediates, effectors and memory cells. Science. 2000;290:92–7.
3. Lanzavecchia A, Sallusto F. Regulation of T cell immunity by dendritic cells. Cell. 2001;106: 263–6.

2
Gut-oriented immune responses and oral tolerance to dietary antigens

O. ALPAN

Oral tolerance is an old field of study. It dates back to the early 1980s when R. Dakin questioned the efficacy of the practice of preventing painful skin rashes from poison ivy contact by prior chewing of the leaves of the plant. In history, one can find this practice among American Indians and habitants of Central Asia. Amazingly, this is still practiced today by some patients to prevent recurrences of the skin disease caused by poison ivy. It was not until the early 1900s that the field entered the scientific literature through experiments by Wells *et al.*, who demonstrated that anaphylactic reactions to OVA in guinea pigs could be eliminated by prior feeding of OVA[1]. Chase later described the immunologic nature of this protection in 1946, using contact-sensitizing agents and showing that the effect is antigen specific[2]. Since then, our knowledge of the field has substantially increased and the following review will focus on how oral antigens affect the body's immune system.

IMMUNE ARCHITECTURE OF THE GUT

More that 50% of the immune system is in the gastrointestinal tract in the form of an organized gut-associated lymphoid tissue (GALT) or in the lamina propria and the intraepithelial compartment. The organized GALT includes ~30 000 scattered solitary B-cell follicles and approximately 7–8 large lymphoid cells aggregated along the gut, named as Peyer's patches[3]. Although Peyer's patches resemble lymph nodes, there are several important differences. First is the presence of specialized epithelial M cells within the epithelium that covers the luminal surface of the Peyer's patches. M cells are identified by their sparse and short microvilli, abundant mitochondria, basally oriented nucleus and extensions, which form pockets in which cells of the immune system nestle[4]. They are MHC Class II negative and are thought to function in the transit of micro-organisms and soluble antigens to the underlying lymphoid tissue[4]. Second is the presence of a subepithelial dome, which is rich in lymphoid and immature dendritic cells. The Peyer's patch microenvironment is thought to play a crucial role in the generation of an IgA response against antigens and micro-organisms entering through the gut[5].

Of the lymphoid cells that populate the lamina propria, approximately 60% are B cells that secrete IgA, and the rest is dendritic cells and various populations of T cells. Approximately 95% of these T cells have the $\alpha\beta$ TCR and have an activated phenotype (e.g. expressing IL2R). They make IL-2, IL-4 and IL-5 and low levels of IFN-γ, a cytokine secretion pattern that facilitates the differentiation of B cells into IgA-producing cells[6]. T cells that express $\gamma\delta$ TCR has been shown to be important in intestinal IgA responses since mice lacking these cells fail to produce secretory IgA to mucosal vaccination using cholera toxin or tetanus toxoid[7]. In the layer above the lamina propria, intraepithelial lymphocytes (IEL) constitute the first immune cell line of defence in the gut.

LOCAL EFFECTS OF INGESTED ANTIGEN

The majority of the ingested antigen is broken down by stomach acidity before it reaches the duodenum. This digestion continues as proteins enter the small intestine within the alkaline environment. Therefore, only a very small fraction of intact antigen becomes available for absorption and can gain access to the mesenteric lymphatics and the blood stream. The initial response to dietary antigen is the production of IgA[8]. The IgA-secreting B cells are generated in the germinal centres throughout the gut and transfer IgA into the gut lumen with the aid of secretory piece via the epithelial cells that line the villi. Although IgA has been long thought to function by binding and preventing the absorption of intact antigens and micro-organisms, its demonstration in the M cells as antigen–antibody complex, raises the possibility of re-entering into the body through these cells. The precise mechanism of how the antigen becomes available to B cells to produce antibodies is still not known. It could go through or between epithelial cells or it can use the M cell. In mice, milk-borne retroviruses exclusively use the M cell to gain entry since mice that lack M cells cannot be infected via the gut[9]. Alternatively, Salmonella can gain entry both via the M cell or by CD18-positive dendritic cells that crawl between epithelial cells to pick up luminal pathogens[10]. Protein antigens possibly do not use M cells as the sole route of entry since, in their absence, they can enter even more efficiently[11].

SYSTEMIC EFFECT OF INGESTED ANTIGEN

Besides the local effect, fed antigen can have a systemic effect on the immune response. Systemically, the typical response to fed antigen is characterized by a decrease in both delayed type hypersensitivity (DTH) and T-helper cell proliferation upon a subsequent immunization with the same antigen[12]. Other characteristics of the systemic T-cell response depend on the dose of fed antigen. High doses can lead to deletion of the antigen-specific T cells within Peyer's patches[13] whereas low doses can lead to a state in which the immune response has switched from the production of a DTH/Th1 response to the production of Th2/Th3 type responses and, in some cases, the production of IgA[14]. In addition,

T cells from animals fed low doses can be adoptively transferred to depress the DTH and proliferative responses of normal naive recipients. In the original host, fed T cells have suppressive bystander effects on DTH responses to new antigens when given together in an immunization with the original fed antigen. Both the transferable suppression and the bystander effect have been associated with Th3 cells producing TGF-β, as well as with Th2 cells that produce IL-4 and IL-10, though subsequent high-dose feeding may change these characteristics. Thus the response to fed antigen, whether called 'oral vaccination' (because it produces IgA and protects against pathogens) or 'oral tolerance' (because it reduces systemic DTH responses and ameliorates the symptoms of experimental autoimmune diseases), appears to differ in well-defined characteristics from responses induced at other sites[14].

WHAT REGULATES GUT-ORIENTED IMMUNITY?

The intestinal environment might influence an immune response in several ways. First, the cells of the gut itself produce TGF-β, vasoactive intestinal peptide (which controls the secretory piece of IgA) and other immunologically relevant molecules. Second, dendritic cells within the gut may serve as a specialized set of APCs to induce tolerance to or drive immune responses towards particular effector classes. To test whether the dendritic cells of the gut play a role in inducing a gut-oriented immune response, we fed pigeon cytochrome C (PCC) to B10.A mice by adding it to their drinking water, harvested the mesenteric lymph nodes (MLNs) on day 4, and purified the $CD11c^+$ dendritic cells by positive selection using magnetic columns[14]. We then irradiated these dendritic cells and used them as APCs *in vitro* for a monoclonal population of naive TCR Tg T cells specific for PCC (5CC7 TCR Tg bred onto a B10.A $Rag2^{-/-}$ background), and compared them with APCs from the MLN of unfed mice or from popliteal nodes (pLN) from mice immunized in the footpads to pigeon cytochrome C or from control mice. MLN dendritic cells from the fed mice induced the naive T cells to make higher levels of IL-4 and IL-10 and less IFN-γ than did APCs from control mice or APCs draining a peripheral site injected with PCC. In contrast, APCs from the popliteal lymph nodes of mice injected at the footpad with PCC induced strong IFN-γ production, low level IL-10 production and no IL-4.

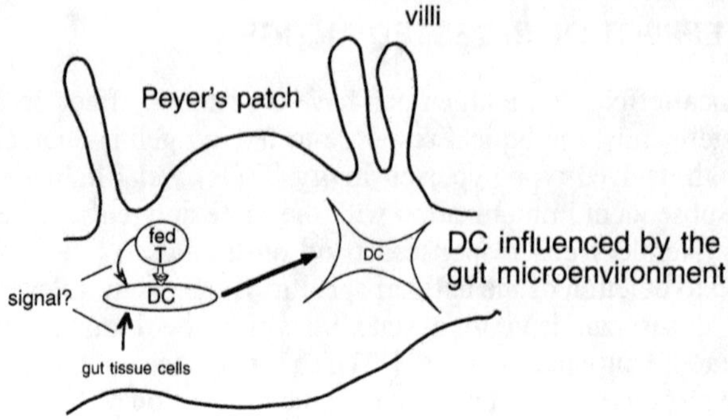

Various cells in the gut could be responsible for inducing gut-oriented immune responses. Gut epithelial cells are unlikely candidates. Although these express MHC Class II constitutively,[15] they are not professional APCs[16] and should therefore induce deletion rather than activation of T cells. They are thus apt to be involved in the antigen-specific deletion of T cells that occurs after high-dose administration of oral antigen. This leaves us with macrophages and DCs. The observation that oral tolerance is enhanced by *in-vivo* treatment with Flt3 ligand (which expands the number of DCs) supports the view that, as with other responses, the immune response to oral antigens is most likely initiated by dendritic cells[17].

But the initiation of the response is not the whole story. Gut-oriented immune responses are characterized by a particular class of effector function, such as IgA, TGF-β, IL-4 and IL-10, that are known alternatively as oral tolerance or immune deviation. What gives rise to these qualities? The gut-oriented immune response is neither tolerance nor deviation. It is simply an immune response tailored to the environment of the gut, which has specific immunological needs (the production of IgA) as well as certain sensitivities (it can be harmed by a DTH response[18]. In these respects, it is similar to the eye[19]. To protect itself, and to ensure that a local immune response is nevertheless effective, the gut suppresses DTH responses and enhances IgA production. It appears that it may not do this through specialized antigen handling, nor through cytokines produced by B or M cells, but via the conditioning (or education) of DCs.

It has recently been shown that DCs from naive Peyer's patches induce T cells to make IL-6, IL-10 and IL-4, but only very low levels of IFN-γ *in vitro*[20], suggesting that the effector class of the local Peyer's patch response may be controlled by the resident DCs. Our data show that the systemic T-cell response to fed antigen might also be influenced by DCs, but regulated at a different lymph node rather than the Peyer's patches. We have demonstrated that DCs from the MLNs of fed animals had the startling capacity to elicit IL-4 production from naive T cells in primary cultures. They also induced high secondary levels of TGF-β, but little IFN-γ, whereas DCs from the MLN of mice that were not fed antigen did not elicit these responses[14]. The fed DCs are equally active at inducing this Th2/Th3 response regardless of whether they were derived from WT animals or from those lacking B cells, M cells and Peyer's patches. Thus DCs draining the gut of antigen-fed animals seem to carry class-specific instructions with them regardless of the existence of an organized GALT microenvironment.

It is not know whether the MLN DCs are a separate population or whether they are influenced by local signals as they traffic through the gut. It has been shown in other systems that the effector function of DCs can be altered by interactions with helper T cells[21] or by signals, such as PGE2[22] which is produced by many different tissues. We think, therefore, that the most likely scenario is that gut-oriented immune responses, like those occurring elsewhere, are initiated by activated local professional APCs, such as dendritic cells, and that resident T cells in the gut, or the cells of the gut itself, set the effector class by educating the DC, as well as by producing such immunomodulatory cytokines as TGF-β and VIP. In this way, a tissue may control several aspects of a response. It initiates the response by sending danger signals to activate local APCs[23] and it also influences the class of response in order to enhance efficacy and to ensure its own safety.

References

1. Wells PW, Pass DA, Eyre P. Acute systemic immediate hypersensitivity in the pig. Res Vet Sci. 1974;16:347–50.
2. Faria AM, Weiner HL. Oral tolerance: mechanisms and therapeutic applications. Adv Immunol. 1999;73:153–264.
3. Zarzaur BL, Kudsk KA. The mucosa-associated lymphoid tissue structure, function, and derangements. Shock. 2001;15:411–20.
4. Neutra MR, Mantis NJ, Kraehenbuhl JP. Collaboration of epithelial cells with organized mucosal lymphoid tissues. Nat Immunol. 2001;11:1004–9.
5. Hein WR. Organization of mucosal lymphoid tissue. Curr Top Microbiol Immunol. 1999;236: 1–15.
6. MacDonald TT. Effector and regulatory lymphoid cells and cytokines in mucosal sites. Curr Top Microbiol Immunol. 1999;236:113–35.
7. Fujihashi K, McGhee JR, Kweon MN *et al.* Gamma/delta T cell-deficient mice have impaired mucosal immunoglobulin A responses. J Exp Med. 1996,183:1929–35.
8. Richman LK, Graeff AS, Yarchoan R, Strober W. Simultaneous induction of antigen-specific IgA helper T cells and IgG suppressor T cells in the murine Peyer's patch after protein feeding. J Immunol. 1981;126:2079–83.
9. Golovkina TV, Shlomchik M, Hannum L, Chervonsky A. Organogenic role of B lymphocytes in mucosal immunity. Science. 1999;286:1965–8.
10. Neutra MR, Pringault E, Kraehenbuhl JP. Antigen sampling across epithelial barriers and induction of mucosal immune responses. Annu Rev Immunol. 1996;14:275–300.
11. Gonnella PA, Waldner HP, Weiner HL. B cell-deficient (mu MT) mice have alterations in the cytokine microenvironment of the gut-associated lymphoid tissue (GALT) and a defect in the low dose mechanism of oral tolerance. J Immunol. 2001;166:4456–64.
12. Weiner HL. Oral tolerance: immune mechanisms and treatment of autoimmune diseases. Immunol Today. 1997;7:335–44.
13. Chen Y, Inobe J, Reinhard M, Gonella P, Kuchroo YJ, Weiner HL. Peripheral deletion of antigen-reactive T cells in oral tolerance. Nature. 1995;376:177–80.
14. Alpan O, Rudomen G, Matzinger P. The role of dendritic cells, B cells, and M cells in gut-oriented immune responses. J Immunol. 2001;166:4843–52.
15. Farstad IN, Halstensen TS, Fausa O, Brandtzaeg P. Heterogeneity of M cell associated B and T cells in human Peyer's patches. Immunology. 1994;66:457–64.
16. Bland PW, Whiting CV. Differential control of major histocompatibility complex class II I-Ek alpha protein expression in the epithelium and in subsets of lamina propria antigen-presenting cells of the gut. Immunology. 1993;79:107–11.
17. Viney JL, Mowat AM, O'Malley JM, Williamson E, Fanger NA. Expanding dendritic cells *in vivo* enhances the induction of oral tolerance. J Immunol. 1998;160:5815–25.
18. Strober W, James SP. The immunopathogenesis of gastrointestinal and hepatobiliary diseases. J Am Med Assoc. 1987;258:2962–9.
19. Streilein JW. Regional immunity and ocular immune privilege. Chem Immunol. 1999;73:11–38.
20. Everson MP, Lemak DG, McDuffie DS, Koopman WJ, McGhee JR, Beagley KW. Dendritic cells from Peyer's patch and spleen induce different T helper cell responses. J Inter Cyto Res. 1998;18:103–15.
21. Ridge JP, Di Rosa F, Matzinger P. A conditioned dendritic cell can be a temporal bridge between a CD4+ T-helper and a T-killer cell. Nature. 1998;393:474–8.
22. Kalinski P, Schuitemaker JH, Hilkens CM, Kapsenberg ML. Prostaglandin E2 induces the final maturation of IL-12-deficient CD1a+CD83+ dendritic cells: the levels of IL-12 are determined during the final dendritic cell maturation and are resistant to further modulation. J Immunol. 1998;161:2804–9.
23. Matzinger P. An innate sense of danger. Semin Immunol. 1998;10:399–415.

3
Role of molecular mimicry in viral and autoimmune liver disease

D. VERGANI, K. CHOUDHURI, D. P. BOGDANOS and G. MIELI-VERGANI

INTRODUCTION

The immune system has evolved to discriminate between endogenous or 'self' tissues and exogenous and neoplastic components collectively termed 'non-self'. A dominant selective pressure in this process has been the threat to self-integrity posed by infectious pathogens. The virtually infinite antigenic variety of pathogens that the immune system must respond to has resulted in an innate set of responses, that allow the triggering of immunity to commonly encountered pathogens, and an adaptive system, that adopts an anticipatory approach in responding to more antigenically exotic or complex challenges.

The central problem for the adaptive immune system is to generate T- and B-lymphocytes, its two most important components that can specifically recognize a potentially infinite number of non-self antigens without any prior information as to their structure. This is achieved by randomly generating a large number of T- and B-cell specificities (via their respective antigen receptors – the T-cell receptor (TCR) and the antibody) that are then able to clonally expand and recruit effector mechanisms on recognition of their specific antigen. It is, however, becoming clear that even this system cannot cope with the extent of non-self antigenic diversity, and, in the past decade, convincing evidence for crossreactivity as an inherent property of immune ontogeny has emerged. This has been studied primarily in the context of T-lymphocytes, where it is clear that altered peptide ligands (APL), peptides similar in structure to the peptide antigen which are initially encountered, are able to induce both stimulatory and inhibitory T-cell responses and, indeed, endogenous APLs operate in selecting the T-cell repertoire in the thymus[1]. This implies that a single T-cell, rather than responding to a single antigen specificity, is able to crossreactively respond to a number of antigens, thus expanding the antigenic specificities of the immune system to a level that reflects the antigenic diversity of the external environment.

MOLECULAR MIMICRY

This inherent potential for crossreactivity, whilst allowing efficient responses to a vast array of pathogens, also imbues the immune system with the potential to crossreact with self, leading to autoimmunity. This concept has been termed 'molecular mimicry', where immune responses to external pathogens become directed towards structurally similar self components[2]. Molecular mimicry has been demonstrated to be a dominant mechanism in the pathogenesis of autoimmune disease both in experimental models and in the human setting at the level of both T- and B-cells[3–6]. We and others have described immunological crossreactivity between pathogen and self to operate in the aetiopathogenesis of auto-immune liver disease and autoimmunity associated with chronic viral hepatitis[7–12].

LIVER–KIDNEY MICROSOMAL TYPE 1 ANTIBODIES AND MOLECULAR MIMICRY

Autoimmune hepatitis type 2 (AIH2) is characterized by seropositivity for liver–kidney microsomal type 1 (LKM1) antibody[13]. The target of this autoantibody is cytochrome P4502D6, a member of the hepatic P450 enzyme family[14]. Due to the very strong association between LKM1 antibodies and AIH2, and in view of a recent report demonstrating surface expression of CYP2D6 on hepatocytes (rendering them amenable to recognition by these antibodies), LKM1 antibodies are thought to be involved in the pathogenesis of AIH2[15]. Intriguingly, LKM1 antibodies are also found in up to 10% of patients with hepatitis C virus (HCV) infection, and appear to correlate with increased disease severity and adverse reactions to IFN treatment[16]. Moreover, a minority of LKM1+ AIH2 patients are also infected with HCV, although the significance of HCV infection in this setting is unclear[17]. There are important clinical reasons for differentiating those with LKM1+ AIH2 and those with LKM1+ HCV infection, as immunosuppression, the first line treatment for AIH2, may be harmful if administered to patients infected with HCV[18]. Conversely, IFN may potentiate autoimmune disease if administered to patients with autoimmune hepatitis[19].

LKM1 antibodies recognize linear regions of CYP2D6 in a hierarchical manner in AIH2. The principal linear B-cell epitope, $CYP2D6_{257–269}$, is recognized by 85% of patients, $CYP2D6_{321–351}$ by 53% of patients, and two additional minor epitopes, $CYP2D6_{373–389}$ and $CYP2D6_{410–429}$, recognized by 7% and 13% respectively[20]. In addition, we have identified $CYP2D6_{193–212}$ as a major B-cell epitope recognized by 93% of patients with AIH2 and 50% of those with LKM1+ HCV infection[6]. This is in a partial agreement with Klein *et al.* who described reactivity to $CYP2D6_{196–218}$ in 68% of patients with AIH2 but in only 18% of the LKM1+ HCV-infected patients[21]. We further demonstrated crossreactive antibody recognition of homologous regions of HCV (NS5B $HCV_{2985–2990}$) and CMV (EXON $CMV_{130–135}$) antigens in LKM+ HCV-infected patients recognizing CYP2D6 ($CYP2D6_{204–209}$). Others have also invoked crossreactive mechanisms to explain the aetiology of LKM1 antibodies. Manns *et al.* suggested that reactivity to the major epitope of CYP2D6 recognized by LKM1 antibodies may arise through a crossreactive response to HCV or HSV, as the aa 310–324 of E1 HCV and aa 156–170 of IE175 HSV1 share sequence homology with the immunodominant region, aa 254–271, of CYP2D6[11]. Although attractive, there has been little experimental evidence to support this hypothesis. We have recently demonstrated highly specific simultaneous antibody reactivity to both $CYP2D6_{254-271}$ and E1 $HCV_{310-324}$ in LKM1+ HCV-infected patients[6]. Competition studies suggest this 'double-reactivity' to be crossreactive (Bogdanos *et al.*, manuscript in preparation).

MULTI-HIT HYPOTHESIS

As LKM1 antibodies appear to crossreact with homologous regions of CYP2D6, HCV and HSV, and CMV, a 'multi-hit' mechanism for the generation of these antibodies and possibly AIH2 may be envisaged. In this model, multiple exposures to CMV or HSV, common viral pathogen, may establish permissive immunological conditions, by priming a crossreactive subset of T-cells, in the genetically predisposed host. Chronic infection with HCV may then provide the final impetus for the generation of LKM1 autoantibodies through crossreactive mechanisms. Depending on the degree of immunological priming, the degree of genetic susceptibility (particularly at the HLA locus and coding regions for 'innate' components of immunity), and antigenic dose of the infecting pathogens, a minority of individuals may progress to autoimmune disease. It is therefore conceivable that an as-yet-unknown virus infection may be at the origin of the autoimmune attack in AIH, in agreement with the concept expressed by Rolf Zinkernagel that an autoimmune disease is a viral disease in which the virus is unknown[22].

OTHER EXAMPLES OF MOLECULAR MIMICRY

Aspects of this model are not without precedent as, in rheumatic carditis, multiple exposure to group A streptococcus leads to a spectrum of immunological responses based on molecular mimicry between pathogen and cardiac myosin and laminin[23]. Multiple exposure to this pathogen in the susceptible host leads to progressive valvular damage mediated by crossreactive antibodies. Neither does the initial pathogenic insult need to be closely temporally related to the manifestation of autoimmune disease. This is well illustrated in Chagas' disease caused by the *Trypanosoma cruzi*. Acute infection with *T. cruzi* causes a transient myocarditis which resolves completely. Decades later, an autoimmune myocarditis, histologically characterized by mononuclear cell infiltration, in the absence of detectable parasites, develops in the susceptible host, leading eventually to dilated cardiomyopathy. Molecular mimicry between the B13 antigen of *T. cruzi* and cardiac myocytes is thought to be responsible for the development of the autoimmune response[24]. This system illustrates the 'hit and run' model for the development of autoimmunity following infection[2]. These models taken together provide conceptual insights into mechanisms that may operate in leading to autoimmunity and autoimmune liver disease[6,9].

References

1. Sloan-Lancaster J, Allen PM. Altered peptide ligand-induced partial T cell activation: molecular mechanisms and role in T cell biology. Annu Rev Immunol. 1996;14:1–27.
2. Oldstone MB. Molecular mimicry and immune-mediated diseases. Faseb J. 1998;12:1255–65.
3. Wucherpfennig KW, Strominger JL. Molecular mimicry in T cell-mediated autoimmunity: viral peptides activate human T cell clones specific for myelin basic protein. Cell. 1995;80:695–705.
4. Gross DM, Forsthuber T, Tary-Lehmann M *et al.* Identification of LFA-1 as a candidate autoantigen in treatment-resistant Lyme arthritis. Science. 1998;281:703–6.
5. Zhao ZS, Granucci F, Yeh L, Schaffer PA, Cantor H. Molecular mimicry by herpes simplex virus-type 1: autoimmune disease after viral infection. Science. 1998;279:1344–7.
6. Bogdanos DP, Choudhuri K, Vergani D. Molecular mimicry and autoimmune liver disease: virtuous intentions, malign consequences. Liver. 2001;21:225–32.
7. Gregorio GV, Choudhuri K, Ma Y, Vegnente A, Mieli-Vergani G, Vergani D. Mimicry between the hepatitis B virus DNA polymerase and the antigenic targets of nuclear and smooth muscle antibodies in chronic hepatitis B virus infection. J Immunol. 1999;162:1802–10.
8. Choudhuri K, Gregorio GV, Mieli-Vergani G, Vergani D. Immunological cross-reactivity to multiple autoantigens in patients with liver kidney microsomal type 1 autoimmune hepatitis. Hepatology. 1998;28:1177–81.
9. Bogdanos DP, Mieli-Vergani G, Vergani D. Virus, liver and autoimmunity. Dig Liver Dis. 2000; 32:440–6.
10. Shimoda S, Nakamura M, Ishibashi H, Hayashida K, Niho Y. HLA DRB4 0101-restricted immunodominant T cell autoepitope of pyruvate dehydrogenase complex in primary biliary cirrhosis: evidence of molecular mimicry in human autoimmune diseases. J Exp Med. 1995;181: 1835–45.
11. Manns MP, Griffin KJ, Sullivan KF, Johnson EF. LKM-1 autoantibodies recognize a short linear sequence in P450IID6, a cytochrome P-450 monooxygenase. J Clin Invest. 1991;88:1370–8.
12. Kammer AR, van der Burg SH, Grabscheid B *et al.* Molecular mimicry of human cytochrome P450 by hepatitis C virus at the level of cytotoxic T cell recognition. J Exp Med. 1999;190: 169–76.
13. Homberg JC, Abuaf N, Bernard O *et al.* Chronic active hepatitis associated with antiliver/kidney microsome antibody type 1: a second type of 'autoimmune' hepatitis. Hepatology. 1987;7: 1333–9.
14. Gueguen M, Meunier-Rotival M, Bernard O, Alvarez F. Anti-liver kidney microsome antibody recognizes a cytochrome P450 from the IID subfamily. J Exp Med. 1988;168:801–6.
15. Muratori L, Parola M, Ripalti A *et al.* Liver/kidney microsomal antibody type 1 targets CYP2D6 on hepatocyte plasma membrane. Gut. 2000;46:553–61.
16. Vergani D. LKM antibody: getting in some target practice. Gut. 2000;46:449–50.
17. Lenzi M, Ballardini G, Fusconi M *et al.* Type 2 autoimmune hepatitis and hepatitis C virus infection. Lancet. 1990;335:258–9.
18. Muratori L, Lenzi M, Cataleta M *et al.* Interferon therapy in liver/kidney microsomal antibody type 1-positive patients with chronic hepatitis C. J Hepatol. 1994;21:199–203.
19. Vergani D, Mieli-Vergani G. Type II autoimmune hepatitis: the conundrum of cytochrome P450IID6. Clin Exp Immunol. 1993;92:367–8.
20. Yamamoto AM, Cresteil D, Boniface O, Clerc FF, Alvarez F. Identification and analysis of cytochrome P450IID6 antigenic sites recognized by anti-liver–kidney microsome type-1 antibodies (LKM1). Eur J Immunol. 1993;23:1105–11.
21. Klein R, Zanger UM, Berg T, Hopf U, Berg PA. Overlapping but distinct specificities of anti-liver–kidney microsome antibodies in autoimmune hepatitis type II and hepatitis C revealed by recombinant native CYP2D6 and novel peptide epitopes. Clin Exp Immunol. 1999;118:290–7.
22. Aichele P, Bachmann MF, Hengartner H, Zinkernagel RM. Immunopathology or organ-specific autoimmunity as a consequence of virus infection. Immunol Rev. 1996;152:21–45.
23. Galvin JE, Hemric ME, Ward K, Cunningham MW. Cytotoxic mAb from rheumatic carditis recognizes heart valves and laminin. J Clin Invest. 2000;106:217–24.
24. Cunha-Neto E, Coelho V, Guilherme L, Fiorelli A, Stolf N, Kalil J. Autoimmunity in Chagas' disease. Identification of cardiac myosin-B13 Trypanosoma cruzi protein crossreactive T cell clones in heart lesions of a chronic Chagas' cardiomyopathy patient. J Clin Invest. 1996;98: 1709–12.

4 Autoantibodies in autoimmune hepatitis

W. B. STORCH

With regard to the general and specific significance of autoantibodies in autoimmune hepatitis, beliefs in the 20th century can be divided into three periods:

1. 1900–approx. 1950: Non-existence, better: non-acceptance of autoantibodies.
2. 1950–approx. 1975: Autoantibodies exist; they express, however, a pathological process.
3. Since approx. 1975: Autoantibodies are ubiquitous. They are present in healthy and sick people. Therefore, they are deemed to be predominantly physiological in nature.

Period 1. As early as in 1908, Fiessinger[1] suspected autoantibodies to be a pathogenetic principle of chronic liver diseases. However, these findings were described only in a doctoral dissertation. Paul Ehrlich's dogma of 'horror autotoxicus'[2] seems to have prevented their publication in a journal.

Period 2. At the beginning of the 1950s, the existence of autoantibodies, in particular of antibodies against thyroglobulin[3], was indisputably proven, e.g. by Roitt, Doniach and colleagues[3]. Nevertheless, autoantibodies were still regarded as an expression (cause or consequence) of a pathological process. This may be explained, on the one hand, by the still prevailing impact of 'horror autotoxicus' and, on the other hand, by the influence of Burnet's clonal selection theory (the latter was based on the assumption that 'self-reacting clones' cannot survive the embryonal period). Thus, there was the idea that the existence or development of autoantibodies against thyroglobulin could be explained by the assumption that thyroglobulin had no access to the immune system during the embryonal period, so that 'self-reacting clones' could not be removed and autoantibodies could develop. This hypothesis continued to prevail up to the fourth quarter of the 20th century, partly even up till now, though modified on the basis of so-called forbidden clones or break of tolerance.

Period 3. Since the end of the 1960s, we have found several types of autoantibodies in nearly all humans, whether healthy or ill, and we believed and continue to believe that autoimmunity in general and the majority of autoantibodies are physiological (and necessary) at least in view of the organism's integrity. This idea is increasingly gaining acceptance, particularly after inauguration of the term 'autogene' (in analogy to oncogene)[4]; but also since the existence of so-called 'natural autoantibodies' has been proved and accepted[5,6].

Thus, the attitude of the medical community towards autoantibodies depends on the respective point of view and the predominant school of thought. Let me discuss the problem with help of a black-and-white painting by the artist M. C. Escher. In his picture, Escher was able to link the complementarity of Angel and Devil. The Devil (painted in black) represents the bad, i.e. the pathological, pathogenetic principle, while the Angel (painted in white) symbolizes the good, protecting or helpful principle. From a teleological view of the problem, we must also consider a third possibility: indifferent, insignificant and trivial things. Thus, a so-called epiphenomenon may also be present. Grabar pointed out this fact as early as in the 1950s when he highlighted the clearing function of autoantibodies.

Therefore, considering the great variety of detectable autoantibodies, we should assess their respective relevance for the individual case. Meanwhile, the diagnostic value of autoantibodies is beyond doubt. In fact, diseases are increasingly defined and classified according to the presence of autoantibodies. It also does not matter at all whether one uses the term diagnostic aid, expression, marker, witness, indicator, or reporter of an autoimmune process. We have already very early pointed to the fact that autoantibodies can be very helpful for diagnosis, e.g. of autoimmune hepatitis, if several parameters are employed (Table 1, from Reference 7). These criteria were recently mentioned in a somewhat modified form[8].

In cases of autoimmune hepatitis, too, a multitude of autoantibodies may be involved. Table 2 (see also Reference 9) contains a selection of them in chronological order. Based on this table, let me discuss early and recent findings, although special attention will be paid only to the exact type of autoantibodies, e.g. to the fluorescence pattern observed.

Table 1 Parameters for assessing the diagnostic relevance of autoantibodies

1. Exact autoantibody type.
2. Titre (the amount of autoantibodies circulating in the serum).
3. Reaction with autogenous material to be examined (the presence of a real autoantibody is more probable if it also reacts with autogenous tissue).
4. Uniformity of evidence in repeated tests, possibly depending on the course of the disease or therapy.
5. Immunoglobulin class or subclass of the antibody.
6. Complement fixation in question.
7. Simultaneous occurrence of other antibodies, possibly in a characteristic combination.
8. *In-vivo* deposition in the affected organ.

From Reference 7.

Table 2 Autoantibodies in autoimmune hepatitis

Autoantibody against	*First description*
Nuclear material (ANA)	1957 Friou *et al.*
Bile ducts (BDA)	1964 Paronetto *et al.*
Smooth muscle (SMA)	1965 Johnson *et al.*
Mitochondria (AMA)	1965 Walker *et al.*
Bile canaliculi (BCA)	1969 Diederichsen *et al.*
Endoplasmic reticulum (AER, LKM)	1973 Storch; Rizzetto *et al.*
Liver cell membranes (LMA)	1973 Storch
Cytosol (LCA)	1975 Storch
Liver ribosomes (LRA)	1979 Storch and Wohlgemuth
Connective tissue type 3 (CTA-3) (so-called endomysium) (EMA)	1979 Storch
Mononuclear cells (so-called ANCA)	1981 Storch *et al.*
Auerbach's plexus (AAPA)	1993 Storch
Podocytes (APA)	1995 Storch
Calreticulin	1996 Kreisel *et al.*
Calpastatin	1998 Storch

After Reference 9.
Abbreviations: ANA = antinuclear antibodies; BDA = bile duct antibodies; SMA = smooth muscle antibodies; AMA = antimitochondrial antibodies; BCA = bile canaliculi antibodies; AER = antibody against endoplasmic reticulum; LKM = liver kidney microsomal antibody; LMA = liver membrane antibody; LCA = liver cytosol (or cytoplasm) antibody; LRA = liver ribosomal antibody; CTA-3 = connective tissue antibody, type 3; EMA = endomysial antibody; ANCA = anti-neutrophil-cytoplasmic-antibody; AAPA = anti-Auerbach' plexus-antibody; APA = anti-podocyte-antibody.

Antibodies against nuclear material (ANA)

At present, we can distinguish more than 100 different antibodies. Nevertheless, we have not found a 'specific', or better, pathognomomic antibody for autoimmune hepatitis so far. As a rule, antibodies against nuclear material are still 'screened' today by means of immunofluorescence. The Hep 2 cell (a cultivated laryngeal carcinoma cell, which allows for easy distinction between different dividing phases, the so-called mitotic phases, besides the resting or interphase cells) serves as antigenous substrate. Homogeneous fluorescence images of the nuclei indicate the presence of antibodies against native DNA. They are found predominantly in acute lupus erythematodes disseminatus, but are also observed in so-called lupoid hepatitis, i.e. classical autoimmune hepatitis. The findings obtained can be confirmed by means of specific tests, such as radioimmunoassay, ELISA or a special immunofluorescence test using flagellates, e.g. crithidiae luciliae.

Two types of antibodies against so-called 'nuclear dots' can be distinguished, those that cause staining of only a 'few dots' and those with staining of 'multiple nuclear dots'. Their presence strongly indicates the clinical picture of primary biliary cirrhosis. It should be noted that the mitotic phases are nearly always negative (see Reference 9).

However, in the case of antibodies against so-called centromeres (more correctly, kinetochores: see Reference 9), the mitotic phases are always similarly positive. Such antibodies occur mainly with the so-called CREST syndrome (calcinosis, Raynaud's phenomenon, oesophagus dysmotility, sclerodactyly and teleangiectasias). This syndrome may be associated with, for example, primary biliary cirrhosis. In our experience, this type of antibody is also found in autoimmune hepatitis and the so-called overlap syndromes.

Antibodies against bile ducts (BDA)

These were first described by Paronetto *et al.* in 1964 (see Reference 9) and (wrongly) called an artefact by some authors. Even today, they are considered to be of no diagnostic value. However, we have occasionally observed in autoimmune hepatitis not a diffuse cytoplasmatic fluorescence of the bile ducts but apical emphasis (see Reference 9).

Anti-smooth-muscle antibodies (SMA, ASMA)

These form an extremely heterogeneous group. Up to now, more than 200 antibodies have been detected. These antibodies are best called antibodies against the cytoskeleton. Of particular diagnostic relevance for autoimmune hepatitis is the antibody against actin, which characteristically stains the muscularis, the muscularis mucosae, the media in blood vessels, the so-called septa between glands and the parietal cells in gastric sections. In the kidney, three types of anti-smooth-muscle antibodies can be differentiated: types SMA-V, -G and -T. The SMA-V type reacts only with the blood vessels (V = vessel) while the SMA-G type reacts additionally with the glomerules (G = glomerule). Only the SMA-T type (T = tubuli), which also reacts with the brush border, especially of the proximal renal tubuli and the peritubular fibrillae, is characteristic for autoimmune hepatitis. If the titre is above 1 : 640 and if it is an IgG antibody, then, in my opinion, autoimmune hepatitis (possibly developing) can be suspected even if other characteristic signs of autoimmune hepatitis are absent. Thus, the antibody picture is largely pathognomonic for the disease. As already mentioned, besides antibodies against actin, there is a huge variety of antibodies against the cytoskeleton, e.g. against cytokeratines, which were recently described in literature[10]. For diagnosing autoimmune hepatitis, such antibodies are, however, of little significance in my opinion, although they may be sometimes useful for differential diagnosis.

Antimitochondrial antibodies (AMA)

These are also a heterogeneous group. Type 2 is undoubtedly associated with primary biliary cirrhosis (or a preliminary stage of it). Individual antimitochondrial antibodies seem also to be linked to autoimmune hepatitis. They are only rarely observed. Let me mention here type 8 after Storch. We described this type as early as in 1981 (see References 9 and 11). Type 8 antimitochondrial antibodies react nearly exclusively with the distal renal tubuli. They should be distinguished from, for example, cold agglutinins and also from antibodies against the proteolytic enzyme cathepsin D (see Reference 11), which can produce a similar picture. Besides the by-then-detected six, we described another four antimitochondrial antibodies. Also, type 8 after Storch has nothing to do with type 8 after Berg. Berg's nomenclature was published later than Storch's (see Reference 9).

For the sake of completeness, let me mention that, unaware of our nomenclature, another so-called type 10 antimitochondrial antibody was described in 1999[12].

Antibodies against bile canaliculi (BCA)

These were first described by Diederichsen *et al.* in 1969[9]. They had the same fate as the antibodies against bile ducts. In my opinion, they do not represent an artefact. Good evidence is limited, however, to isolated bovine liver cells. The pictures observed vary on other substrates. Their antigen does not seem to be known so far[9,13].

Antibodies against endoplasmatic reticulum (AER, LKM)

These are the more recently detected LKM (liver and kidney microsomal antibodies). Three research teams described them at nearly the same time: Homberg in Paris, Doniach in London and myself in Leipzig[9,14]. Their common characteristic is strong fluorescence of hepatocyte cytoplasma and a somewhat weaker fluorescence, particularly of the cytoplasma of the third segment of proximal murine renal tubuli. The second segment of proximal tubular cells reacts less strongly. With the first segment, hardly any reaction is observed. Homberg was the first author to point to this fact. Distal tubular cells, the preferred sites of reaction of antimitochondrial antibodies, are always clearly negative. The currently valid classification (see Reference 9) distinguishes at least six different types. Only the so-called type 1 with a high titre (1 : 320 or higher) is typical for a still idiopathic autoimmune hepatitis, called type 2 autoimmune hepatitis. Most of its antigens are known; they are mainly isoenzymes of cytochrome P 450.

Antibodies against liver cell membranes (LMA)

These antibodies, which are very interesting, are probably irrelevant for diagnosis. It is still unclear, even today, whether individual subtypes might be suitable for differential analysis[15,16].

Anticytosol antibodies (LCA)

Great effort is being made towards their study. They show considerable heterogeneity and their assignment, their names and antigens are under dispute (see, for example, References 9, 13, 17). To mention them in passing, argininosuccinate lyase[18] and formiminotransferase cyclodeaminase[19] are antigens of anticytosol antibodies, as are probably other proteins, such as a still largely unknown 58-kDa protein[20]. Glutathione-S transferase[21,22] and, more importantly, proteins of the UGA serin tRNA protein complex were recently characterized as antigens of anticytosol antibodies[23–25]. Even more proteins might be involved such as a 40-kDa protein[26].

Anti-liver-ribosomal antibodies (LRA)

In my experience, these antibodies are characteristic of a specific, though infrequently occurring, clinical picture, namely the so-called virus-associated autoimmune hepatitis. They are characterized by intralobular emphasis on cytoplasmic fluorescence of hepatocytes, meaning that it is mainly the cytoplasma around the central veins that reacts. Hepatocytes around the portal fields are mostly negative (see Reference 9).

Anti-connective tissue antibodies (CTA, EMA)

In autoimmune hepatitis, only a few specimens representative of this type of antibody have been closely examined[9,27]. These antibodies should be differentiated from the so-called type 3 anti-connective-tissue antibody, which was erroneously seen as being directed against endomysium. Having identified tissue transglutaminase as the main target antigen of this antibody, the search for other antigens in autoimmune hepatitis as well as in coeliac disease is being continued[27,28].

Antibodies against mononuclear cells (ANCA)

These were described especially for hepatitis C as early as in 1981 (see Reference 9). In my mind, the nomenclature employed at present should be revised; this is one of the reasons why discussion of this heterogeneous group of antibodies will be dispensed with.

Antibodies against Auerbach's plexus (AAPA)

In closing, let me shed some light on two antibodies detected recently, which were observed also in autoimmune hepatitis (see Reference 9). Cytoplasmic fluorescence, with the nuclei being left free, is typical for antibodies against Auerbach's plexus. It should be noted that different nerves are stained synchronously in nearly every instance. This can be illustrated by counterstaining using Evan's blue, which results in red staining of the connective tissue and facilitates allocation. These antibodies should not be mistaken for antibodies against the cytoplasma of smooth muscles, which are sometimes found simultaneously! Antibodies against the plexus myentericus, too, show considerable heterogeneity. (Additionally, antibodies against other nerve plexuses such as Meissner's and Schabadach's plexus should be considered.) Individual antibodies react, e.g. with the 68-kDa protein of the neurofilament, as we were able to demonstrate by means of double immunofluorescence.

Autoantibodies against renal podocytes (APA)

Figure 1 shows a typical picture. The green colour is produced by the human autoantibody, while mouse monoclonal antibodies against podocytes causes the red colour. The yellow colour of Figure 1c points only to the identical intensity of the green and red fluorescences. The white colour (Figure 1d) of this laser scanning fluorescence record in the case of artificial colouring (white) proves the identical localization of the green and red fluorescences. This means that the antigen is really located in podocytes (this fact was confirmed by immunoelectron microscopy).

In conclusion, a huge variety of autoantibodies is involved in autoimmune hepatitis. An 'International Autoimmune Hepatitis Group'[29,30] has accepted, in the first place, antibodies against nuclear material, smooth muscles and endoplasmic reticulum (LKM) and suggested that a distinction should be made

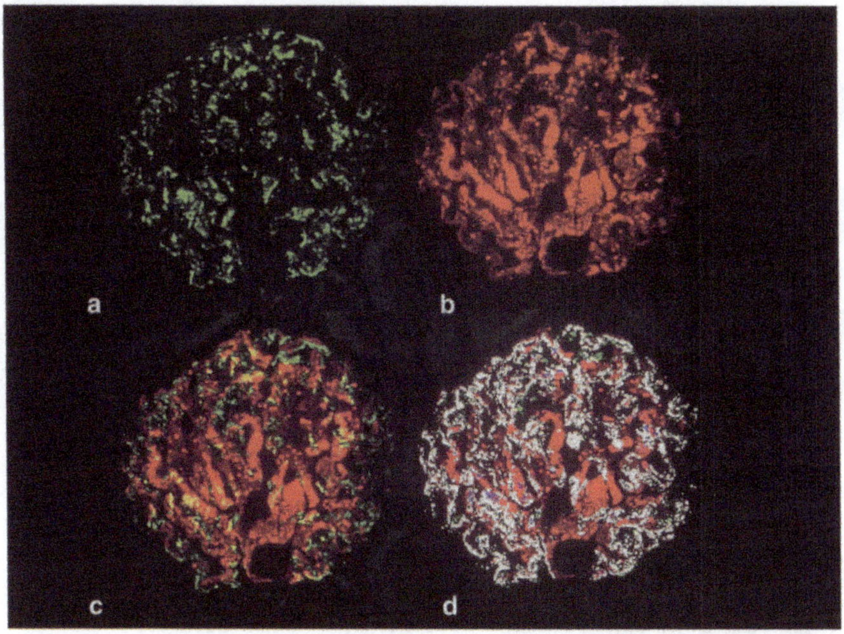

Figure 1 Antibodies against podocytes. Rat kidney antigen. Double immunofluorescence. First incubation with a mixture of diluted patient serum and of mouse monoclonal antibodies against a 44-kDa protein of podocytes. Second incubation with a mixture of the working dilution of the luminescent green, fluorescein isothiocyanate-marked antibody against human immunoglobulin G and luminescent red Cy-3-marked anti-mouse-immunoglobulin. Confocal laser scanning–microscopic record.

(a) Stimulation at 488 and 568 nm with representation of green fluorescence of the human autoantibody when red fluorescence is blocked. (b) Stimulation at 568 nm with representation of red fluorescence of the mouse monoclonal antibody against podocytes. (c) Stimulation at 488 and 568 nm with double exposure. The yellow colour signals sites of identical intensity. (d) As (c) but artificial (white) representation of identical localization of green and red fluorescences. (After Reference 9, by courtesy of Birkhäuser Publishing Company.)

between two types of autoimmune hepatitis, so-called type 1 with antibodies against nuclear material and/or against smooth muscles, and type 2 with antibodies against endoplasmic reticulum (so-called LKM). An interesting discussion is going on concerning antibodies against cytosol at present, with special focus on their antigens.

Due to limited time, consideration of recent findings concerning other autoantibodies, e.g. against lactoferrin[31,32], carboanhydrase[33,34], chromatin[35,36], enolase[37] and arginase[38,39], was omitted.

References

1. Fiessinger N. Histogenèse des processus de cirrhose hépatique. Lésion parenchymateuse et cirrhose. In: Etude Histologique Expérimentale et Pathologique, ed. by Maloine A. Thesis, Paris 1908.
2. Ehrlich P. Die Schutzstoffe des Blutes. Dtsch Med Wschr. 1901;27:913–16.

3. Roitt IM, Doniach D, Campell PN, Hudson RV. Autoantibodies in Hashimoto's disease. Lancet. 1956;II:820–1.
4. Storch WB. Gene hypothesis of autoimmunity and autoimmune disease. In: Mestecky J *et al.*, editors, Advances in Mucosal Immunology. New York: Plenum Press, 1995:1213–15.
5. Marrack P, Kappler J, Kotzin BL. Autoimmune disease: why and where it occurs. Nature Med. 2001;7:899–905.
6. Davidson A, Diamond B. Autoimmune disease. N Engl J Med. 2001;345:340–50.
7. Storch W. Immunpathogenese chronischer Hepatitiden. Leipzig: JA Barth, 1978.
8. Cjaja AJ, Homburger HA. Autoantibodies in liver disease. Gastroenterology. 2001;120:239–49.
9. Storch WB. Immunofluorescence in Clinical Immunology. A Primer and Atlas. Basel, Boston, Berlin: Birkhäuser, 2000.
10. Murota M, Nishioka M, Fujita J *et al.* Anti-cytokeratin antibodies in sera of the patients with autoimmune heaptitis. Clin Exp Immunol. 2001;125:291–9.
11. Storch WB. Immunfluoreszenz. In: Luppa H, Ambrosius H, Storch W: Immunreaktionen in der Histochemie. Handbuch der Histochemie, ed. by Graumann W and Neumann K, Band IV Proteine, Chapter 2. Stuttgart, New York: G Fischer, 1986:189–297.
12. Johanet C, Dubel L, Chazouillères O. Auto-anticorps en hépatologie. Pathol Biol Paris. 1999;47:997–1003.
13. Storch W. Autoimmune Hepatitiden: Autoantikörper als diagnostische Marker. Der Bayrische Internist. 1992;12:30–8.
14. Storch WB. Antikörper gegen endoplasmatisches Retikulum: Welche Bedeutung haben sie? (Editorial). Leber Magen Darm. 1997;27:194–6.
15. Matsuo I, Ikuno N, Omagari K *et al.* Autoimmunity reactivity of sera to hepatocyte plasma membrane in type 1 autoimmune hepatitis. J Gastroenterol. 2000;35:252–3.
16. Sasaki M, Yamauchi K, Tokushige K *et al.* Clinical significance of autoantibody to hepatocyte membrane antigen in type 1 autoimmune hepatitis. Am J Gastroenterol. 2001;96:846–51.
17. Storch W. Virus and Autoimmunität. Eine Odyssee am Beispiel der autoimmunen Hepatitis (Editorial). Leber Magen Darm. 1992;22:5–9.
18. Pelli N, Fensom AH, Slade C, Boa F, Mieli-Vergani G, Vergani D. Argininosuccinate lyase: a new autoantigen in liver disease. Clin Exp Immunol 1998;114:455–61.
19. Lapierre P, Hajoui O, Homberg J-C, Alvarez F. Formiminotransferase cyclodeaminase is an organ-specific autoantigen recognized by sera of patients with autoimmune hepatitis. Gastroenterology. 1999;116:643–9.
20. Muratori L, Cataleta M, Muratori P, Lenzi P, Bianchi FB. Liver/kidney microsomal antibody type 1 and liver cytosol antibody type 1 concentrations in type 2 autoimmune hepatitis. Gut. 1998;42:721–6.
21. Wesierska-Gadek J, Grimm R, Hitchman E, Penner E. Members of glutathione S-transferase gene family are antigens in autoimmune hepatitis. Gastroenterology. 1998;114:329–35.
22. Wesierska-Gadek J, Lindner H, Hitchman E, Sarg B, Penner E. Anti-SLA seropositive autoimmune hepatitis sera recognize distinct subunits of glutatione S-transferase: High prevalence of the Ya autoantigen. Cell Mol Biol. 2002;48:301–7.
23. Costa M, Rodriguez-Sanchez A, Czaja J, Gelpi C. Isolation and characterization of cDNA encoding the antigenic protein of the human tRNP (Ser) Sec complex recognized by autoantibodies from patients with type-1 autoimmune hepatitis. Clin Exp Immunol. 2000;121:364–74.
24. Wies I, Brunner, S, Henninger J *et al.* Identification of target antigen for SLA/LP autoantibodies in autoimmune hepatitis. Lancet. 2000;355:1510–15.
25. Volkmann M, Martin L, Bäurle A *et al.* Soluble liver antigen: Isolation of a 35-kd recombinant protein (SLA-p 35) specifically recognizing sera from patients with autoimmune hepatitis. Hepatology. 2001;33:591–6.
26. Duclos-Vallee J-C, Johanet C, Bach JF, Yamamoto AM. Autoantibodies associated with acute rejection after liver transplantation for type-2 autoimmune hepatitis. J Hepatol. 2000;33:163–6.
27. Dieterich W, Storch WB, Schuppan D. Serum antibodies in celiac disease. Clin Lab. 2000;46: 361–4.
28. Storch WB, Schloeder U. A new autoantibody in celiac disease. Clin Lab. 2002;48:19–23.
29. International Autoimmune Hepatitis Group report. Review of criteria for diagnosis of autoimmune hepatitis. J Hepatol. 1999;31:29–38.
30. McFarlane IG. Autoimmune hepatitis: clinical manifestations and diagnostic criteria. Can J Gastroenterol. 2001;15:107–13.

31. Ohano M, Okazaki K, Hajiro K, Uchida K. Antilactoferrin antibodies in autoimmune liver diseases. Am J Gastroenterol. 1998;93:1334–9.
32. Muratori L, Muratori P, Zauli D *et al.* Antilactoferrin antibodies in autoimmune liver disease. Clin Exp Immunol. 2001;124:470–3.
33. Invernizii P, Battezzatti PM, Crosignani A *et al.* Antibody to carbonic anhydrase II is present in primary biliary cirrhosis (PBC) irrespective of antimitochondrial antibody status. Clin Exp Immunol. 1998;114:448–54.
34. Comay D, Cauch-Dudeck K, Hemphill D, Diamandis E, Wanless I, Heathcote EJ. Are antibodies to carbonic anhydrase II specific for anti-mitochondrial antibody-negative primary biliary cirrhosis? Dig Dis Sci. 2000;45:2018–21.
35. Li L, Chen M, Huang DY, Nishioka M. Frequency and significance of antibodies to chromatin in autoimmune hepatitis type I. J Gastroenterol Hepatol. 2000;15:1176–82.
36. Mackay IR. Antinuclear (chromatin) autoantibodies in autoimmune hepatitis. J Gastroenterol Hepatol. 2001;16:245–7.
37. Gitlis VM, Toh BH, Sentry JW. Disease association, origin, and clinical relevance of autoantibodies to the glycolytic enzyme enolase. J Invest Med. 2001;49:138–45.
38. Mafune N, Kobayashi K, Nishioka M, Watanabe M, Sasaki M. Autoantibody to the liver arginase in sera of patients with autoimmune hepatitis and chronic hepatitis. Autoimmunity. 1999;30:147–55.
39. Kimura M, Tatsumi, KI, Tada H *et al.* Enzyme immunoassay for autoantibodies to human liver-type arginase and its clinical application. Clin Chem. 2000;46:112–17.

Section II
Pathology and clinical manifestations of autoimmune liver disease

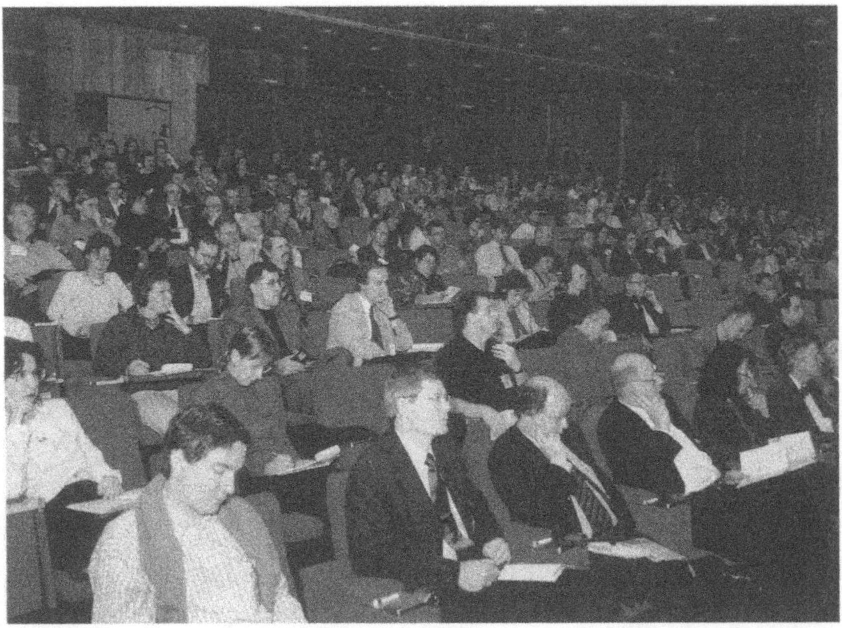

5
The pathology of autoimmune hepatitis

D. S. HUFF

INTRODUCTION

The pathologist has three objectives in the management of autoimmune hepatitis: 1. to help establish the diagnosis; 2. to assess the severity of the lesion; and 3. to monitor the results of treatment. The pathologist can accomplish these objectives through interpretation of liver biopsies even though autoimmune hepatitis has no pathognomonic pathological features. The pathology of autoimmune hepatitis is non-specific chronic hepatitis, which has many causes. Recent textbooks provide a wealth of up-to-date clinical and pathological details and extended bibliographies[1–4].

Autoimmune hepatitis is a diagnosis both of inclusion and exclusion and is established by a combination of clinical and pathological findings. The diagnosis is suspected when an appropriate clinical presentation is accompanied by liver function studies which favour hepatocellular damage over cholestasis and ductal damage and by serological studies demonstrating an appropriate autoantibody profile. The diagnosis is strengthened by a liver biopsy demonstrating non-specific chronic hepatitis compatible with autoimmune hepatitis. The diagnosis is established when the other causes of chronic hepatitis are excluded by immunohistochemical studies on the liver biopsy, by the clinical history, and by appropriate laboratory studies. The other causes of chronic hepatitis which must be excluded include chronic viral hepatitis, especially hepatitis B and hepatitis C viruses, drug-induced liver disease, toxic liver injury, hypoxic–ischaemic injury, Wilson's disease, α_1-antitrypsin deficiency and primary sclerosing cholangitis. A thorough clinical–pathological work-up is usually sufficient to establish or exclude the diagnosis of autoimmune hepatitis.

However, in some cases, the diagnosis remains in doubt. The International Autoimmune Hepatitis Group has established a semiquantitative system for scoring many clinical, laboratory and histopathological features to more accurately and objectively categorize a given case as definite, probable or inconclusive autoimmune hepatitis[5]. This system is useful in inter-institutional clinical trials and in comparisons between different studies but has not gained acceptance in routine diagnosis.

The clinical presentation ranges from acute fulminant hepatitis to chronic hepatitis with varying degrees of active hepatocellular damage with or without a small liver and splenomegaly. Less commonly, the illness is non-specific and the hepatic origin is revealed only by laboratory examination. The presenting histopathology may be submassive necrosis which obscures the underlying chronic hepatitis. More commonly, it is a picture of chronic hepatitis with variable degrees of hepatocellular necrosis, inflammation, fibrosis and structural change which may be commensurate with the severity of the clinical disease. The pathology of Type I autoimmune hepatitis (smooth muscle antibody and antinuclear antibody positive) is identical to that of Type II (liver kidney microsomal 1 antibody positive).

PATHOLOGY OF CHRONIC HEPATITIS

The histological lesions of non-specific chronic hepatitis are divided into three geographical sites: portal, interface and lobular, and two histological types: necroinflammatory (necrosis and inflammation) and structural (fibrosis and cirrhosis). The early portal lesions called triaditis are mild inflammation, enlargement, also

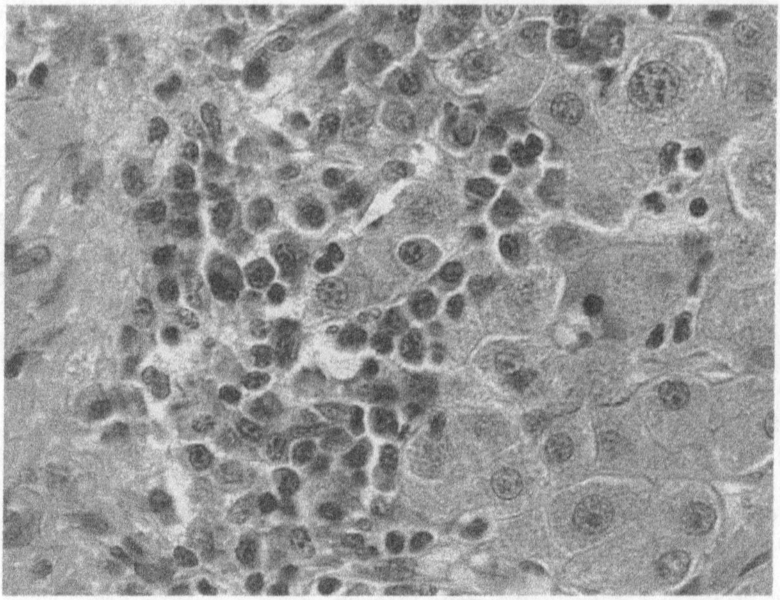

Figure 1 Interface lesion. The periphery of the portal tract is along the left edge of the photograph. An intense lymphoplasmacytic infiltrate invades through the limiting plate to surround periportal hepatocytes in the middle third of the photograph. Disorganized hepatocytes occupy the right third of the photograph. Just to the left of centre, the tip of the arrow points to two lymphocytes invading a hepatocyte (emperipolesis), and the tail of the arrow points to an apoptotic body. A large hepatocyte demonstrating ballooning degeneration is seen in the upper right hand corner. H&E stain; 60×.

referred to as expansion, and fibrosis. The inflammatory infiltrate is predominantly lymphoplasmacytic with a variable number of neutrophils and eosinophils. Bile ducts are usually spared, although mild swelling and stratification of bile duct epithelium and an occasional intraepithelial lymphocyte may be seen, as in acute hepatitis. Cholestasis is not a feature of autoimmune hepatitis. With increasing severity, the intensity of the inflammatory infiltrate and the expansion and fibrosis of portal tracts increase.

Interface lesions develop along mesenchymal–parenchymal junctions, such as portal–parenchymal or septal–parenchymal interfaces. The characteristic portal interface lesions, previously called piecemeal necrosis, consist of a few foci around the perimeter of the portal tracts in which the portal infiltrate invades through the limiting plate into the periportal parenchyma. Immune-mediated parenchymal damage to the limiting plate and adjacent parenchyma ensues with lymphocytic emperipolesis, ballooning degeneration, and apoptotic cell death of hepatocytes. With increasing severity, more of circumference of the portal tracts becomes involved. Tongues of portal inflammation break through the limiting plate to surround islands of periportal parenchyma (Figure 1). Foci of periportal hepatocytic death lead to reticulin collapse, further portal expansion and 'maple leaf' distortion of portal tracts (Figure 2). Damaged and regenerating hepatocytes surrounded by the interface necroinflammatory lesions undergo 'hepatitic' tubulo-acinar formation. Uncommonly, the interface necrosis completely surrounds a portal tract, a picture referred to as sleeve necrosis.

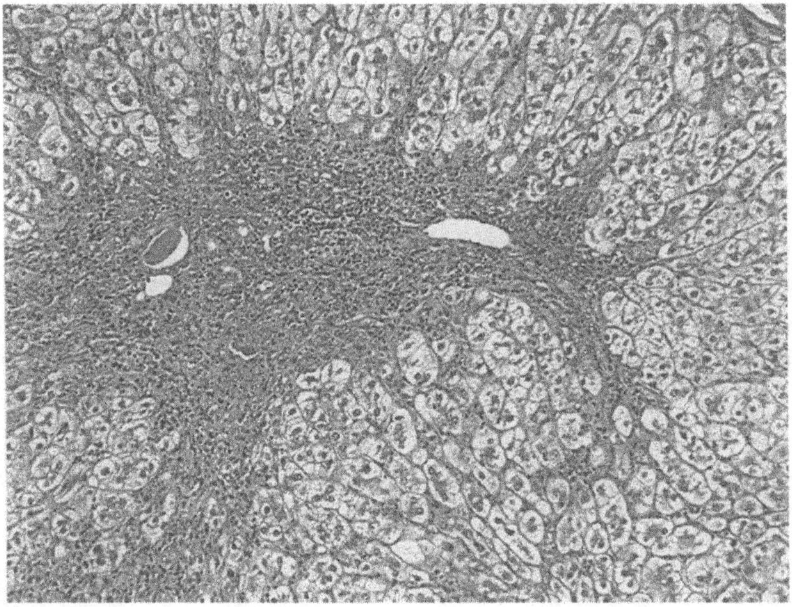

Figure 2 'Maple leaf' expansion of portal tract. Previous sites of interface inflammation and necrosis have been replaced by fingers of reticulin collapse and fibrosis extending out from the periphery of the portal zone. H&E stain; 10 ×

Foci of necrosis and inflammation of the lobule are referred to as lobulitis. Mild lobulitis consists of a few small foci of inflammation associated with lymphocytic emperipolesis and apoptosis of hepatocytes. Apoptosis of hepatocytes in both the interface and lobule is also referred to as single cell necrosis or pyknotic necrosis. The remnant of an apoptotic hepatocyte is a round or oval brightly eosinophilic body called a Councilman body which is a characteristic feature of chronic hepatitis and many other liver injuries. The lesions may be prominent around central veins. Ballooning degeneration and giant cell transformation may be prominent in the lobule as well as in the interface lesions. With increasing severity the foci of lobular necrosis increase in size, and bands of necrosis linking portal zones to portal zones, central zones to central zones, and central zones to portal zones are referred to as portal–portal, central–central, and central–portal bridging necrosis, respectively. These bands of necrosis may be replaced by reticulin collapse and fibrosis to form portal–portal, central–central, and central–portal bridging fibrosis, also referred to as inactive septa. The chronicity of the septa can be established by demonstrating mature collagen and reticulin fibres in the septa using trichrome and elastic stains. Both types of fibres take some time to appear. These fibrous bridges constitute additional mesenchymal–parenchymal interfaces. They may become inflamed, and interface necroinflammatory lesions may develop along them. Inflamed septa with interface lesions are referred to as active septa. Bridging necrosis and fibrosis lead to extensive structural alteration and cirrhosis.

DIFFERENTIAL DIAGNOSIS OF CHRONIC HEPATITIS

The lesions of chronic hepatitis described above are non-specific but their presence establishes the diagnosis of autoimmune hepatitis when accompanied by the appropriate clinical and serological findings if the other causes of chronic hepatitis and hepatitis-like lesions have been excluded. The combination of the pathological and clinical features is usually required to exclude the other causes of chronic hepatitis and diseases that may mimic chronic hepatitis. Specific pathological features may favour one or another cause. Less frequently, a special stain or immunohistochemical stain may positively establish a diagnosis.

Chronic hepatitis may be difficult to differentiate from acute hepatitis. Extensive involvement of the central areas, inconspicuous involvement of portal areas, and cholestasis all favour acute hepatitis. Prominent portal and interface lesions favor chronic hepatitis. The presence of mature collagen and elastic fibres in bridging septa by trichrome and elastic stains confirms the diagnosis of chronic hepatitis and excludes acute hepatitis.

Once the diagnosis of chronic hepatitis is established by the pathologist, specific features that favour one or another cause are evaluated. A heavy plasma cell infiltrate at any age, giant cell transformation in the older child or adolescent, and prominent interface and lobular necroinflammatory lesions all raise the suspicion of autoimmune hepatitis. The viral cytopathic effects of hepatocyte sanded nuclei and ground glass cytoplasm with peripheral halos raise the suspicion of chronic hepatitis B virus infection which can be confirmed histologically by positive immunohistochemical stains for hepatitis B surface and core antigens.

The presence of portal lymphoid follicles with or without germinal centres and macrovesicular fatty change raises the suspicion for chronic hepatitis C virus infection which can be confirmed histologically by positive immunohistochemical stain for hepatitis C cytoplasmic antigen. A prominent eosinophilic and neutrophilic inflammatory infiltrate and epithelioid granulomata somewhat favour drug-induced hepatitis, but drug-induced hepatitis is best suspected or excluded by the clinical history. Prominent pericentral necroinflammatory lesions with inconspicuous interface and lobular lesions may occur in autoimmune hepatitis but raise the more likely possibilities of toxic, hypoxic–ischaemic or haemodynamic injuries or of acute hepatitis. The presence of periportal hepatocytic eosinophilic cytoplasmic globules which are PAS positive and diastase resistant raises the possibility of α_1-antritrypsin deficiency disease which can be confirmed histologically by positive immunohistochemical staining for α_1-antritrypsin. Wilson's disease may mimic chronic hepatitis clinically and pathologically. It is best excluded by clinical and laboratory findings. Rhodamine stain, demonstrating increased copper in sections of the liver biopsy, may support the diagnosis, although increased copper is not specific for Wilson's disease, and negative results do not exclude it. Cholestasis, extensive bile duct lymphocytic infiltrates, extensive bile duct epithelial damage, concentric periductal lymphocytic infiltrate or fibrosis, disappearance of ducts, or ductal proliferation with a cholangitic picture on a background of chronic hepatitis suggest primary sclerosing cholangitis. The same changes with an additional periductal granulomatous inflammation suggests primary biliary cirrhosis. Both diseases can be confirmed by clinical, laboratory and serological findings.

Some diseases may co-exist with autoimmune hepatitis. Excessive iron, demonstrated by Prussian blue stain, raises the possibility of co-existing haemochromatosis. Chronic hepatitis C infection may co-exist with autoimmune hepatitis and can be identified by the histopathological findings outlined above and by diagnostic serological findings.

Clinical, serological and pathological features of primary sclerosing cholangitis or primary biliary cirrhosis may co-exist with those of autoimmune hepatitis. Also, an illness with classical clinical, laboratory, serological and pathological features of autoimmune hepatitis may transform into one with the classical clinical, laboratory, serological and pathological features of primary sclerosing cholangitis or *vice versa*. The pathologist must be alert to these variant and overlap syndromes which may require adjustments in treatment.

SEVERITY OF CHRONIC HEPATITIS

Elaborate quantitative scoring systems for documenting the severity of autoimmune hepatitis have been devised[6,7]. These are useful in clinical trials, especially those involving multiple centres, or in comparing the results of different studies but have not gained wide acceptance in routine diagnostic pathology. The systems are divided into grades – the severity of portal/interface and lobular necroinflammatory lesions – and stages – the severity of fibrosis and structural alteration. Some practicing pathologists indicate the grade and stage as mild, moderate or severe, rather than using one of the cumbersome numerical systems.

When evaluating sequential pre- and post-treatment biopsies, direct comparison of the current with previous biopsies and documentation of the changes in the pathology report is preferable to a numerical system.

SUMMARY

The pathology of autoimmune hepatitis is non-specific. The diagnosis is one of both inclusion and exclusion, utilizing clinical, laboratory, serological and histopathological findings. The pathologist plays an active role in establishing the diagnosis of chronic hepatitis compatible with autoimmune hepatitis, excluding other causes of chronic hepatitis, assessing the severity of the lesions, and monitoring the results of treatment.

References

1. Czaja AJ, Carpenter HA. Autoimmune hepatitis. In: Mac Sween RNM, Burt AD, Portmann BC, Ishak KG, Scheuer PJ, Anthony PP, editors, Pathology of the Liver. London: Churchill Livingstone, 2002:415–33.
2. Ferrell LD, Theise ND, Scheuer PJ. Acute and chronic hepatitis. In: Mac Sween RNM, Burt AD, Portmann BC, Ishak KG, Scheuer PJ, Anthony PP, editors, Pathology of the Liver. London: Churchill Livingstone, 2002:313–62.
3. Scheuer PJ. Chronic hepatitis. In: Scheuer PJ, Lefowitch JH, editors, Liver Biopsy Interpretation. London: WB Saunders, 2000:151–72.
4. Alvarez F. Autoimmune hepatitis. In: Suchy FJ, Sokol RJ, Balistreri WF, editors, Liver Disease in Children. Philadelphia: Lippincott Williams and Wilkins, 2001:429–41.
5. Alvarez F, Berg PA, Biandin FB *et al.* International autoimmune hepatitis group report: review of criteria for diagnosis of autoimmune hepatitis. J Hepatol. 1999;31:929–38.
6. Ishak K, Baptista A, Bianchi L *et al.* Histologic grading and staging of chronic hepatitis. J Hepatol. 1995;22:696–99.
7. Scheuer PJ. Classification of chronic hepatitis: A need for reassessment. J Hepatol. 1991;13: 372–4.

6
Autoimmune hepatitis and sclerosing cholangitis

G. MIELI-VERGANI and D. VERGANI

INTRODUCTION

Autoimmune liver disorders are inflammatory liver diseases characterized histologically by a dense mononuclear cell infiltrate in the portal tract and serologically by the presence of non-organ and liver specific autoantibodies and increased levels of immunoglobulin G (IgG), in the absence of a known aetiology. They usually respond to immunosuppressive treatment, which should be instituted as soon as the diagnosis is made. The onset of these conditions is often ill-defined, frequently mimicking acute hepatitis. The previously accepted requirement of a six-month duration of symptoms before a diagnosis of autoimmune disease could be made has been abandoned[1]. Liver disorders in which the liver damage is likely to arise from an autoimmune attack include autoimmune hepatitis (AIH), autoimmune sclerosing cholangitis (ASC), and *de-novo* autoimmune hepatitis after liver transplant, which is described in Section III.

AUTOIMMUNE HEPATITIS

Clinical features

Two types of AIH are recognized according to seropositivity for smooth muscle and/or antinuclear antibody (SMA/ANA, type 1 AIH) or liver kidney microsomal type 1 antibody (LKM1, type 2 AIH). There is a female predominance in both. LKM1-positive patients tend to present more acutely, at a younger age and commonly have immunoglobulin A (IgA) deficiency, while duration of symptoms before diagnosis, clinical signs, family history of autoimmunity, presence of associated autoimmune disorders, response to treatment and long-term prognosis are similar in the two groups[2,3].

In our retrospective review of 52 children with AIH seen between 1973 and 1993, 32 had ANA and/or SMA, and 20 had LKM. Three clinical patterns of disease were observed[3].

Pattern 1. In 50% of patients with ANA/SMA and 65% of patients with LKM1, the presentation was indistinguishable from that of an acute viral hepatitis. Non-specific symptoms of malaise, nausea/vomiting, anorexia and abdominal pain followed by jaundice, dark urine and pale stools characterized this pattern. Six children, including 5 with LKM1, developed acute liver failure with grade II–IV hepatic encephalopathy between two weeks and two months from onset of symptoms (median interval one month). In the remaining children, the duration of disease before diagnosis ranged from ten days to five months (median interval 1.8 months).

Pattern 2. Twenty-five per cent of children with LKM1 and 38% with ANA/SMA had an insidious onset with an illness characterized by progressive fatigue, relapsing jaundice, headache, anorexia and weight loss, lasting from six months to two years before diagnosis (median interval nine months).

Pattern 3. In six children, including two with LKM1, there was no history of jaundice, and the diagnosis followed presentation with complications of chronic liver disease, including haematemesis from oesophageal varices, bleeding diathesis, chronic diarrhoea, weight loss and vomiting. Clearly, the mode of presentation of AIH in childhood is variable, and the disease should be suspected and excluded in all children presenting with symptoms and signs of prolonged or severe acute liver disease.

Laboratory features

Children with LKM1 have higher median levels of serum bilirubin and aspartate aminotransferase (AST) than children with ANA/SMA[3]. In our study, however, these differences were not significant when the six patients with acute hepatic failure were excluded. Severe impairment of hepatic synthetic function, as reflected in a prolonged prothrombin time and hypoalbuminaemia, tended to be more common in patients with ANA/SMA than in those with LKM1 (53% vs. 30%).

The majority of patients (80%) had increased serum levels of IgG, but 10, including 5 with LKM1, had normal levels for age[3]. Three of these latter patients had presented with acute liver failure. These findings indicate that a normal serum IgG value in children, albeit a rare finding, does not exclude the diagnosis of AIH. As reported also in another study[4], a partial serum IgA deficiency was more common in children with LKM1 than those with ANA/SMA (45% vs. 9%).

The frequency of human leukocyte antigen (HLA) DR3 was significantly higher in patients with ANA/SMA than in control subjects[3]. This difference was not seen in patients with LKM1, a finding that suggests that the two types of AIH have different immunopathogenic mechanisms. Further studies are needed to confirm this hypothesis in larger numbers of children.

Histological features

The severity of portal tract inflammation, lobular activity, and interface hepatitis at diagnosis is similar in both groups[3]. Cirrhosis on initial biopsy evaluation is more frequent in patients with ANA/SMA than in those with LKM1 (69% vs. 38%). Notably, 57% of children who had cirrhosis at diagnosis presented with a clinical picture reminiscent of a prolonged acute viral hepatitis. Multi-acinar or panacinar collapse suggestive of an acute liver injury was present in 8 children, including 5 with LKM1. Progression to cirrhosis was noted in 4 of 7 children with ANA/SMA and 2 of 5 children with LKM1 at follow-up biopsies performed 17–56 months after diagnosis[3]. Overall, 74% of patients with ANA/SMA and 44% of patients with LKM1 showed evidence of cirrhosis on initial or follow-up histological assessment. This finding indicates that, apart from the greater tendency to present as acute liver failure, the disease associated with LKM1 is of similar severity to that associated with ANA/SMA.

Treatment

Autoimmune hepatitis responds well to immunosuppression unless it presents as acute liver failure. In the latter circumstance, urgent liver transplantation is usually required.

Prednisolone, 2 mg kg^{-1} day^{-1} (maximum dose 60 mg/day), is the typical initial treatment. The dose is gradually decreased over a period of 4–8 weeks if there is a progressive improvement of the serum aminotransferase level. The patient is then maintained on the minimal dose of prednisolone necessary to keep the serum aminotransferase level normal (usual maintenance dose 2.5–5 mg/day, depending on age). During the first 6–8 weeks of treatment, liver function tests are checked weekly to allow a constant and frequent fine-tuning of the treatment, avoiding severe steroid side-effects. If a progressive normalization of the liver function tests is not obtained over this period of time or if too high a dose of prednisolone is required to maintain normal transaminases, azathioprine is added at a starting dose of 0.5 mg kg^{-1} day^{-1} which, in the absence of signs of toxicity, is increased up to a maximum of 2 mg $kg^{-1}$$day^{-1}$ until biochemical control is achieved. We never use azathioprine as first-line treatment because of its hepatotoxicity, particularly in severely jaundiced patients.

Although an 80% decrease of the initial transaminase levels is obtained within 6 weeks in most patients, the complete normalization of the liver function may take several months. In our own series, normalization of transaminase levels occurred at a median of 0.5 years (range 0.2–7) in ANA/SMA-positive children and of 0.8 years (range 0.02–3.2) in LKM1-positive ones[3]. Relapse while on treatment is common, affecting about 40% of the patients and requiring a temporary increase of the steroid dose. The risk of relapse is higher during puberty or if steroids are administered on an alternate-day schedule, often instituted in the unsubstantiated belief that it has a smaller negative effect on the child's growth. Small daily doses should be used, since they are more effective in maintaining disease control, minimizing the need for high-dose steroid pulses during relapses, with attendant more severe side-effects. If, after one year of normal liver function tests, a liver biopsy shows minimal or no inflammatory changes, cessation of treatment should be considered. In 13 children (4 with LKM1), the only ones fulfilling these criteria in our series, discontinuation of treatment was attempted. This was successful in 6, all ANA/SMA positive, after a median duration of 3.2 (range 1–11) years of treatment. All 6 have remained in remission for a period of 9–13 years. The remaining children (3 ANA/SMA and

4 LKM1 positive) relapsed between 1 and 15 months (median 2 months) after immunosuppression was discontinued. They all responded to re-introduction of treatment. These data indicate that most children with AIH, and particularly those who are LKM1 positive, are likely to require life-long immunosuppressive treatment. Despite the efficacy of current treatment, severe hepatic decompensation may develop even after many years of apparent good biochemical control. Thus, four of our patients who responded satisfactorily to immunosuppression ultimately required transplantation from 8 to 14 years after diagnosis. Overall, in our series, 46 of the 47 patients treated with immunosuppression were alive between 0.3–19 years (median 5) after diagnosis, including 5 after liver transplant.

Sustained remission of AIH has been reported in adult patients maintained on azathioprine alone[5]. Following this observation, we have attempted to stop prednisolone, maintaining azathioprine, in 5 children, 2 ANA/SMA and 3 LKM1 positive: while the attempt was successful in ANA/SMA-positive cases, all LKM1-positive children relapsed and required reinstitution of steroid treatment.

In a recent report[6], remission was achieved in 25 of 32 children with AIH treated with cyclosporin A alone for 6 months, followed by combined low-dose prednisone and azathioprine for one month, after which cyclosporin was stopped and the other two drugs continued. Cyclosporin A side-effects were mild and high-dose steroid side-effects avoided. Disadvantages of this schedule are that remission was achieved in only 78% of the patients compared with 94% using standard immunosuppression[3] and that all patients were eventually treated long term with the prednisone/azathioprine combination, while, using the conventional treatment schedule, about a third of the children can maintain remission with very low-dose steroids alone. In addition, longer follow-up of the patients is necessary to detect possible long-term toxicity of cyclosporin.

Mycophenolate mofetil (MMF) has been successfully used in adult patients with type 1 AIH who were either intolerant of or not responsive to azathioprine[7]. Mycophenolate mofetil is an inhibitor of purine nucleotide synthesis, and it has a mechanism of action similar to that of azathioprine[8]. It is not hepatotoxic or nephrotoxic, and its main side-effects are diarrhoea, vomiting and bone marrow suppression. In our experience, the drug was able to resolve laboratory abnormalities in 5 of 12 children who did not tolerate or respond to azathioprine. In four others, it reduced serum aminotransferase levels to a degree that allowed a decrease in the dose of prednisolone. Only 3 patients did not respond to MMF, and the side-effects were minor apart from severe nausea and dizziness in one of these 3 children.

SCLEROSING CHOLANGITIS

Sclerosing cholangitis in childhood is a heterogeneous condition, with different aetiopathogeneses. Recognized variants are: neonatal sclerosing cholangitis and sclerosing cholangitis associated with primary or secondary immunodeficiencies, with Langerhans cell histiocytosis, or with cystic fibrosis. In contrast to the experience in adults, sclerosing cholangitis occurring as an idiopathic disease (primary sclerosing cholangitis) is rare in paediatrics. The most common type of sclerosing cholangitis in childhood is autoimmune sclerosing cholangitis.

Autoimmune sclerosing cholangitis (ASC)

Clinical, laboratory and histological features

An overlapping syndrome between AIH and sclerosing cholangitis has been anecdotally reported in children[9–11] and adults[12–14]. A retrospective study from our Unit has shown that 40% of children with sclerosing cholangitis have clinical, biochemical, immunological and histological features that are indistinguishable from those of AIH[10]. In both AIH and sclerosing cholangitis, the serum IgG level is commonly increased and non-organ specific ANA and/or SMA are frequently present. Both diseases also commonly have portal tract inflammation and interface hepatitis. Indeed, most of the reported cases of overlap were originally diagnosed as AIH[12–15]. Typically, the overlap with sclerosing cholangitis was not recognized until years later when biliary features on follow-up liver biopsy examination led to the performance of a cholangiography. The sequence of diagnoses was then interpreted as an evolution from AIH to sclerosing cholangitis, but the concurrence of these diseases had not been excluded by cholangiographic studies performed at presentation.

In a prospective study over a period of 16 years, we have found that 27 of 55 children who presented with clinical and/or laboratory evidence of AIH had evidence of sclerosing cholangitis when assessed by liver biopsy examination, cholangiography, sigmoidoscopy and rectal biopsy at presentation[16]. Bile duct abnormalities on cholangiography were both intra- and extrahepatic in two thirds of patients and intrahepatic in one third.

Of the 27 patients with ASC, 26 were seropositive for ANA and/or SMA, and one for LKM1[16]. Fifty-five per cent were girls, and the mode of presentation was similar to that of 28 patients with typical AIH. Symptoms were those of acute hepatitis or chronic liver dysfunction. In some instances, symptoms were absent, and the diagnosis was revealed after the incidental discovery of abnormal liver tests. Inflammatory bowel disease was present in 44% of children with cholangiopathy compared with 18% of those with typical AIH, and more than 75% of children with ASC had greatly increased serum IgG levels. Perinuclear antineutrophil cytoplasmic antibodies (pANCA) were present in 74% of individuals with ASC compared with 36% of patients with typical AIH.

There was only a partial concordance between the histological and radiological findings, six patients having histological features more compatible with AIH than sclerosing cholangitis[16]. Interestingly, all patients fulfilled the criteria for the diagnosis of 'definite' or 'probable' AIH established by the International Autoimmune Hepatitis Group[1]. Indeed, the diagnosis of sclerosing cholangitis was possible only because of the cholangiographic studies.

Treatment

Children with ASC respond to the same immunosuppressive treatment described above for typical AIH[16]. The liver test abnormalities resolved in almost 90% of our patients within a median of 2 months after starting treatment. This good response is in contrast to the outcome in adults with primary sclerosing cholangitis (PSC) who have no beneficial effects from corticosteroid treatment[17,18]. The PSC of adults, however, is usually diagnosed at an advanced stage, and it may be the result of various aetiologies. Disappointing results with immunosuppressive agents have been reported in a small number of children with sclerosing cholangitis associated with autoimmune features, but these children may have had a more advanced disease than those recruited into our prospective study[11].

Ursodeoxycholic acid (UDCA) was added to our treatment schedule in 1992 following preliminary reports of its value in the treatment of adult PSC[19,20]. The small number of patients and the relatively short follow-up period do not allow us to determine whether treatment with UDCA from the onset is successful in arresting the progression of ASC. In adults with well-established PSC, UDCA treatment has been disappointing, possibly because of its advanced stage at the time of diagnosis[21].

Follow-up liver biopsy assessments in our series have shown no progression to cirrhosis, although one patient did develop a vanishing bile duct syndrome. Follow-up endoscopic retrograde cholangiograms have shown static bile duct disease in half of our patients with ASC and progression of the bile duct abnormalities in the other half. Interestingly, one of the children with AIH who was followed prospectively developed sclerosing cholangitis 8 years after presentation despite treatment with corticosteroids and no biliary changes on several follow-up liver biopsy specimens. This experience suggests that AIH and ASC are part of the same pathogenetic process and that prednisolone and azathioprine may not be as effective in controlling the bile duct component of the disease.

The medium-term prognosis of ASC is good[16]. All patients in our series were alive after a median follow-up of 7 years. Four patients with ASC, however, required liver transplantation after 2–11 years of observation (median interval of follow-up, 7 years). In contrast, liver transplantation has not been required by any of the 28 children with typical AIH who have been followed for this same time.

Pathophysiology

It is unclear if the juvenile autoimmune form of sclerosing cholangitis and AIH are two distinct entities or different aspects of the same condition. Akin to AIH, liver-specific autoantibodies, including antibodies to liver-specific lipoprotein, asialoglycoprotein receptor, alcohol dehydrogenase and soluble liver antigen are found in ASC[22–24]. The HLA DR3, DR13 and DR15 occur as commonly in patients with ASC as in healthy control subjects, but HLA DR4 occurs less commonly. This HLA profile has been associated with susceptibility to PSC in adults[25], and a shared genetic predisposition between AIH and PSC may facilitate the expression of a hybrid syndrome.

References

1. International Autoimmune Hepatitis Group. International Autoimmune Hepatitis Group report: review of criteria for diagnosis of autoimmune hepatitis. J Hepatol. 1999;31:929–38.
2. Maggiore G, Veber F, Bernard O *et al.* Autoimmune hepatitis associated with anti-actin antibodies in children and adolescents. J Pediatr Gastroenterol Nutr. 1993;17(4):376–81.
3. Gregorio GV, Portmann B, Reid F *et al.* Autoimmune hepatitis in childhood: a 20-year experience. Hepatology. 1997;25(3):541–7.
4. Homberg JC, Abuaf N, Bernard O *et al.* Chronic active hepatitis associated with antiliver/kidney microsome antibody type 1: a second type of "autoimmune" hepatitis. Hepatology. 1987;7(6): 1333–9.

5. Johnson PJ, McFarlane IG, Williams R. Azathioprine for long-term maintenance of remission in autoimmune hepatitis [see comments]. N Engl J Med. 1995;333(15):958–63.
6. Alvarez F, Ciocca M, Canero-Velasco C *et al.* Short-term cyclosporine induces a remission of autoimmune hepatitis in children. J Hepatol. 1999;30(2):222–7.
7. Richardson PD, James PD, Ryder SD. Mycophenolate mofetil for maintenance of remission in autoimmune hepatitis in patients resistant to or intolerant of azathioprine. J Hepatol. 2000;33(3): 371–5.
8. Dhawan A, Mieli-Vergani G. Mycophenolate mofetil – a new treatment for autoimmune hepatitis? J Hepatol. 2000;33(3):480–1.
9. Debray D, Pariente D, Urvoas E, Hadchouel M, Bernard O. Sclerosing cholangitis in children. J Pediatr. 1994;124(1):49–56.
10. el-Shabrawi M, Wilkinson ML, Portmann B *et al.* Primary sclerosing cholangitis in childhood. Gastroenterology. 1987;92(5 Pt 1):1226–35.
11. Wilschanski M, Chait P, Wade JA *et al.* Primary sclerosing cholangitis in 32 children: clinical, laboratory, and radiographic features, with survival analysis. Hepatology. 1995;22(5):1415–22.
12. Gohlke F, Lohse AW, Dienes HP *et al.* Evidence for an overlap syndrome of autoimmune hepatitis and primary sclerosing cholangitis. J Hepatol. 1996;24(6):699–705.
13. McNair AN, Moloney M, Portmann BC, Williams R, McFarlane IG. Autoimmune hepatitis overlapping with primary sclerosing cholangitis in five cases. Am J Gastroenterol. 1998;93(5): 777–84.
14. Rabinovitz M, Demetris AJ, Bou-Abboud CF, Van Thiel DH. Simultaneous occurrence of primary sclerosing cholangitis and autoimmune chronic active hepatitis in a patient with ulcerative colitis. Dig Dis Sci. 1992;37(10):1606–11.
15. Sisto A, Feldman P, Garel L *et al.* Primary sclerosing cholangitis in children: study of five cases and review of the literature. Pediatrics. 1987;80:918–23.
16. Gregorio GV, Portmann B, Karani J *et al.* Autoimmune hepatitis/sclerosing cholangitis overlap syndrome in childhood: a 16-year prospective study. Hepatology. 2001;33(3):544–53.
17. Czaja AJ. Frequency and nature of the variant syndromes of autoimmune liver disease. Hepatology. 1998;28(2):360–5.
18. Lee YM, Kaplan MM. Primary sclerosing cholangitis. N Engl J Med. 1995;332(14):924–33.
19. Beuers U, Spengler U, Kruis W *et al.* Ursodeoxycholic acid for treatment of primary sclerosing cholangitis: a placebo-controlled trial. Hepatology. 1992;16(3):707–14.
20. Lebovics E, Salama M, Elhosseiny A, Rosenthal WS. Resolution of radiographic abnormalities with ursodeoxycholic acid therapy of primary sclerosing cholangitis. Gastroenterology. 1992;102: 2143–7.
21. Lindor KD. Ursodiol for primary sclerosing cholangitis. Mayo Primary Sclerosing Cholangitis-Ursodeoxycholic Acid Study Group [see comments]. N Engl J Med. 1997;336(10):691–5.
22. Ma Y, Bogdanos BP, Williams R, Mieli-Vergani G, Vergani D. Anti-SLA antibody is a marker of severity of liver damage in patients with autoimmune liver disease. J Hepatol. 2001;34(Suppl 1):212.
23. Ma Y, Gaken J, McFarlane BM *et al.* Alcohol dehydrogenase: a target of humoral autoimmune response in liver disease. Gastroenterology. 1997;112(2):483–92.
24. Mieli-Vergani G, Lobo-Yeo A, McFarlane BM, McFarlane IG, Mowat AP, Vergani D. Different immune mechanisms leading to autoimmunity in primary sclerosing cholangitis and autoimmune chronic active hepatitis of childhood. Hepatology. 1989;9(2):198–203.
25. Donaldson P, Manns MP. Immunogenetics of liver disease. In: Bircher J BJ-P, McIntyre N, Rizzetto M, Rhodes J, editors. Oxford Textbook of Clinical Hepatology. Oxford: Oxford University Press; 1999:173–88.

7 Primary biliary cirrhosis

U. LEUSCHNER

Primary biliary cirrhosis is an autoimmune disease of the liver. Together with autoimmune cholangitis and primary sclerosing cholangitis, it belongs to primary biliary liver diseases. Until now primary biliary cirrhosis (PBC) has been described in adults only, but, in 2001, two cases of affected children were reported. In a 15-year-old girl, PBC took an aggressive course accompanied by extrahepatic manifestations, such as significant peripheral neuropathy characterized by numbness in the upper and lower extremities as well as frequent falls. A nerve biopsy showed severe chronic axonal neuropathy with a marked loss of myelinated fibres. The mother of this girl suffered from a PBC/autoimmune hepatitis overlap syndrome and had undergone liver transplantation. The second patient was a 17-year-old girl with PBC, Raynaud's phenomenon, but no other symptoms of CREST syndrome. She had a mild course of the disease, similar to PBC in many adults. Both children had a stage II primary biliary cirrhosis. The authors came to the conclusion that, with increased awareness, further paediatric cases of PBC will be discovered[1].

PRIMARY BILIARY CIRRHOSIS (PBC)

Epidemiology and clinical features

Primary biliary cirrhosis, primary sclerosing cholangitis and overlap syndromes are classified as vanishing bild duct syndromes (Table 1). According to a modern classification of autoimmune liver diseases, we have to differentiate between cholestatic and hepatitic diseases. Autoimmune hepatitis (AIH) type 1 (ANA/SMA positive) and type 2 (LKM positive), as well as autoimmune hepatitis in patients with autoimmune poliendocrine syndrome type 1 (APS-1), are classified under hepatitic autoimmune disease, whereas primary biliary cirrhosis, autoimmune cholangitis and primary sclerosing cholangitis are classed as cholestatic diseases. Simultaneous existence of cholestatic and hepatitic criteria in one patient is called overlap syndrome (OLS)[2,3]. In some patients, diagnosis may change from one autoimmune disease to another (Table 2).

Table 1 Vanishing bile duct syndromes

Autoimmune	Primary biliary cirrhosis Primary sclerosing cholangitis Overlap syndromes
Alloimmune	Allograft rejection Graft vs. host disease
Others	Sarcoidosis Chronic hepatitis C Drug reactions

Table 2 Classification of autoimmune liver diseases

Cholestatic	Cholestatic, hepatitic	Hepatitic
Primary biliary cirrhosis Autoimmune cholangitis Primary sclerosing cholangitis*	Overlap syndromes Changing diagnosis	Autoimmune hepatitis Type 1 and 2 AIH in APS-1**

*Autoimmunity questionned; **APS = Autoimmune polyendocrine syndrome type 1

Primary biliary cirrhosis is a non-suppurative destructive cholangitis that leads to hepatic cirrhosis. PBC is considered a rare autoimmune disease of the liver, but, because of improved diagnostic procedures, it is found more often now than in previous years. In 1987, the prevalence of PBC amounted to 14/100 000 inhabitants, but, in 1994, to 25/100 000 and, in 2000, to 40.1/100 000[4]. In a study from England, 94/100 000 women suffered from primary biliary cirrhosis[5] because PBC is predominantly seen in women (f : m = 9 : 1). These figures will continue to rise and today we can no longer consider primary biliary cirrhosis to be a rare disease.

By means of histology, we can differentiate 4 stages of PBC. However, for clinical use, it is sufficient to differentiate early stage from advanced and late-stage disease. There are no characteristic symptoms. Uncharacteristic abdominal complaints, gas formation and weakness are typical for cholestatic diseases. Pruritus and fatigue are more characteristic symptoms and pruritus can be experienced by the patients months or even years before the correct diagnosis is established. AST and ALT are mildly elevated and, as usual in cholestatic liver diseases, a greater increase of alkaline phosphatase (AP) and γ-glutamyl transpeptidase (GGT) is to be seen. The evidence of antimitochondrial antibodies (AMA) is pathognomonic and found in more than 90% of all patients. AMA are directed against PDH (pyruvate dehydrogenase), BCKD (branched chain keto-dehydrogenase) and KGD (keto glutarate dehydrogenase) enzyme complexes. The enzyme complexes are located on the inner mitochondrial membrane[6–8]. In the 5–10% of patients without AMA antinuclear antibodies (ANA), atypical p-ANCA and other antibodies are to be found (Table 3). Furthermore, serum concentrations of immunoglobulin M are increased. Immunogenetically, PBC is associated with DR8 but the association is only of marginal significance.

Table 3 Autoantibodies in primary biliary cirrhosis

AMA	Against	PDH-E_2, -$E_1\alpha$, -$E_1\beta$, protein X	95%
		BCKD-E_2, -$E_1\alpha$, -$E_1\beta$	50–60%
		KGD-E_2, -E_1, -E_3	40–90%
ANA: MND	Nuclear envelope		
Nuclear ring staining	Nuclear envelope		40%
Atypical p-ANCA	Blood cell antigens		15%
ANCA-BPI (also in systemic vasculitis)			>90%
EClpP		*E. coli* proteases	30%*

PDH: Pyruvate dehydrogenase; BCKD: branched chain keto-dehydrogenase; KGD: ketoglutarate dehydrogenase; MND: multiple nuclear dots; BPI: bacterial/permeability increasing protein IgG; * of AMA-positive patients

Table 4 Extrahepatic manifestations in PBC

Autoimmune thyroiditis, M. Basedow	15–20%
Sicca syndrome	50–70%
Sjögren syndrome	60–90%
CREST syndrome	15%
Arthritis	
Coeliac disease	6–20%
Inflammatory bowel disease	
Diabetes mellitus	
Osteoporosis	25–35%
Urinary tract infections	20%
Others	

Since PBC is an autoimmune disease in more than 80% of patients, extrahepatic concomitant phenomena exist, such as keratoconjunctivitis, arthropathies, thyreoiditis and others (Table 4). Forty per cent of the patients present with two extrahepatic manifestations simultaneously.

Pathology and prognosis

Histologically, the non-suppurative destructive cholangitis is characterized by dense inflammatory infiltrates in the periportal tracts. CD4 lymphocytes predominate over CD8 cells at a ratio of 4:1 Immunocompetent cells infiltrate the bile duct epithelia and, within months or years, induce complete destruction. Bile ducts vanish and cholestasis develops. When the disease progresses, the inflammatory cells invade the hepatic parenchyma, and bundles of fibres of connective tissue divide the liver lobules into irregularly shaped areas, but, at the stage of cirrhosis, inflammation and bile ducts have almost vanished[9–11]. PBC is a focal disease, which means that different stages of the disease can be present simultaneously in the same organ. This renders staging rather difficult.

Table 5 Primary biliary cirrhosis: survival in relation to serum bilirubin

Bilirubin		*Expected survival*	*Bilirubin before liver transplant*		*1-year survival after liver transplantation (%)*
(mg%)	*(μmol/L)*	*(months)*	*(mg%)*	*(μmol/L)*	
<2	<34	49	<11	<187	75
≥6	≥102	25	11–19	188–335	63
>10	>170	17	>19	>335	45

The prognosis of primary biliary cirrhosis is relatively benign. The mean life expectancy of untreated PBC patients is 12 years. But there are also asymptomatic courses that take up to 20 years and more. Bilirubin has been accepted as the best prognostic marker. The survival in relation to serum bilirubin is given in Table 5. The question is still unresolved whether primarily symptomatic patients have a poorer prognosis than those who are primarily asymptomatic. Data from studies from Scandinavia suggest that asymptomatic patients have the less favourable course of the disease; others suggest the opposite.

Influence of PBC on pregnancy

There are only a few observations concerning the relationship between PBC and pregnancy. As in some other non-hepatic autoimmune diseases, pregnancy may improve the disease. In a study with 206 pregnant PBC patients, pruritus developed in only 9%; further complications were not observed. Eighty-two per cent of pregnancies in PBC mothers ended with a regular delivery[12–14]. In our own PBC patients with early stages of the disease (stage I, II), pregnancy improved AP, GGT, AST and ALT. These values remained at a low level, increased after delivery and shortly thereafter dropped to the pre-pregnancy level[15]. In patients with late-stage PBC (stage III, IV), in whom pregnancy is extremely rare, pregnancy might result in deterioration of primary biliary cirrhosis.

OVERLAP SYNDROMES (OLS)

The simultaneous occurrence of two autoimmune or chronic liver diseases in one patient is called overlap syndrome. These overlap syndromes include autoimmune hepatitis (AIH), primary biliary cirrhosis (PBC), autoimmune cholangitis (AIC) and primary sclerosing cholangitis (PSC). Since patients with so-called overlap syndromes require adequate treatment, an awareness of OLS is important, even if, in future, there will be many changes in the definition and therapy of these new variants of autoimmune liver disease[3,16]. At present, there is no unequivocal definition of overlap syndromes or 'atypical manifestations of autoimmune hepatitis'.

According to the prevalence of serological and morphological features, the overlap syndrome AIH/PBC is seen in about 8% of all patients with chronic

Table 6 Overlap syndromes – prevalence of serological, morphological and immunogenetic features (% of autoimmune chronic liver disease)

AIH/PBC	AMA, ANA/SMA Histology AIH, PBC HLA-DR3, -DR4	8%
AIC*	ANA/SMA Histology: PBC, no overlap with AIH histology	10%
AIH/PSC	ANA, p-ANCA Histology AIH, PSC HLA-?	6% and more

*Second variant of AIH/PBC OLS, separate disease or outlier syndrome?

autoimmune liver diseases[3]. The OLS AIH/AIC is seen in 10% and AIH/PSC in 6% (Table 6).

AIH/PBC OLS

This OLS can be divided into two variants. The first shows mainly the histological criteria of autoimmune hepatitis but, serologically, there is AMA positivity. IgG is rather low, IgM, characteristic for PBC, is seen in higher concentrations. As in autoimmune hepatitis, ANA and smooth muscle antibodies (SMA) can be found. Immunogenetically, the AIH/PBC OLS is associated with HLA DR3 and DR4, as in autoimmune hepatitis. AIH/PBC OLS seems to respond favourably to ursodeoxycholic acid/glucocorticoid combination therapy.

The second variant is characterized by the histological features of classic primary biliary cirrhosis; histological overlapping does not occur[17,18]. Serologically, antimitochondrial antibodies are absent. In a recent study, AMA were positive when more sensitive methods were used. IgG is rather low and ANA and SMA titres are higher than in PBC. The immunogenetics show DR3 and DR4 as seen in autoimmune hepatitis, but, in addition, DR8, which is typical of primary biliary cirrhosis. This overlap syndrome responds excellently to UDCA monotherapy.

This variant is also called autoimmune cholangitis (AIC). Some aspects suggest that autoimmune cholangitis is nothing but a variant of PBC: there are no histological differences between the two diseases, PDC-E2 is expressed on bile duct cells, the course of the disease is identical to that of PBC and treatment with ursodeoxycholic acid is successful in most patients[19].

Others believe autoimmune cholangitis to be a separate liver disease: AST is higher and IgM lower than in PBC; in contrast to PBC, patients express carboanhydrase II-antibodies; the ANA, SMA titres at 1 : 160 are rather high; there are antibodies against glycogen phosphorylase and against nuclear envelope. Furthermore, the lymphocytes of AIC patients express Vβ5.1 T-cell receptors and, as already mentioned, the HLA risk factors are different from those of PBC.

Since, at present, it is not possible to define autoimmune cholangitis as a variant of PBC, a separate disease or an overlap syndrome between PBC and autoimmune hepatitis, AIC is also called an outlier syndrome[3] (Table 7). Recently an OLS of PBC and primary sclerosing cholangitis has been described in a 40-year-old female[20].

Table 7 Atypical manifestations of autoimmune hepatitis

Overlap syndromes (two diseases in one liver)
AIH/PBC
AIH/PSC
AIH/AIC

Outlier syndromes (cannot be classified)
AIC (AMA neg. PBC?, OLS?, separate disease?)
Cryptogenic chronic hepatitis

Changing diagnosis
PBC to AIH
AIH to PSC

Table 8 Ursodeoxycholic acid therapy in patients with PBC

Drug	*Statistically proven results*
Ursodeoxycholic acid (UDCA) (10–15–20 mg kg^{-1} day^{-1})	Improves laboratory tests Improves liver histology Reduces progression to cirrhosis Reduces risk of oesophageal varices Prolongs life expectancy
UDCA plus glucocorticoids	AIH/PBC OLS (not proven in larger studies)

Changing diagnosis

There have been a few reports on patients with a well-defined and suitably treated autoimune liver disease in whom a change of diagnosis has occurred after several years[2]. In these cases the serological and histological picture may alter completely or only partially. Such cases with transitional syndromes are rare but show that a patient with one autoimmune disease is at high risk of another one. Not all changes in laboratory parameters, however, are evidence of a new diagnosis. Only careful evaluation of biochemical and morphological criteria will confirm the change and justify a change of therapy.

Therapy

In PBC, therapeutic trials have been performed with D-penicillamine, glucocorticoids, colchicine, azathioprine, methotrexate, cyclosporin, chlorambucil and many other substances. All data published suggest no substantial positive effect.

In 1985, we introduced ursodeoxycholic acid (UDCA, 10–15 mg kg^{-1} day^{-1}) to the therapy of primary biliary liver diseases (PBC; PSC) after we had shown that UDCA results in a significant improvement of laboratory values in cholestatic chronic active hepatitis[21,22]. Over the following 15 years, it has been shown that UDCA retards disease progression from one stage of fibrosis to the next, slows down the development of oesophageal varices, prolongs the interval free of transplantation, improves life expectancy in PBC and represents basic therapy of the so-called overlap syndromes[23] (Table 8).

References

1. Dahlan YM, Smith L, Simmonds D *et al.* Pediatric onset primary biliary cirrhosis. Hepatology. 2001;34:369A.
2. Heathcote J. Overlap syndromes and changing diagnosis. In: Manns MP, Paumgartner G, Leuschner U, editors. Immunology and Liver. Dordrecht, Boston, London: Kluwer, 2000: 288–95.
3. Czaja AJ. The variant forms of autoimmune hepatitis. Ann Intern Med. 1996;125:588–9.
4. Kim WR, Lindor KD, Locke III GR *et al.* Epidemiology and natural history of primary biliary cirrhosis in a U.S. community. Gastroenterology. 2000;119:1631–6.
5. James OFW, Bhopal R, Howel D *et al.* Primary biliary cirrhosis once rare, now common in the United Kingdom? Hepatology. 1999;30:390–4.
6. Gershwin ME, Mackay IR. Primary biliary cirrhosis: paradigm or paradox for autoimmunity. Gastroenterology. 1991;100:822–33.
7. Berg PA, Doniach D, Roitt IM. Mitochondrial antibodies in primary biliary cirrhosis. I. Localization of the antigen to mitochondrial membranes. J Exp Med. 1967;126:277–90.
8. Suhr CD, Danner DJ, Ahmed A *et al.* Reactivity of PBC sera with a human fetal liver cDNA clone of branched chain keto acid dehydrogenase (BCKD) dihydrolipoamide acyltransferase, the 52 kD mitochondrial autoantigen. Hepatology. 1988;9:63–8.
9. Popper H, Schaffner F. Non-suppurative destructive chronic cholangitis and chronic hepatitis. In: Popper H, Schaffner F, editors. Progress in Liver Diseases. Vol. III, New York: Grune and Stratton, 1970:336–54.
10. Ludwig J, Dickson ER, McDonald GS. Staging of chronic non suppurative cholangitis (syndrome of primary biliary cirrhosis). Virchows Arch (A). 1978;379:103–12.
11. Hübscher SG. Histological classification of autoimmune cholestatic liver diseases. In: Manns MP, Paumgartner G, Leuschner U, editors. Immunology and Liver. Dordrecht, Boston, London: Kluwer, 2000:223–43.
12. Olsson R, Loof L, Wallerstedt S *et al.* Pregnancy in patients with primary biliary cirrhosis. A case for discussion? Liver. 1993;13:316–18.
13. Rabinovitz M, Appasamy R, Finkelstein S. Primary biliary cirrhosis diagnosed during pregnancy. Does it have a different outcome? Dig Dis Sci. 1995;40:571–4.
14. Podda M, Crosignani A, Larghi A *et al.* Female sex hormones and primary biliary cirrhosis. In: Reyes HB, Leuschner U, Arias IM, editors. Pregnancy, Sex Hormones and the Liver. Dordrecht, Boston, London: Kluwer, 1996:179–86.
15. Schlichting JK, Leuschner MS, Caspary WF *et al.* Ursodeoxycholic acid does not impair primary biliary liver diseases and pregnancy. Does pregnancy improve primary biliary liver diseases? Hepatology. 2000;32:509A.
16. Alvarez F, Berg PA, Bianchi FB and members of the IAIHG. International Autoimmune Hepatitis Group Report: review of criteria for diagnosis of autoimmune hepatitis. J Hepatol. 1999;31:929–38.
17. Woodward J, Neuberger J. Autoimmune overlap syndromes. Hepatology. 2001;33:994–1002.
18. Czaja AJ, Carpenter HA, Santrach PJ *et al.* Autoimmune cholangitis within the spectrum of autoimmune liver disease. Hepatology. 2000;31:1231–8.
19. Ishibashi H. Are primary biliary cirrhosis and autoimmune cholangitis reflective of the pendulum of a clock and therefore represent a "phase" of the same disease? J Gastroenterol Hepatol. 2001;16:121–3.
20. Burak KW, Urbanski SJ, Swain MG. A case of coexisting primary biliary cirrhosis and primary sclerosing cholangitis. A new overlap of autoimmune liver disease. Dig Dis Sci. 2001;46: 2043–7.
21. David R, Kurtz W, Leuschner U. Die Wirkung von Ursodesoxycholsäure bei chronischen Leberkrankheiten. Z Gastroenterol. 1985;23:420(abstr.).
22. Leuschner U, Fisher H, Kurtz W *et al.* Ursodeoxycholic acid in primary biliary cirrhosis: results of a controlled double blind trial. Gastroenterology. 1989;97:1268–74.
23. Poupon RE. Ursodeoxycholic acid for primary biliary cirrhosis: Lessons from the past – issues for the future. J Hepatol. 2000;32:685–8.

Section III
Treatment and complications

8
Paediatric liver transplantation. Geneva experience from 1989 to 2001

C. LE COULTRE, P. MAJNO, G. MENTHA,
PH. BUGMANN and D. BELLI

INTRODUCTION

Over the last 20 years, paediatric orthotopic liver transplantation (OLT) has witnessed remarkable progress.

In the 1980s, children were dying on waiting lists (16–25%) because of the shortage of organs of appropriate size, namely from paediatric donors. For the same reason, they reached transplantation too late. Furthermore, the technical complexities of the surgical act and the problems of peri- and postoperative care were unresolved. While these aspects are still a challenge to any team who is involved with these small patients in terminal liver failure, most of these problems have been resolved, providing these children with optimal chances of leading a normal life.

To palliate the organ shortage, Bismuth and Houssin[1] developed the technique of reduced liver transplantation in 1981: a whole liver from an adult cadaveric donor is reduced to the desired size to fit the infant. This technique is founded on a precise knowledge of the internal anatomy of the liver, that is divided into lobes and segments that have their own separated vascular and biliary pedicles. However, this technique reduces the availability of organs for the adults on waiting lists. In 1988, Pilchmayr and Bismuth[2–5] introduced the technique of split liver transplantation: one donor organ providing two grafts, one for an adult and one for a child. This procedure can be performed *ex situ* (after retrieving the organ, division of the liver into two parts is done on the bench table at 4°C), with an obvious lengthening of the cold ischaemic time, or *in situ*, during the retrieval operation in the cadaveric donor with the two halves of the liver still perfused (technically more challenging, this method requires excellent surgical skill, a good stability of the donor and prolongs the waiting time for teams involved in the transplantation of other organs).

With the *in-situ* technique, split liver transplantation offers the same results as OLT with whole or reduced organs. This technique permits transplantation to the children without depleting the pool of organs for adult recipients.

In 1989, Raia and then Strong[6–10] initiated the use of the left lobe of the liver from a living related donor to transplant to a child. Over 1000 of such cases have been performed worldwide with excellent results, similar to the best series of split liver and whole organ transplantation. And this technique has led to a decrease in mortality while on the waiting list and allowed transplantation of children more electively, before their general condition deteriorates. However, to the best of our knowledge, at least 2 donors have died after liver donation for a child.

Overall, the results of liver transplantation for children are excellent[11,12], both in terms of survival and of quality of life. The most recent series report 5-year survival rates of 95% for metabolic diseases, 85% for biliary atresia (BA) and 75% for fulminant hepatitis[13–15].

The aim of this review is to discuss several important issues in paediatric liver transplantation.

THE PROGRAMME OF PAEDIATRIC LIVER TRANSPLANTATION IN GENEVA

Our programme started in 1989, one year after the first adult liver transplantation, and is a combined adult–paediatric programme. Geneva is the only referral centre for paediatric liver transplantation in our country. Children are hospitalized at the Children's Hospital, under the care of the paediatricians, paediatric hepatologist and surgeons from the paediatric and adult transplantation team.

From 1989 to July 2001, we performed 48 transplantations in 44 children (4 retransplantations, 2 for primary non-function of the graft, 2 for chronic rejection). The indications are similar to other series in the literature (Table 1). No child was refused transplantation on the basis of age, weight or anatomy (i.e. preduodenal portal vein, polysplenia, malrotation, absence of vena cava). In two cases, transplantation was refused by the parents, one because of a cardiac defect that would have required open heart surgery before OLT, and one, early in our experience, because the parents refused conventional treatment. Eight patients

Table 1

Cholestatic diseases	
Biliary atresia	25
Sclerosing cholangitis	2
Alagille's syndrome	1
Metabolic diseases	
α_1-Antitrypsine deficiency	2
Tyrosinaemia	2
Wilson's disease	2
a-beta-Lipoproteinaemia	1
Crigler–Najar's disease	1
Others	
Fulminant hepatitis	4
Cryptogenic cirrhosis	4

died on the waiting list, six before 1997, and two afterwards from other causes: one from a head trauma complicated by abnormal clotting, and the other from a strangulated small bowel obstruction.

CHOICE OF ORGANS

In our series, we could use a whole liver in only 13 children (of a total of 48 liver grafts). The donors of whole livers were aged 9 months to 15 years (mean 5.76 years).

From 1989 to the end of 1998, most of the livers we used were adult-size organs that had to be reduced to fit the size of the paediatric recipients (24 reduced livers of a total of 37 transplantations). Donors during this period were aged 5 to 66 years, with a mean of 26.4 years. From 1999 to July 2001, only 4 livers were reduced (of a total of 11 transplantations), and all of these were paediatric size organs that had to fit the size of a smaller recipient. Donors were aged 5 to 13 years (mean of 8 years). No adult liver was reduced from the beginning of 1999. We performed 3 split liver transplantations *ex vivo* early in our experience (until the end of 1998), with a cold ischaemic time of 10.66 hours, and, since 1999, 4 *in-situ* splits, with a mean cold ischaemic time of 4.3 h. We encountered two biliary complications with the *ex-situ* technique and one minor biliary complication with the *in-situ* technique. Four additional biliary complications were seen in the rest of the series. In our experience, the split technique, especially *in situ*, was not associated with more problems with biliary reconstruction. No vascular complications could be attributed to the split technique (one arterial thrombosis early in the series).

In our group, we started a programme of living related donors in 1998 (as a mixed adult–paediatric programme). Of the 21 children placed on a waiting list from April 1998 (19 transplantations performed since that time), 12 parents offered to donate. With the policy of splitting any suitable organ, this was not necessary. During the same time, 5 transplantations were successfully performed in adults with a living related donor. Because of the increasing shortage of organs, however, the parents of two children have undergone the preliminary work-up, in case no organ becomes available in due time.

RESULTS

The overall survival rate of our series is 91%.

Although this series is relatively small, the survival rate allows to comment on some of the aspects of the programme.

Mortality

There were 4 deaths in this series: the first patient of the programme, after 8 months on the waiting list, in very poor condition at the time of OLT, was transplanted at the beginning of our learning curve. Patient number 11, aged 19 months and weighing 6 kg, received our first split, the right liver being given to an adult with fulminant hepatitis (donor and both recipients were in our centre).

Both experienced primary non-function, and both were re-transplanted 2 days later, again with the *ex-vivo* split technique. The adult survived, but the child had arterial thrombosis and died of multiple organ failure after three months. Patients 18 and 42, aged 2 years and 7 months, respectively, had fulminant hepatic failure. The first was transferred when already in a hepatic coma, with a prothrombin time of less than 10%. She died shortly after the OLT with a functioning graft, from cardiac deficiency and multiple organ failure. Postmortem examination revealed a generalized mitochondrial disease. The other patient had a primary non-function, and neurological deterioration contraindicated retransplantation.

All four deaths in the series occurred in the early postoperative period (within three months).

Survival

The 40 remaining children are all doing well and all but two lead a normal life. Several points contributed to these results and deserve comment:

- This is a common adult–paediatric programme. For a small country like Switzerland, where the need for liver transplantation in children is 5–8 per year, such a joint programme is the only way to gather enough experience and surgical skill, both for the paediatric and the adult surgeons.
- Children are hospitalized in the Children's Hospital, experienced in paediatric intensive care and in all paediatric specialties. In our institution, there is an active programme of cardiac surgery (3 cases of open heart surgery per week for congenital malformations) and a large neonatal unit. We have a paediatric trauma centre for patients from the region and from nearby France. Transplanted children are hospitalized in the same intensive care facilities and benefit from the same high level of knowledge.
- A single paediatric waiting list allows the best patient-to-graft match.
- Distances in Switzerland are short, and visits to the centre are easy and encouraged (housing facilities are available for the parents when the children are hospitalized for the transplantation and for check-ups).
- High priority is given to communication with the referring hospital and home physicians, allowing anticipation of many pre- and post-transplantation problems.

Management of the children in the programme has four different phases, each with its own specificities:

1. Pretransplant preparation:
    - Nutrition is the key factor. Any patient who is unable to feed correctly, receives enteral feeding through a nasogastric tube (at home, with the help of the paediatrician of the child and a visiting nurse). Except for the two small children who eventually died early in our series, all our children continued to gain weight while on the waiting list.
    - An active programme of immunization is performed.

- Children are regularly reviewed to determine the optimal time for transplantation, a compromise between weight gain and progression of the liver disease.

2. Transplantation:
   Technical improvements have allowed us to overcome different problems:

   - The portal vein is often underdeveloped in biliary atresia and cannot provide adequate flow. Most of the anastomoses are performed between the portal vein of the graft[16] and the recipient's spleno-mesenteric junction. If necessary, we do not hesitate to interpose a venous graft to facilitate the portal vein anastomoses. Two portal vein thromboses occurred early in the series and were saved by immediate reoperation.
   - We shortened the length of the hepatic veins of the graft. This makes anastomoses technically more difficult but reduces the risks of malpositioning and kinking and has virtually resolved the problem of postoperative ascites which is due in part to outflow obstruction.
   - For artery anastomoses, microvascular techniques are used as appropriate, with liberal use of the techniques used in the care of the premature and newborn. The four arterial complications occurred at the beginning of this series.
   - All vascular anastomoses since 1998 have been checked by intraoperative ultrasound – Doppler examination, allowing correction of technical faults, malpositioning and spontaneous systemic shunts that can divert portal flow from the graft. This technique has resulted in a series of 17 paediatric and 56 adult consecutive transplantations in the programme with no vascular complications.

Surgical complications were the cause of graft loss and mortality in only one patient.

3. Early post-transplant care:

   - Twice-daily multidisciplinary rounds take place at the bedside as long as the child is in ICU. Although this is time consuming, it allows consensual decisions, taking care of all aspects of management and avoiding multiple changes in treatment.
   - An echo-Doppler is performed at the bedside twice a day to monitor the graft.
   - Immunosuppression is tailored to the clinical situation and the infectious risks of the patient on an individual basis, with a low incidence of septic episodes and steroid-resistant rejection. The standard regimen is cyclosporine A, azathioprine and steroids. Tracrolimus (FK 506) is used as a rescue therapy in case of resistant rejection or retransplantation for chronic rejection (3 cases) or for severe side-effects of cyclosporine (hypertrichosis, gingival hyperplasia). Poly/monoclonal anti-T cell antibodies are used only occasionally. This regimen is progressively decreased and, after 2 years, most children are on cyclosporine monotherapy.

- On the ward, with the help of the nurses, parents are encouraged to take over progressively the treatment of their child.
- Families can adjust to outpatient life in the housing facilities near the hospital before returning home.

4. Long-term follow-up:
   Children are followed regularly with special emphasis on chronic post-transplant problems, with the help of the referring physicians. Several long-term studies have been possible thanks to the high level of care and compliance that can be expected in our country.

Kidney function

Twenty-eight patients, aged 7 months to 14 years at the time of transplantation, have been studied for creatinine clearance, tubular phosphate reabsorption (TRP), calcium/creatinine ratio, sodium excretion fraction, and proteinuria, with a follow-up of 60 months after OLT. The effects of CsA trough levels, cumulated dose, and the effect of antihypertensive drugs on creatinine clearance over nine years, were evaluated. We also looked at how the group with metabolic diseases and an underlying tubulopathy differed from the group with liver disease only. Results showed that both glomerular and tubular functions improved significantly following liver transplantation in both groups of patients. Overall, creatinine clearance was correlated with CsA trough levels, suggesting that CsA does not have a 'sclerosing' effect in the medium term. Patients treated for hypertension had lower creatinine clearance values, although this was not statistically significant. Combined antihypertensive therapy using nifedipine and enalapril seemed to be the optimal choice. The liver diseases group had greater calciuria following OLT. The group with an underlying tubulopathy showed rapid improvement in TRP following OLT.

Bone densitometry after OLT

In our series, 8 fractures were encountered in 6 children. This inclined us to study the modifications in bone density. Fifty-one mineralometries were performed in 29 children, at the level of vertebrae L2–L4 and of the femoral neck. This was compared with normal values for age by the Z-score, and the analysis provided a mean of 58 months of follow-up after OLT. The femoral Z-score improved markedly over the long term, as opposed to the Z-score for vertebrae. The femoral Z-score was significantly different between the periods 0–12 months and 18–36 months post-OLT. The progression of the Z-score (femoral and vertebral) was correlated with catch-up of height growth. Currently, all children are followed up with mineralometry, and a programme of monthly injections of biphosphonates is instituted whenever necessary.

Growth

Our studies show catch-up growth especially in the second and third year after OLT, when steroids are withdrawn.

Psychomotor development

In patients with retarded psychomotor development, we could see an improvement or the gain of a normal status in 77%. In the remaining children, the psychomotor status remained the same in 15% and 8% showed a temporary deterioration. Two children in the series are neurologically handicapped; both of them were too young and encephalopathic for optimal evaluation at the time of transplantation.

CONCLUSIONS

Overall, of the 40 children who have been successfully transplanted, 38 live a normal life, with catch-up growth. They go to normal school or kindergarten, and have normal leisure and sporting activities.

The four deaths in this series occurred during the first 3 months after OLT (3 during the first 2 days). No death was observed after that time.

FUTURE PROSPECTS

Alternatives to whole-organ transplantation for children with metabolic liver diseases are being investigated in our unit and in other centres. Hepatocyte transplantation is gaining credit. Gene transduction to correct the liver enzymatic deficiency opens up new therapeutic fields. This could be done by transplantation of human allogenic-hepatocytes (from a donor liver), encapsulated to avoid rejection. It is, however, more interesting to use autologous hepatocytes (isolated from the native liver), manipulated genetically, and re-infused in the patient. Our research laboratory is conducting experiments showing that transplantation of normal rat hepatocytes improves bilirubin levels in rats with a congenital defect of bilirubin metabolism (a model for Crigler–Najar's disease, normally treated with whole-organ transplantation). New experiments show that it is even possible to treat the same disease by isolating the abnormal hepatocytes, treating them with the virus encoding for the gene, and transplanting the cells thus modified, therefore correcting the enzymatic defect and the hyperbilirubinaemia, without having to use antirejection treatment. Eventually, it may be possible to inject a modified virus encoding for the deficient gene directly in the portal vein, correcting the metabolic disease.

References

1. Bismuth H, Houssin. Partial resection of liver grafts for orthotopic or heterotopic liver transplantation. Transplant Proc. 1985;17:279–83.
2. Pilchmayr R, Ringe B, Gubernatis G *et al.* Transplantation einer Spenderleber auf zwei Empfanger (Splitting-Transplantation): Eine neue Methode in der Weiterentwicklumg der Lebersegmenttransplantation. Langenbecks Arch Chir. 1988;373:127–30.
3. Boillot O, Boudjema K. Progrès techniques en transplantation hépatique. Ann Chir. 1996;3: 231–40.
4. Rela M, Vougas V, Muiesan P *et al.* Split liver transplantation. Ann Surg. 1998;227:282–8.
5. Azoulay D, Astarcioglu I, Bismuth H *et al.* Split liver transplantation. Ann Surg. 1996;224: 737–48.

6. Raia S, Nery JR, Mies S. Liver transplantation from live donors. Lancet. 1989;ii:497–8.
7. Strong RW, Lynch SV, Ong TH *et al.* Successful liver transplantation from a living donor to her son. N Engl J Med. 1990;322:1505–7.
8. Broelsch C, Whitington P, Emond J *et al.* Liver transplantation in children from living related donors. Ann Surg. 1991;214:428–39.
9. Broelsch C, Burdelski M, Rogiers X *et al.* Living donor for liver transplantation. Hepatology. 1994;20:49S–55S.
10. Boillot O, Dawahra M, Porcheron J *et al.* Transplantation hépatique pédiatrique et donneur vivant apparenté. Ann Chir. 1993;47:577–85.
11. de Ville de Goyet J, Reding R, Van Obbergh L *et al.* Pediatric liver transplantation: from the full-size liver graft to the reduced, split, and living related liver transplantation. Ped Surg Int. 1998;13:308–18.
12. Otte JB, de Ville de Goyet J, Reding R *et al.* Living related donor liver transplantation in children: the Brussels experience. Transpl Proc. 1996;28:2378–9.
13. Lopez-Santamaria M, Gamez M, Murcia J *et al.* Long-term follw-up of patients with biliary atresia successfully treated with hepatic portoenterostomy. The importance of sequential treatment. Pediatr Surg Int. 1998;13:327–30.
14. Otte J-B, de Ville de Goyet J, Reding R. Sequential treatment of biliary atresia with Kasai portoenterostomy and liver transplantation: a review. Hepatology. 1994;20:41S–8S.
15. Le Coultre C, Battaglin C, Bugmann P *et al.* Biliary atresia and orthotopic liver transplantation. 11 years of experience in Geneva. Swiss Surg. 2001;5:199–204.
16. Saad S, Tanaka K, Inomata Y *et al.* Portal vein reconstruction in pediatric liver transplantation from living donors. Ann Surg. 1998;227:275–81.

9
Patient management after paediatric liver transplantation

M. BURDELSKI, R. GANSCHOW, M. LYONS, A. VENZKE, E. GRABHORN, E. HARPS, H. H. HELLWEGE, D. BROERING, K. HELMKE and X. ROGIERS

INTRODUCTION

Liver transplantation has come of age after an almost exponential development in the last decade. This phenomenon was stimulated by simultaneous use of innovative surgical techniques, such as living-related and split-liver transplantation, improvements in immunosuppression, intensive care management and progress in diagnostic and therapeutic tools in bacterial, viral and fungal infections[1,2]. Thus, transplantation is an excellent example of the power of interdisciplinary cooperation.

From 1968 to 2001, a total of 4675 paediatric liver transplantations has been performed in Europe, the actual 10-year survival rates being 73%[3] (Figure 1). The actual short-term survival is approaching even 90%. Compared with the initial results obtained during the first years of transplantation, these figures reflect satisfactory progress[4].

Management aims to either avoid or recognize as early as possible surgical and medical complications and to use an optimized intensive care and normal care protocol.

SURGICAL PROBLEMS

Surgical problems may derive from many sources since liver transplantation is one of the most complex surgical procedures, requiring surgery of the liver, vessels and bowel. There are recipient-related and donor-organ-related aspects which have to be taken into account. The typical paediatric liver transplant recipient in our centre is suffering from multiorgan disease, and weighs between 6 and 10 kg, indicating severe malnutrition since the median age is 40 months[5]. At the beginning of transplantation, severe malnutrition, a body weight below 10 kg, or vascular malformations, for instance preduodenal portal vein in combination with aplasia of the inferior vena cava and azygos continuation, were considered as contraindications. Today, the only contraindications are active bacterial, viral or fungal infections and pulmonary hypertension[2]. Even systemic metabolic disorders, such as cystic fibrosis, mitochondriopathies or other metabolic disorders, are accepted in special cases[6].

Mortality on the waiting list may be abolished despite the extension of indications by using, apart from full-size organs, all technical variants such as split-liver, living-related and, in rare cases only, reduced size organs[7]. In contrast to the other techniques, split-liver and living-related liver transplantation provides paediatric patients with grafts without affecting the limited donor pool for adult recipients (Figure 2)[8]. All these technical variants, however, may increase the risk of surgical complications, such as bleeding and biliary leakage from the cut surface, leakages from bile duct reconstructions, and initial poor or non-function.

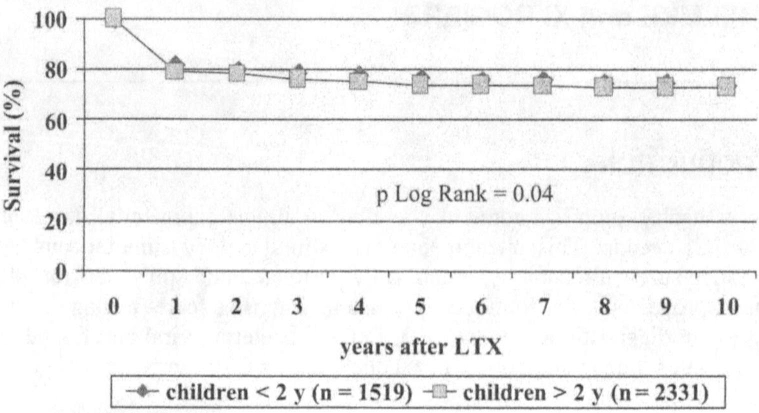

Figure 1 Results of paediatric liver transplantation of patients aged 0–2 and 2–16 years in the years 1968–2000. Modified from Reference 3.

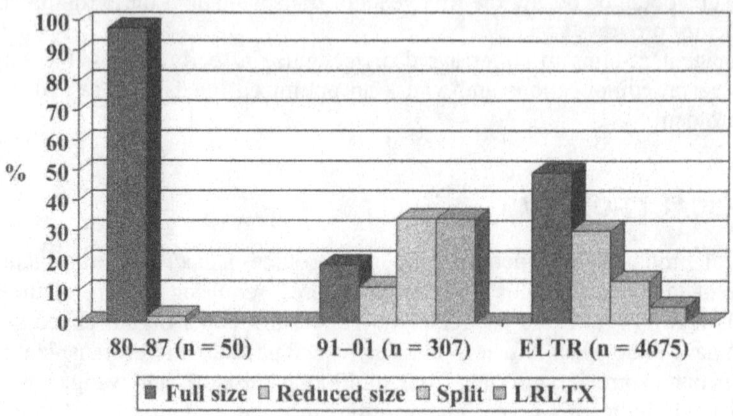

Figure 2 Surgical techniques used in 1980–1987, 1991–2001 in Hannover and Hamburg respectively and in ELTR 1968–2000. Modified from Reference 3 and own data.

Therefore, the optimized management of any paediatric transplant recipient aims to detect these potential surgical complications as early as possible. The surgical procedure itself has been optimized by using magnifying glasses, special suture materials, and new perfusion solutions, such as the University of Wisconsin or the Brettschneider solution.

After the introduction of intraoperative Doppler ultrasound, many grafts were rescued by immediate surgical correction, either by repositioning the organ or by reanastomosing the portal vein or hepatic artery in cases with impaired flow of hepatic artery, portal or hepatic vein (Figure 3). Since split techniques and living-related transplantation have steadily improved due to the growing experience gained in transplantation, a significant decrease in surgical complications has been observed in recent years (Figure 4). The monitoring of clotting factors, under the use of heparin, and the close observation of the abdominal drain secretions

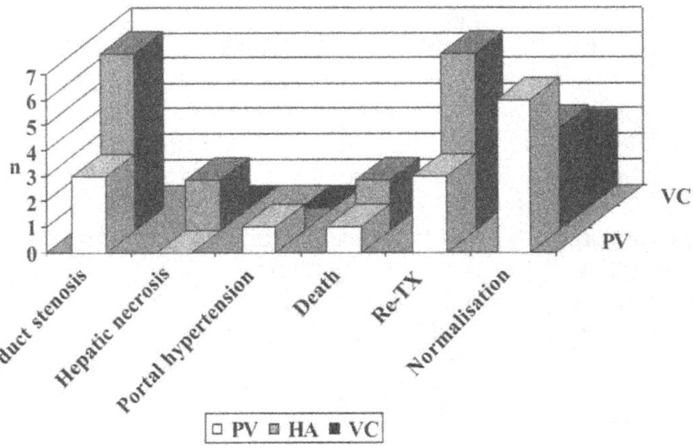

Figure 3 Results of ultrasound-detected intraoperative perfusion damage and immediate surgical repair with regard to complications, retransplantation, normalization and death (own data).

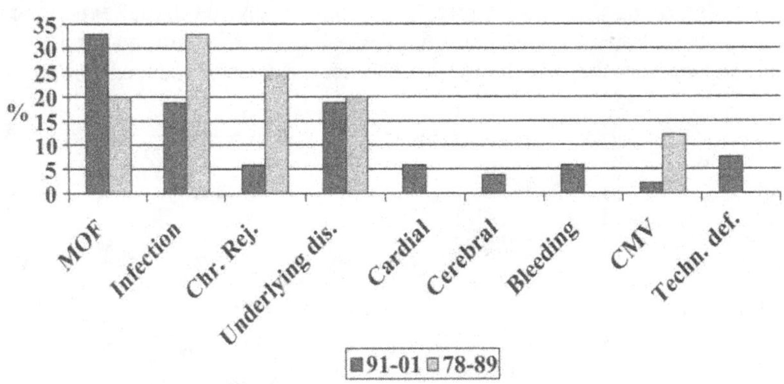

Figure 4 Causes of patient losses after paediatric liver transplantation. Comparison between 1978–1989 and 1991–2001. Modified from Reference 3 and own data.

help to detect bleeding from any surgical source and identification of any leakage from the bile duct system or the intestine as soon as possible. Increased bilirubin or bile acid concentrations in the ascites surpassing the serum concentrations are strong indicators of a biliary leak, whereas the additional increase of amylase concentration in these fluids indicates a leak from the intestine. These complications are managed either conservatively by drains or by immediate reoperation.

MEDICAL PROBLEMS

Medical problems include initial poor or non-function, infections and rejections, together with drug-induced complications. The incidence of poor or non-function is between 5 and 8%; the infection rate is much higher, reaching 50%, although the rejection rate was cut to 17% after the introduction of interleukin-2 receptor antibody in the pannel of immunosuppressive drugs[9]. This progress is remarkable since the infection rate did not increase.

Initial poor function is indicated by the need for further substitution of clotting factors, increase in serum bilirubin, and high serum transaminases above 2000 U/L. Initial non-function is characterized by severe acidosis, coma, complete breakdown of the clotting system and rapid development of multiorgan failure. Living-related liver tranplantation provides excellent organ quality; only in cases with extremely small-for-size organs is poor organ function observed. The minimum organ size for the recipient is calculated to be 0.8% of the recipient's body weight[10].

These problems in liver transplantation are present in the very first hours and days after transplantation, followed by infections between post-op days 3 and 10, and rejections between days 5 and 15. However, after the introduction of interleukin-2 receptor antibody into the immunosuppressive protocol with consequent reduction of rejection from 50 to 16%, the manifestation of rejection has been postponed in most cases from days 5–7 post-operation to days 21–25[11].

Surgical and medical complications are the major causes of organ and patient losses observed in the first weeks after transplantation. The analysis of the causes of death in our series shows that multiorgan failure ranks first, followed by infection and underlying diseases (Figure 4). Compared with the initial experience in paediatric liver transplantation, the number of cases of multiorgan failure has increased, whereas the infection-related losses have been reduced[12]. The large

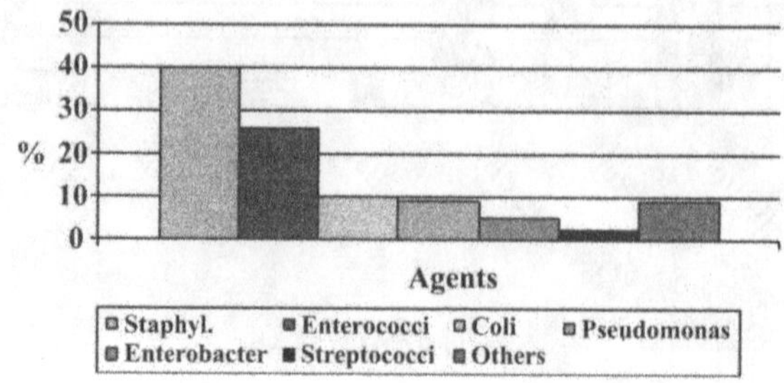

Figure 5 Bacterial agents causing infections after paediatric liver transplantation 1991–1996. Modified from Reference 12.

number of multiorgan failures includes losses after retransplantation due to initial poor or non-function and patients transplanted in desperate state after acute or chronic liver failure. In consequence, it is essential to emphasize the need for an early referral of patients to a transplant centre in order to avoid these losses.

The relatively large number of infections must be taken as an argument that still too much immunosuppression is applied. Life-threatening bacterial infections are mainly caused by staphylococci, and enterococci (Figures 5 and 6)[12]. Another argument against too much immunosuppression is the observation of toxic side-effects, mainly of calcineurin inhibitors and steroids, which include toxic kidney, liver and central nervous system damage and arterial hypertension (Figure 7).

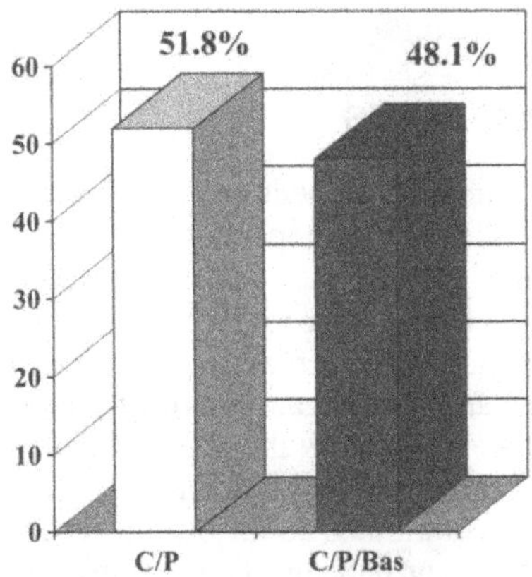

Figure 6 Comparison between infectious complications observed under conventional (C/P) and IL-2 receptor antibody supplemented immunosuppression (C/P/Bas). Modified from Reference 9.

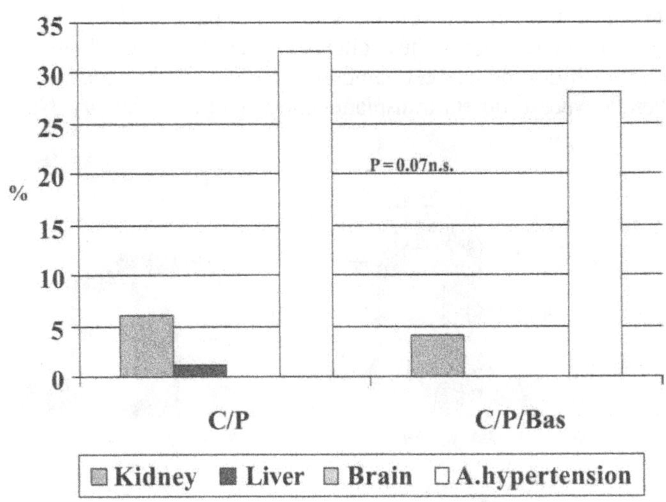

Figure 7 Medical complications under conventional (C/P) and IL-2 receptor antibody supplemented immunosuppression (C/P/Bas). Modified from Reference 9.

Another strong argument for reconsidering high-dose immunosuppression protocols is the fact that there is a clear age-dependent prevalence of acute graft rejection[11]. Infants have the lowest rejection rate with 26.8%, followed by toddlers with 40% and finally children >36 months of age with 71.8%. These figures clearly indicate a need for individualized immunosuppression where age, immunological status and compromized reactivity under infections are considered.

Compared with other centres, we have used a lower dosage immunosuppression protocol from the beginning. In our opinion, this is the main reason for the low rate of post-transplant lymphoproliferative disease (PTLD) of 0.7% which has been observed in our patients. This result is not counteracted by a high rate of chronic rejection. This serious complication was only seen in 1.8% in our patients.

INTENSIVE CARE PROBLEMS

An optimized intensive care management is the prerequisite for a good postoperative course. Therapy of the early postoperative period has changed significantly in our centre: the length of the ICU stay and of ventilation has shortened from 9 to 6.5 days and from 3 to 1 day, respectively[5]. At the same time, the manifestations of pulmonary complications, such as pneumonitis, pleural effusions, bacterial infections, rejections and multiorgan failures, have been reduced (Figure 8). This observation must be explained by the effect of good quality control leading to better management of these multimorbid patients.

All these factors have contributed to an overall result of almost 80% three-year cumulative survival in our patients. This result is comparable to the ELTR data[3], showing that the international standard of paediatric liver transplantation has reached a high level.

Further progress will rely on close cooperation of primary care hospitals and transplant centres in order to ensure early referal of patients. By avoiding multiorgan morbidity of the recipients, the challenge of transplantation should be reduced. Furthermore, multidisciplinary cooperation of all partners in a transplantation centre and even between different transplant centres will be necessary. New tools are

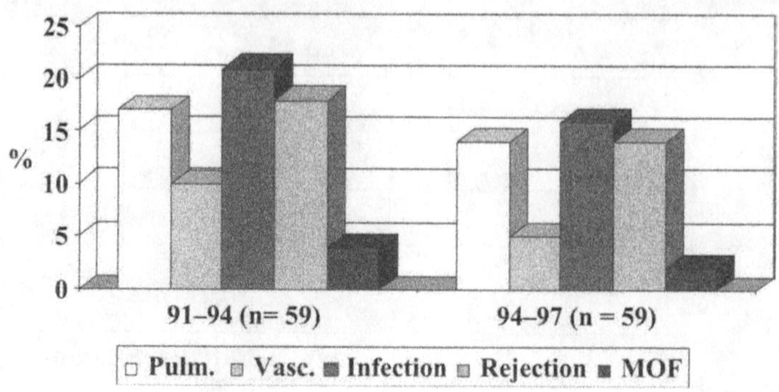

Figure 8 Comparison of serious complications observed during intensive care treatment after paediatric liver transplantation in the years 1991–1994 and 1994–1997. Modified from Reference 5.

needed to evaluate quality of life in children of different age groups. These methods and a high standard of control of quality with regard to results and complications are in progress.

Acknowledgements

We thank all families who agreed to the donation of livers for our patients, and all parents and relatives who donated parts of their livers for living donation to their children.

References

1. Burdelski M, Nolkemper D, Ganschow R *et al.* Liver transplantation in children: long-term outcome and quality of life. Eur J Pediatr 1999;158(Suppl 2):S34–42.
2. Kelly DA. Current results of evolving indications for liver transplantation in children. J Pediatr Gastroenterol Nutr. 1998;27:214–21.
3. European Liver Transplant Registry. Report 2000. Paul Brousse Hospital, 2001.
4. Burdelski M, Schmidt K, Hoyer PF *et al.* Liver transplantation in children. The Hannover experience. Transpl Proc. 1987;19:3277–81.
5. Burdelski M, Ganschow R, Breivik I *et al.* Indication for liver transplantation in children. In: L Flautner, P Kupcsulik, I Rosza, editors. IHPBA, Budapest 1999. Rastignano-Bologna: Monduzzi Editore, 1999:97–108.
6. Burdelski M, Rogiers X. Liver transplantation in metabolic disorders. Acta Gastroenterol Belg. 1999;62:300–5.
7. Otte JB. The availability of all technical modalities for pediatric liver transplant programs. Pediatr Transpant. 2001;5:1–4.
8. Rogiers X, Malago M, Gawad K *et al.* In situ splitting of cadaveric livers. The ultimate expansion of a limited donor pool. Ann Surg. 1996;224:221–241.
9. Ganschow R, Grabhorn E, Burdelski M. Basiliximab in paediatric liver transplantation. Correspondence. Lancet. 2001;357:338.
10. Broering D, Müller, Ganschow R *et al.* Is there still a need for living related liver transplantation in children? Ann Surg. 2001;234:713–722.
11. Ganschow R, Broering DC, Nolkemper D *et al.* Th2 cytokine profile in infants predisposes to improved graft acceptance after liver transplantation. Transplantation. 2001;72:929–34.
12. Drews D, Sturm E, Latta A *et al.* Complications following living related and cadaveric liver transplantation in 100 children. Transplant Proc. 1997;29:421–23.

10
De-novo autoimmune hepatitis after liver transplantation

N. HADZIC, D. VERGANI and G. MIELI-VERGANI

INTRODUCTION

Late graft dysfunction after liver transplantation can be induced by infections, vascular complications, biliary problems, recurrence of the original disease, lymphoproliferative disease, poor compliance leading to cellular rejection, or onset of chronic rejection. We have recently described a novel form of graft dysfunction in the absence of these causes[1]. The characteristic features were strikingly reminiscent of classical autoimmune liver disease (AILD), including hypergammaglobulinaemia, elevated titres of serum autoantibodies, and histological findings of chronic hepatitis with portal and periportal infiltrate with plasma cells and lymphocytes, perivenular cell necrosis, bridging fibrosis and collapse. Furthermore, six out of seven patients have responded to standard treatment of AILD with prednisolone ($2\,mg\,kg^{-1}\,d^{-1}$) and azathioprine ($1.5–2\,mg\,kg^{-1}\,d^{-1}$) within a median of 32 days (range 7–316). Four of the patients fulfilled the international criteria for 'definite' and three for 'probable' autoimmune hepatitis[2]. None of the children was transplanted for AILD and all had serum levels of cyclosporine A or tacrolimus within the therapeutic range at diagnosis. Three patients had low titres of serum autoantibodies before transplantation. During the six-year observation period, the overall incidence of *de-novo* autoimmune hepatitis amongst children transplanted at our centre was 4%[1]. It is noteworthy that five patients had received allografts from donors with HLA DR3/DR4 alleles, known to confer susceptibility to AILD. However, when we compared the HLA alleles of the children who developed *de-novo* autoimmune hepatitis with those of 32 children matched for length of post-transplant follow-up, we could not detect a statistical difference[1].

Several paediatric and adult studies followed our observation, some reporting major complications including progression to cirrhosis, loss of liver grafts and deaths[3–6]. One recent study in adult liver transplant patients reported possession of HLA DRB*0301 or DRB*0401 by either donor or recipient in all individuals diagnosed with *de-novo* autoimmune hepatitis. Unfortunately, no data for control donor–recipient pairs were presented[6].

Since the initial report, we have been routinely monitoring our transplanted patients for emergence of organ specific and non-specific autoantibodies in the serum. Seventy per cent (144/206) of prospectively studied children transplanted between 1996 and 2001 have developed autoantibodies at a titre ≥1/20. The detected antibodies included antinuclear, antismooth muscle, antiliver kidney microsomal, antimitochondrial and antigastric parietal cell antibodies. The patients with a follow-up of >1 and >3 years had an autoantibody prevalence of 76.5% and 87.3%, respectively. It appears that there is a correlation between length of follow-up after liver transplant (and anti-rejection treatment) and emergence of serum autoantibodies. Biochemical graft dysfunction was observed in 16% of the patients with demonstrable autoantibodies.

PATHOGENESIS

The pathophysiology of post-transplant *de-novo* autoimmune hepatitis is unknown. Individuals with various disorders of immune regulation and documented primary or secondary immunodeficiencies frequently have detectable low titres of autoantibodies. Emergence of autoantibodies is often observed after bone marrow transplant for primary immunodeficiencies. These phenomena have no obvious deleterious clinical effects and may be due to ongoing immune dysregulation. In children with no significant immune abnormalities before transplantation, it is conceivable that post-transplant immunosuppression may be responsible for the development of autoantibodies and associated clinical symptoms.

Physiologically, pluripotent stem cells from the bone marrow migrate to the thymus to become T cells following a complex process of intrathymic education. Maturing double positive (CD4/CD8) T cells are subjected to positive and negative selection based on the T-cell receptor affinity for self-peptides presented by self-MHC molecules. T-cells that demonstrate a high self-reactivity are eliminated by apoptosis. Under physiological conditions, this mechanism prevents escape of potentially harmful self-reactive T-cell clones from the thymus into circulation[7].

In animal models, two groups have independently described that cyclosporine A, by preventing IL-2 gene transcription, may interfere with the physiological mechanisms of T-cell maturation in the thymus[8,9]. In a post-bone-marrow transplant rodent model, the emergence of autoaggressive T-cell clones has been described[10]. We postulate that chronic immunosuppression of transplanted patients may lead to overstimulation of bone marrow and to an expanded population of T-cells awaiting intrathymic education and selection. Their number may exceed the capacity of selection mechanisms in the thymus, leading to their emergence in the peripheral circulation (Figure 1a and b). The individuals at risk for autoimmunity either on the basis of their own or grafted liver HLA alleles may then develop graft dysfunction. Akin to other models of autoimmunity, environmental triggers may also play a role[11].

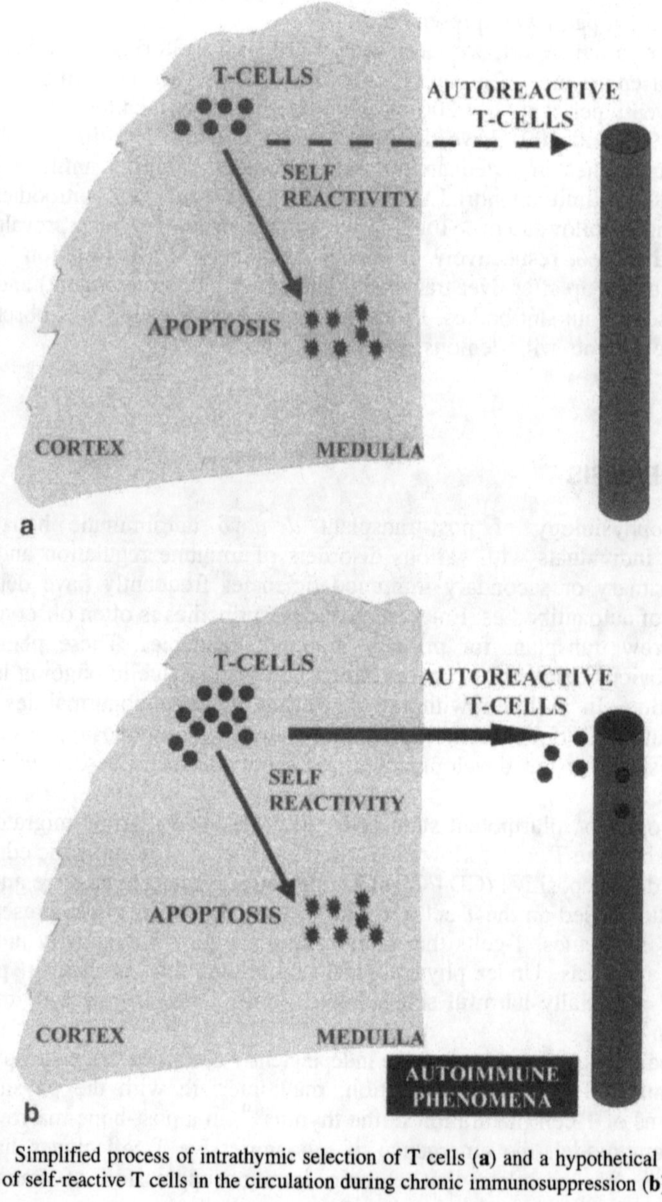

Figure 1 Simplified process of intrathymic selection of T cells (**a**) and a hypothetical mechanism of escape of self-reactive T cells in the circulation during chronic immunosuppression (**b**).

TREATMENT

To control *de-novo* autoimmune hepatitis, we use a similar approach to the treatment of AILD in children[11]. Prednisolone is given at 1–2 mg kg^{-1} d^{-1} (not exceeding 60 mg/day) until improvement of biochemical abnormalities. This dose is then tapered down to a maintenance dose of 5 mg/day within 4–8 weeks. In addition, we also reduce the dose of cyclosporine A or tacrolimus by 20–30%. In the presence of ongoing liver graft dysfunction, azathioprine or mycophenolate mofetil are added at 2 mg/kg and 40 mg kg^{-1} d^{-1}, respectively. If the patient is already taking either of these drugs, the dose is adjusted. We have not seen significant side-effects related to this treatment. If laboratory results remain completely normal, we do not routinely perform follow-up liver biopsies.

NOSOLOGY

The use of the word 'autoimmune' for an entity affecting a transplanted organ has been somewhat contentious. This has led some authors to use complicated alternative terms including 'post-transplant immune hepatitis' or 'graft dysfunction-mimicking autoimmune hepatitis'[5,6]. Of note, recurrences of autoimmune liver disorders after liver transplantation have been reported with no such semantic dilemmas[12,13]. The antigenic targets for liver-specific autoantibodies (e.g. cytochrome P450IID6 for anti-LKM) are species- rather than individuum-specific[11] and therefore shared by both recipient and donor livers. The liver replacement should not change the antigenic targets for T cells. Thus, we believe that the term *de-novo* autoimmune hepatitis is appropriate until elucidation of its pathogenesis is completed.

FURTHER RESEARCH

An obvious question is whether the phenomenon of induction of autoantibodies and organ damage occurs in other settings where long-term use of potent immunosuppressants is indicated. Several recent studies reported emergence of *de-novo* autoantibodies after renal and cardiac transplantation in association with CMV infection, vasculitis and chronic rejection[14–16]. It is important to establish a time scale for the production of serum autoantibodies and the possible development of clinical symptoms in different settings during chronic immunosuppression.

In-vivo information on the effects of cyclosporine A and tacrolimus on peripheral T-cell phenotypes is limited. Serum cytokine levels, immunohistological delineation and target specificity of the inflammatory infiltrate in the affected graft may improve the understanding of the pathogenic mechanisms leading to *de-novo* autoimmune hepatitis.

HLA markers in donor–recipient pairs are routinely determined in the majority of transplant centres. Larger scale studies should test the hypothetical genetic susceptibility to *de-novo* autoimmune hepatitis. If this is confirmed, the recipients 'at risk' should be identified early and more closely scrutinized.

The proposed areas of research may help in understanding the present paradox that cyclosporine A and tacrolimus, potent immunosuppressants sometimes used in the treatment of autoimmune disorders, may also play a role in their pathogenesis.

CONCLUSIONS

Whether post-transplant *de-novo* autoimmune hepatitis represents a distinct entity or a form of atypical rejection in individuals at risk of developing autoimmune phenomena is unclear at present. Further research is urgently needed into the pathogenesis of this clinical phenomenon. Whatever its aetiology, the recognition of this potentially life-threatening syndrome is important since its management differs from standard anti-rejection strategy.

References

1. Kerkar N, Hadzic N, Davies ET *et al.* De-novo autoimmune hepatitis after liver transplantation. Lancet. 1998;351:409–13.
2. Johnson PJ, McFarlane IG. Meeting report: international autoimmune hepatitis group. Hepatology. 1993;18:998–1005.
3. Dubel L, Farges O, Johanet C, Sebagh M, Bismuth H. High incidence of antitissue antibodies in patients experiencing chronic liver allograft rejection. Transplantation. 1998;65:1072–5.
4. Hernadez HM, Kovarik P, Whitington PF, Alonso EM. Autoimmune hepatitis as a late complication of liver transplantation. J Pediatr Gastroenterol Nutr. 2001;32:131–6.
5. Andries S, Casamayuo L, Sempoux C *et al.* Posttransplant immune hepatitis in pediatric liver transplant recipients: incidence and maintenance therapy with azathioprine. Transplantation. 2001;72:267–72.
6. Heneghan MA, Portmann B, Norris SM *et al.* Graft dysfunction mimicking autoimmune hepatitis following liver transplantation in adults. Hepatology. 2001;34:464–70.
7. Delves PJ, Roitt IM. The immune system. First of two parts. N Engl J Med. 2000;343:37–49.
8. Gao E, Lo D, Cheney R, Kanagawa O, Sprent J. Abnormal differentiation of thymocytes in mice treated with cyclosporin A. Nature. 1988;336:176–9.
9. Jenkins MK, Schwartz RH, Pardoll DM. Effects of cyclosporine A on T cell development and clonal deletion. Science. 1988;241:1655–8.
10. Bucy PB, Yan Xu X, Li J, Huang GQ. Cyclosporin A-induced autoimmune disease in mice. J Immunol. 1993;151:1039–50.
11. Mieli-Vergani G, Vergani D. Progress in pediatric autoimmune hepatitis. Semin Liver Dis. 1994;14:282–8.
12. Neuberger J, Portmann B, Calne R, Williams R. Recurrence of autoimmune chronic active hepatitis following orthotopic liver grafting. Transplantation. 1984;37:363–5.
13. Neuberger J, Portmann B, Macdougall BR, Calne RY, Williams R. Recurrence of primary biliary cirrhosis after liver transplantation. N Engl J Med. 1982;306:1–4.
14. Toyoda M, Galfayan K, Galera OA, Petrosian A, Czer LS, Jordan SC. Cytomegalovirus infection induces anti-endothelial cell antibodies in cardiac and renal allograft recipients. Transpl Immunol. 1997;5:104–11.
15. Asif A, Toral C, Diego J, Miller J, Roth D. De novo ANCA-associated vasculitis occurring 14 years after kidney transplantation. Am J Kidney Dis. 2000;35:E10.
16. Ferry BL, Welsh KI, Dunn MJ *et al.* Anti-cell surface endothelial antibodies in sera from cardiac and kidney transplant recipients: association with chronic rejection. Transpl Immunol. 1997;5: 17–24.

11
Ursodeoxycholic acid: its cytoprotective action in liver disease

E. L. RENNER

Cytoprotection in a broad sense means to sustain the vitality of cells in the presence of noxious factors; a cytoprotective substance, thus, increases the resistance of cells against otherwise toxic stimuli. Cytoprotection is therefore a purely descriptive term and does not allow conclusions as to the underlying molecular mechanism(s).

Ursodeoxycholic acid (UDCA), a relatively hydrophobic bile acid with relatively little toxicity, is a major bile acid constituent of the bile of black bears but only a minor component of human bile. Black bear bile was used for centuries in traditional Chinese medicine and UDCA has been shown in controlled trials to produce beneficial effects in liver diseases, especially if cholestatic features prevail.

These beneficial effects are generally attributed to UDCA 'cytoprotection', which has been proposed to be the consequence(s) of one or more of the following pharmacological properties:

1. UDCA therapy expands the bile acid pool, i.e. the fraction of the less-toxic hydrophobic bile acid UDCA increases, while that of more-toxic hydrophilic bile acids, such as chenodeoxycholic acid, decreases. Consequently, in cholestatic liver disease, the total toxicity caused by bile acids retained within the liver may be ameliorated by UDCA therapy.
2. In cell culture and in artificial biomembrane systems, exposure to UDCA has been shown to alleviate cytotoxicity produced by bile acids, such as chenodeoxycholic acid. This has been taken to demonstrate direct cytoprotection by UDCA but may, however, be caused by UDCA-induced changes in the structure and formation of mixed micelles.
3. UDCA is a potent choleretic, undergoes cholehepatic shunting and, thus, leads to extensive biliary secretion of bicarbonate and water. In cholestatic liver diseases, its choleretic properties may improve excretion of toxic biliary constituents through areas of the liver exhibiting still intact biliary drainage and, thus, functionally compensate for other areas where biliary drainage is impaired due to the disease process.

4. In PBC, UDCA has been shown to exert beneficial immunological effects, decreasing the elevated expression of HLA antigens on liver cells towards normal. This may help to limit the autoimmune attack believed to be involved in the pathogenesis of liver damage.
5. Finally, and most importantly perhaps, in animal models of cholestatic liver diseases, UDCA and/or its conjugates have been shown to exert profound effects on intracellular calcium homeostasis and other intracellular signalling pathways, thereby partially restoring expression of biliary excretory proteins in the canalicular membrane and thus biliary excretory capacity, and inhibiting programmed liver cell death. This seems to form the molecular basis of most, if not all, of the beneficial effects of UDCA in cholestatic liver disease described above.

12
Alopecia associated with anti-LKM antibody-positive AIH

D. C. BELLI

The classification of chronic hepatitis in children has become clearer since seroimmunological markers have been developed. Five serological groups can be distinguished: virus-related hepatitis; autoimmune hepatitis with non-organ-specific autoantibodies, divided in type 1, autoimmune hepatitis with smooth muscle antibody, type 2, autoimmune hepatitis with anti-LKM antibodies (also called anti-endoplasmic reticulum antibody), and type 3, autoimmune hepatitis with antisoluble liver antigens (SLA); and chronic hepatitis without markers.

When compared with type 1, type 2 autoimmune hepatitis is characterized by an earlier age at onset of the disease and a quicker spontaneous progression to cirrhosis (80% of cases after 3 years). However, it shows a better response to immunosuppressive therapy. Another feature of type 2 hepatitis is the frequency of associated extrahepatic pathologies in up to 35% of patients. Most of these pathologies, which include diabetes mellitus, vitiligo, thyroiditis, hypoparathyroidism and hereditary polyendocrinopathy, are thought to be of autoimmune origin. More than half of these related diseases can precede hepatitis. Their natural history and especially their response to immunosuppressive therapy is, in most instances, difficult to establish, since they are largely irreversible unless treatment occurs very early in their course. With regards to vitiligo, a good clinical response to hepatitis-related therapy was suggested in one study.

We report a 14-year-old girl presenting with anti-liver–kidney microsome autoimmune hepatitis preceded by alopecia three years earlier. Both pathologies were greatly improved by immunosuppressive therapy. To our knowledge, the association of alopecia with type 2 autoimmune hepatitis has never been reported. Although the aetiology of alopecia remains unclear, an autoimmune cause is suspected because of a higher incidence of organ-specific autoantibodies, especially against the thyroid, and because of a histological infiltrate of T lymphocytes around the hair. Steroid treatment efficacy has been found to be relative and relapses occur commonly when doses are tapered. In our case, the association with hepatic disease and the outstanding response to immunosuppressive therapy strongly suggest that the alopecia was of autoimmune origin.

In summary, this case report suggests that alopecia could be another extrahepatic manifestation related to type 2 autoimmune hepatitis. Therefore, the rare emergence of alopecia in a child could be the first clinical sign raising the suspicion of an autoimmune hepatitis.

13
Acute portal vein thrombosis: treatment by the transjugular approach – A case report

M. RÖSSLE

Acute non-cirrhotic portal vein thrombosis with or without inclusion of the main tributaries, i.e. splenic, superior and inferior mesenteric veins, is a severe disease causing considerable long-term morbidity and mortality. With the exception of a few case reports, larger studies investigating the natural course of the disease are rare. The study by Merkel *et al.*[1] found a cumulative overall 6-year mortality rate of 17% and a cumulative 6-year mortality from bleeding of 14%. The cumulative risk of variceal bleeding was 24%. This shows that variceal bleeding is frequent and the main cause of death after portal vein thrombosis. The considerable morbidity and mortality justifies the search for effective treatments with the aim of thrombus resolution. This can be achieved by local or systemic thrombolysis including the transjugular approach to the portal system.

CASE REPORT

A 13-year-old boy was admitted to KTK – Kindertagesklinik Liestal, Switzerland, with abdominal pain, vomiting, diarrhoea and fever. The blood cultures revealed growth of *Bacteroides fragilis* and an antibiotic treatment was commenced. Sonography showed a thrombus in the portal vein extending into the splenic and mesenteric veins. An abscess formation with a diameter of 5 cm was seen in the right lobe of the liver. After a 2-week treatment period with heparin, the abdominal pain persisted and the patient was transferred to our hospital.

Duplex-sonography confirmed the diagnosis showing absence of flow in the stem of the portal vein, the splenic vein, the mesenteric veins, and the intrahepatic portal branches. The veins were visible but filled with hypoechoic material. Collaterals were seen near the hepatic hilus. The spleen was not enlarged and no ascites was present. Biochemical tests showed slightly elevated liver enzymes and leukocytosis. Apart from slightly decreased concentrations of the proteins C and S, no other thrombophilic abnormalities could be detected.

After detailed information and obtaining written consent, the transjugular intervention was performed the following day as described previously[2]. A puncture needle was advanced transjugularly into a hepatic vein and the (occluded) right intrahepatic portal branch was punctured under sonographic guidance. After successful puncture an angiographic catheter was advanced and angiographies of all major tributaries of the portal vein were performed by gentle hand injection of contrast dye (Figure 1). The following manoeuvres were then performed: (1) All varices seen at angiography were occluded using a mixture of bucrylate and lipiodol (1 : 1, vol/vol, Histoacryl, Braun, Melsungen, Germany, Lipiodol, Byk-Gulden, Constance, Germany). (2) A 10-mm angioplasty balloon catheter was placed into the parenchymal tract and dilated to facilitate access to the portal vein and to allow some flow along the thrombus. (3) An 11 French sheath was advanced into the thrombus; attempts to aspirate parts of the thrombus were made forcefully and aspirated material was sent for bacteriological examination. (4) Two 5 French endhole catheters were placed, one in the splenic and one in the confluence of the splenic and superior mesenteric vein, and thrombolytic treatment was initiated the day after the intervention.

Thrombolytic treatment was started with urokinase (50 000 U bolus injection followed by 75 000 U/h) and heparin with the aim to adjust the plasma fibrinogen concentration to 200 mg/dl and to increase the PTT to 60–80 s, respectively. After 6 days of urokinase plus heparin, urokinase was terminated and r-TPA was given

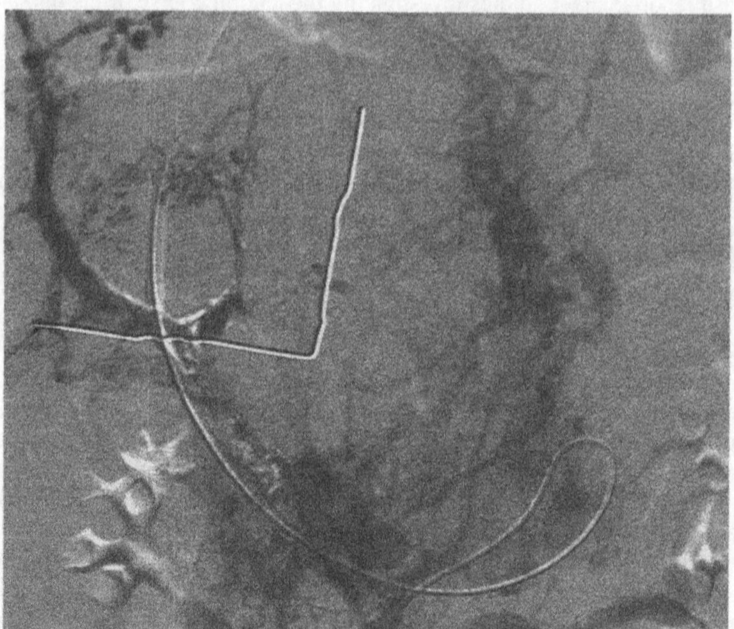

Figure 1 Portal vein thrombosis before thrombolytic therapy. The portal (PV), splenic (SV) and superior mesenteric veins (SMV) are filled with thrombotic material. The intrahepatic branches (IB) of the portal vein are also occluded.

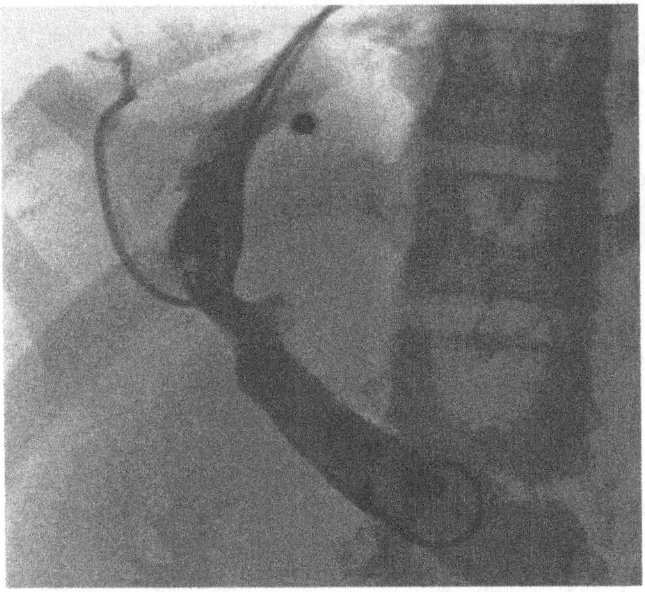

Figure 2 Situation 10 days after beginning the thrombolytic therapy. The splenic and inferior mesenteric veins are free of thrombosis. The portal vein includes residual thrombus which is haemodynamically insignificant. The intrahepatic branches are partially occluded and most of the blood drains through the intraparenchymal channel. Accordingly, pressure in the portal system was normalized (10 mmHg).

instead for another 2 days, resulting in almost complete resolution of the extrahepatic portal system (Figure 2). After a final angiography and measurement of the portosystemic pressure gradient which was 8 mmHg, catheters were removed and systemic anticoagulation initiated. At this time, the intrahepatic abscess was completely organized and the patient had no more fever.

The angiographic result was also documented with duplex-sonography which was then used for further follow-up. It showed patent extrahepatic vessels but occluded intrahepatic branches. The dilatation tract through the liver tissue was patent, draining most of the portal blood. During follow-up of 2 years, the intrahepatic shunt narrowed and occluded within 6 months. Unfortunately, a short and limited portal vein thrombosis recurred without extention into the splenic or mesenteric veins. Large collaterals were formed to bridge the thrombosis.

DISCUSSION

The transjugular treatment in this case can be regarded as a success although portal vein thrombosis recurred. In contrast to the index thrombosis which extended into the main splanchnic veins leading to severe abdominal congestion, the post-treatment thrombus was short, allowing for effective collateral formation. This led to sufficient blood flow through the portal vein collaterals and the liver, with effective reduction of the portal hypertension. A stent resulting in a permanent drainage of the portal system may have prevented recurrence of thrombosis. It was, however, not implanted because of the young age of the patient and the absence of any liver disease.

In comparison with other routes of administration of thrombolytic agents, e.g. percutaneous transhepatic, mesenteric artery, and operative access to the mesenteric vein, the transjugular route may have several advantages. (1) The risk of a bleeding complication during the thrombolytic treatment is low; (2) treatment can be given over a period of up to 10 days; and (3) if thrombolytic treatment of intrahepatic branches cannot be achieved successfully, a stent can be implanted to maintain treatment success and to prevent subsequent portal hypertension.

Using this approach, we have now treated 25 patients between 1994 and 1999[3]. Our preliminary results show an 85% short-term and 50% long-term response to treatment where *restitutio ad integrum* was achieved in 26% of patients. Partial long-term response, defined as patency of the extrahepatic veins but not of intrahepatic portal branches, was found in 34%. In most of these patients, a stent was implanted to maintain long-term treatment effect. It should be emphasized that all of our patients had anticoagulation and about half of them had systemic thrombolytic treatment before the transjugular intervention was attempted. Apart from our own results, a case report by Rivitz *et al.*[4] also described a favorable result in a patient with acute mesenteric venous thrombosis.

A recent study by Condat *et al.*[5] reported on anticoagulation therapy for acute portal vein thrombosis. During a mean follow-up of 30 months, 25 of 31 treated patients improved. Recanalization was complete in 10 patients (30%) and incomplete in 15 patients (48%) while 6 patients did not show a significant effect of treatment. It is important to note that, in the study by Condat *et al.*, only 30% of patients had extended thrombosis and 70% had thrombosis limited to the stem of the portal vein. In this latter group, complete recanalization was seen in 8 of 11 patients while this was achieved in only 2 of 16 patients with extended thrombosis.

In summary, the transjugular thrombolytic treatment of acute portal vein thrombosis with or without implantation of a stent (TIPS) may be a treatment option in the hands of experienced interventionalists. In view of the apparently high efficacy of anticoagulation therapy in patients with limited thrombosis, the transjugular thrombolytic treatment may be reserved for patients with isolated portal vein thrombosis not responding to a short (1–2-week) heparin treatment, or to those with extended portal vein thrombosis.

References

1. Merkel C, Bolognesi M, Bellon S *et al.* Long-term follow-up of adult patients with non-cirrhotic obstruction of the portal system: comparison with cirrhotic patients. J Hepatol. 1992;15:299–303.
2. Rössle M, Haag K, Ochs A *et al.* The transjugular intrahepatic portosystemic stent–shunt procedure for variceal bleeding. N Engl J Med. 1994;330:165–71.
3. Rössle M, Nazary M, Siegerstetter V, Ochs A, Blum HE. Local thrombolytic treatment of acute, non-cirrhotic portal vein thrombosis using a transjugular approach. Gastroenterology. 2000;118 Suppl:A1028.
4. Rivitz SM, Geller SC, Hahn C, Waltmann AC. Treatment of acute mesenteric venous thrombosis with transjugular intramesenteric urikinase infusion. J Vasc Interv Radiol. 1995;6:219–23.
5. Condat B, Pessione F, Denninger MH, Hillaire S, Valla D. Recent portal or mesenteric venous thrombosis: Increased recognition and frequent recanalization on anticoagulant therapy. Hepatology. 2000;32:466–70.

Section IV
Pathology and aetiology of gut autoimmunity

14
Novel perspectives on the possible role of enterocytes in intestinal and systemic autoimmunity

E. M. EISENSTEIN and E. LEBENTHAL

INTRODUCTION

The alimentary tract lining consists of specialized endothelial cells joined together by tight junctions. In the small intestine these cells assume a characteristic morphology and are referred to as enterocytes. The principal function of enterocytes is as a barrier between the intestinal contents and the body. In addition, they serve various roles in gastrointestinal physiology, including digestion and transport of water, electrolytes, and nutrients.

The mucosal immune system is comprised of two distinct components. The former consists mainly of intraepithelial lymphocytes (IEL) bearing γ–δ type T-cell receptors, which recognize antigen in a non-MHC (major histocompatibility complex)-restricted manner. The subject of IEL has recently been reviewed[1,2], and will not be discussed further in this chapter. The latter component consists of mucosal-associated lymphoid tissue (MALT) contained in the lamina propria and underlying Peyer's patches.

The fates of enterocytes and of MALT are intimately intertwined. On the one hand, the enterocyte plays a critical role in determining the nature of mucosal immune responses to enteric antigens. Before encountering the cellular lining of the intestine, antigen must first traverse non-cellular barriers, including peristalsis, mucous, pancreatic enzymes, and secretory IgA. In the rodent intestine, specially adapted highly permeable enterocytes, termed M cells, overly the Peyer's patches and serve to regulate exposure of submucosal lymphoid cells to intestinal antigens[3]. In humans, unlike rodents, relatively few M cells overly Peyer's patches, suggesting that, rather than these cells, enterocytes may be the principal regulators of availability of macromolecules derived from foods and microbes to antigen-presenting cells located in submucosal tissues. In addition, via action of enzymes present on their apical surface, enterocytes can digest and thereby modify antigens, thus altering the form in which they are encountered by cells specializing in antigen presentation such as dendritic cells. Therefore, the enterocyte can be regarded as the prism through which MALT views the world.

On the other hand, the enterocyte is dependent upon protection provided by the mucosal immune system in order to carry out its varied tasks properly. Every day, the gut is exposed to a protean assortment of bacteria and dietary antigens, some of which are essential for normal health, and others of which are potentially harmful. The mucosal immune system must continually discern between antigens which signal the presence of potentially harmful micro-organisms which require elimination, and those to which tolerance is a more appropriate response. Furthermore, when immune responses do occur, they must be carefully regulated in order to limit harm to the body, while at the same time avoiding damage to tissues as a result of an overexuberant inflammatory reaction.

When this symbiotic relationship between enterocytes and MALT is disrupted, intestinal or systemic pathology is often the result. In this chapter, we will examine some novel aspects of enterocyte–immune interactions, and their potential contribution to autoimmunity. To explore them, we will discuss four human conditions, which emphasize a different aspect of these processes: the enterocyte as a victim of abnormal T lymphocytes; the enterocyte as a modifier of antigen; the enterocyte as a modulator of inflammation; and the enterocyte as a portal of entry for immunostimulatory antigens. While more than one of these processes may be involved to varying degrees in many forms of human disease, these examples will serve to highlight the variety of ways in which enterocytes may possibly play a role in the pathogenesis of immune-mediated illnesses.

THE ENTEROCYTE AS A VICTIM OF OVERZEALOUS T LYMPHOCYTES: AUTOIMMUNE ENTEROPATHY IN X-LINKED AUTOIMMUNE SYNDROME WITH ALLERGIC DYSREGULATION (XLAAD)

We will begin by discussing autoimmune enteropathy (AE), an immune-mediated disorder of the small intestine, which occurs mainly[4] but not exclusively[5] in infancy. It is characterized by intractable diarrhoea, villous atrophy, and the presence of infiltrates consisting mainly of CD3+, CD4+, α–β T-cell receptor-bearing lymphocytes in the lamina propria. Antienterocyte antibodies can be demonstrated in the sera of many of these patients, and may be of diagnostic value. However, because these antibodies are also found in some healthy individuals, their pathogenic significance has been questioned.

Autoimmune enteropathy frequently occurs in association with other immune-mediated disorders, including dermatitis, type I diabetes mellitus, thyroiditis, nephritis, hepatitis, haemolytic anaemia, and exaggerated responses to viral infections. A significant proportion of cases of AE are familial, are transmitted by X-linked recessive inheritance, and have been referred to as X-linked autoimmune syndrome with allergic dysregulation (XLAAD) or immune dysregulation, polyendocrinopathy, enteropathy, or X-linked syndrome (IPEX)[6,7].

Understanding of XLAAD has been greatly advanced by studies performed in the scurfy mouse. These animals also present early in life with intractable diarrhoea and wasting, accompanied by autoimmunity and generalized immune activation. Recently, it was found that both XLAAD and the scurfy phenotype are associated with mutations in the gene encoding the T-lymphocyte-specific transcription factor Foxp3[8,9]. Moreover, introduction of wild-type Foxp3 expression into scurfy mice prevents disease[10], thus confirming a causal role for Foxp3 mutations in the murine form of disease, and pointing to the potential utility of these mice for advancing understanding of and developing treatments for XLAAD[11].

The molecular mechanisms by which Foxp3 mutations cause disease are unclear. However, T-lymphocytes obtained from scurfy mice exhibit signs of chronic stimulation, including expression of surface activation molecules CD25 and CD69, as well as overexpression of cytokine genes. Thus, Foxp3 appears to be essential for development of CD4+ T-cell tolerance. This interpretation is supported by studies which show that the Foxp3 gene product, termed scurfin, is a repressor of DNA transcription, and inhibits activation-induced cytokine production in CD4+ T-cell lines[12]. An additional observation, with important clinical implications, is that T-lymphocyte hyperresponsiveness can be suppressed by addition of relatively small numbers of normal T cells. This finding was recently exploited by Baud *et al.*, who performed haploidentical allogeneic bone marrow transplantation to treat an infant with XLAAD. Despite only partial engraftment with mixed chimerism, the child's condition improved greatly, though he eventually succumbed to a rapidly progressive form of haematophagocytic syndrome[13].

Thus, some cases of autoimmune enteropathy appear to be explained by T-cell abnormalities. However, a number of unanswered questions remain. For example, why is the enterocyte among the cells which appear to be selectively targeted by autoreactive T cells? Against which enterocyte-specific or other antigen are these cells directed? Future studies to address these questions may further understanding of XLAAD, and, in addition, may have implications for understanding a number of seemingly unrelated immune-mediated disorders of the intestine.

THE ENTEROCYTE AS A POSSIBLE MODIFIER OF ANTIGEN: COELIAC DISEASE

Coeliac disease (CD) is a systemic disorder, which results from sensitivity to dietary gluten. In contrast to XLAAD, the primary molecular defect in CD has yet to be identified. Moreover, insofar as the coeliac disease does not occur in the absence of dietary gluten, it is not a primary autoimmune disease. However, intestinal inflammation is a prominent feature of active CD, and the disease represents an interesting example of how antigen modification by intestinal cells may contribute to formation of inflammation of the mucosa.

An observation critical to understanding the pathogenesis of CD was made by Ferguson *et al.*, who found that application of unmodified gluten had no effect on mucosal specimens obtained from individuals with CD. However, if gluten was first subjected to proteolytic digestion and then applied to coeliac mucosa, signs of immune activation were observed[14]. The mechanism by which this modification occurs *in vivo* was identified only recently. Remarkably, the process appears to involve antigenic modification through an enzyme possibly made available by the enterocyte itself.

A second observation critical to our current understanding of CD was made by Dietreich *et al.*, who using IgA antibodies obtained from sera of patients with CD, succeeded in immunoprecipitating the enzyme tissue transglutaminase (TGT) from a fibroblast cell line lysate[15]. TGT is found in significant amounts in activated epithelial cells, as well as fibroblasts and macrophages. One of its biochemical functions is to catalyse deamidation of glutamyl residues to form glutamic acid, thereby increasing avidity of glutamyl-containing peptides for MHC-II molecules. Since gluten contains large amounts of glutamine-rich peptides, it was suggested that deamidation of gluten by TGT may be the mechanism by which immunogenicity of gluten is enhanced *in vivo*[16]. This view is supported by studies demonstrating that TGT modifies gluten-derived peptides[17], and exposure of certain peptide sequences found in gluten to TGT augments their immunogenicity for CD lymphocytes[18].

The dividing enterocyte is a rich source of TGT and is in closest proximity to ingested dietary gluten. It therefore appears reasonable that the enterocyte, by producing an enzyme that augments immunogenicity of gluten, actively participates in the immune-mediated process which results in its own destruction, possibly via apoptosis[19].

Whether modification of antigen by enterocytes is important in the pathogenesis of other forms of enteropathy remains speculative. However, it has been suggested that modification of food antigens via endopeptidases, may play a role in food allergy and other conditions.

THE ENTEROCYTE AS A POSSIBLE MODULATOR OF INFLAMMATION: INFLAMMATORY BOWEL DISEASE

The molecular mechanisms which regulate enterocyte–immunocyte interactions are complex and incompletely understood. However, such interactions appear to be essential to the generation of the pronounced and sustained mucosal inflammatory reactions which are the hallmark of inflammatory bowel disease (IBD).

The actions of various T lymphocyte-derived pro-inflammatory and anti-inflammatory cytokines on enterocytes in IBD have been extensively investigated. In particular, recent studies have emphasized the possible importance of dysregulated secretion of cytokines by T lymphocytes. In this regard, T cells isolated from the lamina propria of patients with Crohn disease tend to overproduce Th-1 type cytokines, including interferon-γ, while lamina propria T cells from ulcerative colitis patients overproduce Th-2 type cytokines, such as interleukin-5[20]. It has been suggested that by influencing access of T lymphocytes to various bacterial antigens, enterocytes may influence whether such T-cell-mediated responses are initiated[21]. However, the possible influence of enterocytes on modulating the immune response has been discussed less extensively.

Enterocytes may interact with immunocytes, and thereby influence the nature of the immune response, at several levels. Upon activation, enterocytes are induced to express class II MHC molecules. They therefore may participate, along with follicular dendritic cells located in the Peyer's patches, in presentation

Table 1 Molecules expressed by enterocytes capable of modulating inflammation

Surface adhesion and accessory molecules
ICAM (intercellular adhesion molecule)-1
LFA (lymphocyte function associated antigen)-3
CD47
CD86
E-cadherin
Gp180
CD66a
Chemokines
IL (interleukin)-8
ENA (epithelial-neutrophil activating peptide)-78
Growth regulated oncogene-α
MIP (macrophage inflammatory protein)-1a
MCP (monocyte chemoattractant protein)-1
Cytokines
IL (interleukin)-1α
IL-1β
IL-6
IL-7
IL-10
IL-15
TNF (tumour necrosis factor)-α
TGF (transforming growth factor)-β

Adapted from Pitman and Blumberg, Reference 25.

of antigen to CD4+ T lymphocytes[22]. Enterocytes also express CD1d, a molecule possibly involved in antigen presentation to CD8+ T lymphocytes via a non-classical pathway[23].

In addition to their potential role in antigen presentation, enterocytes both constitutively and inducibly express both soluble and insoluble factors capable of modulating inflammation. These molecules are summarized in Table 1. The chemokines, such as interleukin-8, act to recruit neutrophils and other cell types, and may be particularly important in conditions such as IBD in which neutrophilic infiltration is prominent. Chemokine expression by enterocytes can be inhibited pharmacologically by molecules such as lipoxin analogues[24]. These observations suggest that modulators of enterocyte activation, or compounds that inhibit enterocyte expression of proinflammatory molecules, have the potential to confer therapeutic benefit in inflammatory disorders of the gut.

THE ENTEROCYTE AS A PORTAL OF ENTRY FOR ANTIGEN: REACTIVE ARTHRITIS

In addition to their varied roles in intestinal diseases, enterocytes may play an important role in the pathogenesis of immune-mediated diseases manifest at remote sites in the body. Absorption of macromolecules, such as those derived from food, occurs via endocytosis. Recent studies have shown that, at least in certain circumstances, this process may be facilitated by receptors present on the luminal surface, such as CD23[26]. Furthermore, alteration of the enterocyte barrier by trauma or inflammation has been implicated in the pathogenesis of food allergy[27].

While transport of antigen across the intestinal barrier has received much attention as it pertains to food allergy, we have chosen to focus on another situation in which disease may result from inappropriate transport of antigen across the enterocyte barrier. Specifically, we will examine enterocyte–microbial interactions, and their potential significance for the pathogenesis of rheumatic disease.

Reactive arthritis and certain spondyloarthropathies have been associated with gastrointestinal infection caused by bacteria, including *Yersinia*, *Salmonella*, and *Campylobacter* species. HLA haplotypes, in particular HLA-B27, confer increased risk for these conditions in some individuals. There is evidence that the mechanism of disease involves molecular mimicry of somatic antigens by bacterial-derived epitopes presented by class II HLA molecules[28]. Recently, peptides derived from *Salmonella typhimurium* GroEL heat shock proteins were shown to sensitize murine cells to lysis by cytotoxic CD8+ lymphocytes isolated from Salmonella-infested mice, providing a potential molecular basis for understanding of this phenomenon[29].

Bacterial infection of the gut requires colonization and subsequent pathogenic interaction between microbes and enterocytes. Because of the potential role of bacteria in arthritis, enterocyte–bacterial interactions may have implications for rheumatic conditions.

Salmonella–enterocyte interaction, for example, involves microbial adherence via the epithelial growth factor receptor. Once bound to the enterocyte, these bacteria utilize a specialized 'Type 3' secretion process to transfer proteins into the enterocyte cell membrane. These proteins in turn influence intracellular mediators of signal transduction to facilitate rearrangement of the cytoskeleton, and facilitate entry of the bacterium into the cell[30].

Because of their importance for determining whether or not the systemic immune system is exposed to bacterial antigens, interaction between enteric bacteria and enterocytes may be a critically important step in this process. Further studies of bacterial–enterocyte interactions may lead to better understanding of the mechanisms leading to reactive arthritis.

SUMMARY

Enterocytes may participate in the pathogenesis of autoimmune disorders in numerous ways. At one end of the spectrum, autoimmune enteropathy appears to occur as a result of targeting of enterocytes by autoreactive T cells. In other circumstances, the enterocyte can potentially contribute to the pathogenesis of both local and remote immune-mediated human disease by involvement in processes including antigen processing, antigen absorption and by secreting immunomodulatory factors which influence the nature and possibly the duration of inflammation. It should be emphasized that none of these mechanisms are mutually exclusive, and that, in any given disease state, none or several may be operative. These surprisingly diverse paradigms of the roles enterocytes may play in autoimmune disease derive from their location at the interface between the body and the outside world. Collectively, they illustrate the potential significance of immunocyte–enterocyte interactions for the immune response in general, and for autoimmunity in particular.

References

1. Beagley KW, Husband AJ. Intraepithelial lymphocytes: origins, distribution, and function. Crit Rev Immunol. 1998;18(3):237–54.
2. Ferrick DA, King DP, Jackson KA *et al.* Intraepithelial gamma delta T lymphocytes: sentinel cells at mucosal barriers. Springer Semin Immunopathol. 2000;22(3):283–96.
3. Kucharzik T, Lugering N, Rautenberg K *et al.* Role of M cells in intestinal barrier function. Ann NY Acad Sci. 2000;915:171–83.
4. Mitomi H, Tanabe S, Igarashi M *et al.* Autoimmune enteropathy with severe atrophic gastritis and colitis in an adult: proposal of a generalized autoimmune disorder of the alimentary tract. Scand J Gastroenterol. 1998;33(7):716–20.
5. Russo PA, Brochu P, Seidman EG, Roy CC. Autoimmune enteropathy. Pediatr Dev Pathol. 1999;2(1):65–71.
6. Bennett CL, Yoshioka R, Kiyosawa H *et al.* X-linked syndrome of polyendocrinopathy, immune dysfunction, and diarrhea maps to Xp11.23–Xq13.3. Am J Hum Genet. 2000;66(2):461–8.
7. Powell BR, Buist NR, Stenzel P. An X-linked syndrome of diarrhea, polyendocrinopathy, and fatal infection in infancy. J Pediatr. 1982;100(5):731–7.
8. Wildin RS, Ramsdell F, Peake J *et al.* X-linked neonatal diabetes mellitus, enteropathy and endocrinopathy syndrome is the human equivalent of mouse scurfy. Nat Genet. 2001;27(1): 18–20.
9. Bennett CL, Christie J, Ramsdell F *et al.* The immune dysregulation, polyendocrinopathy, enteropathy, X-linked syndrome (IPEX) is caused by mutations of FOXP3. Nat Genet. 2001; 27(1):20–1.
10. Brunkow ME, Jeffery EW, Hjerrild KA *et al.* Disruption of a new forkhead/winged-helix protein, scurfin, results in the fatal lymphoproliferative disorder of the scurfy mouse. Nat Genet. 2001;27(1):68–73.
11. Patel DD. Escape from tolerance in the human X-linked autoimmunity–allergic disregulation syndrome and the Scurfy mouse. J Clin Invest. 2001;107(2):155–7.
12. Schubert LA, Jeffery E, Zhang Y, Ramsdell F, Ziegler SF. Scurfin (FOXP3) acts as a repressor of transcription and regulates T cell activation. J Biol Chem. 2001;1:1.
13. Baud O, Goulet O, Canioni D *et al.* Treatment of the immune dysregulation, polyendocrinopathy, enteropathy, X-linked syndrome (IPEX) by allogeneic bone marrow transplantation. N Engl J Med. 2001;344(23):1758–62.
14. Ferguson A, MacDonald TT, McClure JP, Holden RJ. Cell-mediated immunity to gliadin within the small-intestinal mucosa in coeliac disease. Lancet. 1975;1(7912):895–7.
15. Dieterich W, Ehnis T, Bauer M *et al.* Identification of tissue transglutaminase as the autoantigen of celiac disease. Nat Med. 1997;3(7):797–801.
16. Schuppan D. Current concepts of celiac disease pathogenesis. Gastroenterology. 2000;119(1): 234–42.
17. Molberg O, McAdam SN, Korner R *et al.* Tissue transglutaminase selectively modifies gliadin peptides that are recognized by gut-derived T cells in celiac disease. Nat Med. 1998;4(6): 713–17.
18. Anderson RP, Degano P, Godkin AJ, Jewell DP, Hill AV. In vivo antigen challenge in celiac disease identifies a single transglutaminase-modified peptide as the dominant A-gliadin T-cell epitope. Nat Med. 2000;6(3):337–42.
19. Ciccocioppo R, Di Sabatino A, Parroni R *et al.* Increased enterocyte apoptosis and Fas–Fas ligand system in celiac disease. Am J Clin Pathol. 2001;115(4):494–503.
20. Fuss IJ, Neurath M, Boirivant M *et al.* Disparate CD4+ lamina propria (LP) lymphokine secretion profiles in inflammatory bowel disease. Crohn's disease LP cells manifest increased secretion of IFN-gamma, whereas ulcerative colitis LP cells manifest increased secretion of IL-5. J Immunol. 1996;157(3):1261–70.
21. Blumberg RS, Strober W. Prospects for research in inflammatory bowel disease. J Am Med Assoc. 2001;285(5):643–7.

22. Hershberg RM, Mayer LF. Antigen processing and presentation by intestinal epithelial cells – polarity and complexity. Immunol Today. 2000;21(3):123–8.
23. Panja A, Blumberg RS, Balk SP, Mayer L. CD1d is involved in T cell-intestinal epithelial cell interactions. J Exp Med. 1993;178(3):1115–19.
24. Gronert K, Gewirtz A, Madara JL, Serhan CN. Identification of a human enterocyte lipoxin A4 receptor that is regulated by interleukin (IL)-13 and interferon gamma and inhibits tumor necrosis factor alpha-induced IL-8 release. J Exp Med. 1998;187(8):1285–94.
25. Pitman RS, Blumberg RS. First line of defense: the role of the intestinal epithelium as an active component of the mucosal immune system. J Gastroenterol. 2000;35(11):805–14.
26. Yang PC, Berin MC, Yu LC, Conrad DH, Perdue MH. Enhanced intestinal transepithelial antigen transport in allergic rats is mediated by IgE and CD23 (FcepsilonRII). J Clin Invest. 2000;106(7):879–86.
27. Heyman M, Desjeux JF. Cytokine-induced alteration of the epithelial barrier to food antigens in disease. Ann NY Acad Sci. 2000;915:304–11.
28. Ebringer A, Wilson C. HLA molecules, bacteria and autoimmunity. J Med Microbiol. 2000; 49(4):305–11.
29. Lo WF, Woods AS, DeCloux A, Cotter RJ, Metcalf ES, Soloski MJ. Molecular mimicry mediated by MHC class Ib molecules after infection with gram-negative pathogens. Nat Med. 2000; 6(2):215–18.
30. Lu L, Walker WA. Pathologic and physiologic interactions of bacteria with the gastrointestinal epithelium. Am J Clin Nutr. 2001;73(6):1124S–30S.

15
Autoimmune enteropathy

E. G. SEIDMAN, G. MARX and C. DESLANDRES

INTRODUCTION

Autoimmune enteropathy can be defined as a clinical disorder generally characterized by severe diarrhoea associated with small bowel villous atrophy and the presence of diagnostic, circulating antienterocyte antibodies[1]. This disorder is typically multisystemic, with autoimmune involvement of a number of other key organs (Table 1). Although autoimmune enteropathy primarily occurs in infants, cases have been reported in adults[2]. Immunosuppressive therapy has dramatically improved the prognosis of this disorder. This review summarizes recent advances in our understanding of the clinical presentations, pathogenesis, and treatment of this potentially fatal condition.

HISTORICAL ASPECTS

In 1968 Avery *et al.*[3] coined the term 'intractable diarrhoea' to refer to unremitting, non-infectious diarrhoea occurring in infants less than 3 months of age, resulting in malnutrition. It was not until a decade later that McCarthy *et al.* reported the first case of total villous atrophy with antienterocyte antibodies[4]. In 1982 Powell and colleagues[5] described an X-linked autoimmune syndrome highlighted by diarrhoea and autoimmune endocrinopathy, associated with fatal infection. It was in 1985 that Unsworth and Walker-Smith first coined the term 'autoimmune enteropathy' to refer to infants presenting with intractable diarrhoea in the presence of antienterocyte antibodies, often in association with other autoimmune manifestations[6]. Although controversial, the absence of antienterocyte antibodies has not precluded some clinicians from classifying cases of severe diarrhoea during infancy as autoimmune enteropathy if accompanied by extraintestinal autoimmune disorders. This is an important consideration, as the diagnosis of this disorder is critically important, given that it is often fatal if not treated with immunosuppression.

Table 1 Autoimmune disorders associated with autoimmune enteropathy

Pancreas: insulin-dependent diabetes – most common; may precede diarrhoea
Renal: nephrotic syndrome; glomerulonephritis (membranous > interstitial): common antigen with intestinal epithelial cells?
Thyroid: thyroiditis + hypothyroidism > thyrotoxicosis
Hepatic: acute/chronic hepatitis, autoimmune hepatitis, sclerosing cholangitis
Intestinal: gluten-sensitive enteropathy (celiac disease)
Haematopoietic system: Coombs positive haemolytic anaemia > neutropenia > thrombocytopenia
Cutaneous: bullous pemphigoid
Systemic: vasculitis, arthritis

Note: In all instances, organ-specific antibodies are more often seen than end-organ involvement.

PATHOGENESIS

In addition to fending off infections the immune system has the monumental task of generating immunocompetent cells able to distinguish self from non-self. This pleiotropic repertoire includes cells able to react with self constituents, resulting in the potential for autoimmune disease. The predisposition to the generation of a destructive immune response against self antigens is due to both genetic and environmental factors. An autoimmune antigenic stimulus may be initiated by molecular mimicry between a microbial and a self antigen. Thus, for example, a potential role for heat-shock protein (Hsp) has been implicated in IBD[7]. Hsp60 in *Yersinia enterocolitica* exhibits 50% homology with human Hsp60. Autoimmune colitis has been shown to develop in mice injected with *Y. enterocolitica* Hsp60[8]. Another experimental model for autoimmune enterocolitis was produced in mice by repeated immunization with homologous colon extracts together with *Klebsiella* 03 lipopolysaccharide, but not in response to either agent alone[9]. Animals developed autoantibodies against columnar epithelium of villi. In humans, Guillain–Barré syndrome and its variant, Miller–Fisher syndrome, are acute, post-infectious autoimmune neuropathies that frequently follow *Campylobacter jejuni* enteritis[10]. The pathogenesis is believed to involve molecular mimicry between sialylated epitopes on *C. jejuni* lipopolysaccharides and neural gangliosides. Serum autoantibodies against gangliosides, found in one-third of patients, are induced by antecedent infection with *C. jejuni*, and subsequently react with nerves, causing damage[11]. A similar mechanism is certainly plausible for autoimmune enteropathies, although the nature of a microbial/mammalian antigen has not been uncovered.

Kobayashi and co-workers in Japan[12] detected a 75-kDa autoantigen which is present throughout the intestine as well as the kidney. Using Western blot analysis they observed that sera from patients with autoimmune enteropathy react with this 75-kDa antigen, perhaps explaining the intestinal and renal damage. In a subsequent study these investigators identified the 75-kDa antigen as a PSD-95/D1g/ZO-1 (PDZ) domain-containing protein expressed in differentiated epithelial cells of the intestine and kidney[13]. More recently the autoimmune enteropathy-associated 75-kDa autoantigen has been implicated to function as a molecular anchor or sorter[14]. The protein has a high homology to the colon cancer tumour suppressor MCC2[14].

It has also been postulated that, irrespective of any putative autoantigen, a fundamental abnormality in immune function is involved in the pathogenesis of autoimmune disorders. This may involve antigen-presenting cells, co-stimulatory signals, or lack of functional elimination of autoreactive T cells[15]. Recently Mais and co-workers[16] reported two cases of autoimmune enteropathy in adults with thymomas, supporting the important role of T cell dysfunction in this disorder. Somewhat paradoxically, immunodeficiency disorders carry an increased risk of autoimmunity. This can occur via the inadequate clearance of microbial antigens, leading to sustained immune activation. Defective immune function may give rise to aberrant, autoimmune responses after certain specific pathogenic infections. It has been observed that the expression of adhesion molecules LFA-1 and ICAM-1 is increased in autoimmune enteropathy[17]. It remains unproven whether this finding is specific for autoimmune enteropathy. Murch and co-workers reported a case of autoimmune enteropathy in association with a T cell activation defect[18]. Thus, infants presenting with intractable diarrhoea merit an extensive immune work-up in addition to testing for autoimmune enteropathy[15,19].

Finally, certain forms of autoimmune enteropathy may be associated with specific genetic mutations. Thus, the immune dysregulation, polyendocrinopathy (neonatal diabetes mellitus), enteropathy, X-linked syndrome (IPEX) has been shown to be caused by mutations of the human gene *FOXP3*, the orthologue of the gene mutated in scurfy mice[20,21]. Mutations invariably impair the seemingly essential forkhead domain of the POXP3 protein, affecting its function. Bone marrow transplantation is a potential cure for this syndrome, which is usually lethal in the first year of life in affected males[22].

DIAGNOSTIC ELEMENTS

The diagnosis should be suspected in patients, particularly infants, presenting with a severe, usually secretory diarrhoea unresponsive to elimination diets and even to total parenteral nutrition with bowel rest. The disease is more common in boys, and usually presents within the first 6 months of life[1]. The disorder may be observed in older children, usually with less severe bowel involvement[23]. Small bowel biopsies typically reveal subtotal to total villous atrophy with marked inflammatory infiltrates of the lamina propria. The latter generally consist of lymphocytes, plasma cells as well as neutrophils. Depletion of mucous cells, lymphocytic infiltration of crypts and foci of epithelial cell necrosis may occur, resulting in a histological appearance resembling graft-versus-host disease[1]. The infiltrating lymphocytes are predominantly of a $CD4^+$ phenotype. Varying degrees of crypt hyperplasia may be observed. However, hypoplastic crypts may also be encountered, with few mitoses. Most cases also have colonic involvement[24], characterized microscopically as a non-specific, mixed acute and chronic inflammatory cell type colitis. Mild focal antral gastritis is another common histological finding[1].

The hallmark diagnostic test is the detection of antienterocyte antibodies in the patient's serum (Figure 1). This is determined using indirect immunofluorescence on normal small bowel mucosa. Staining is typically observed in a linear fashion, mainly along the apical, and at times more discretely, along the basolateral, border of the epithelial cells[1]. The antibodies are usually IgG, complement-fixing, but

(a)

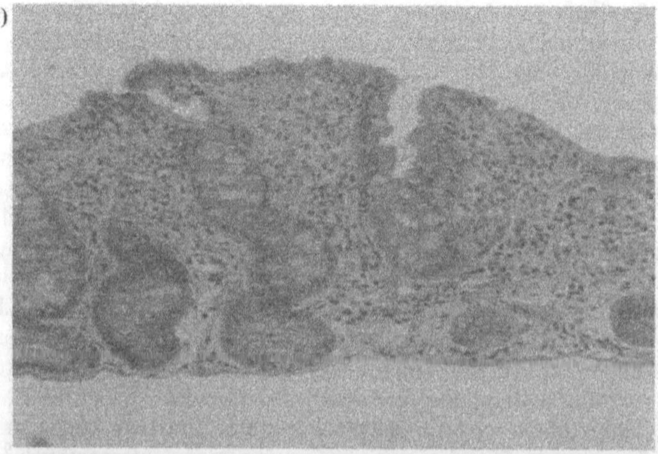

(b)

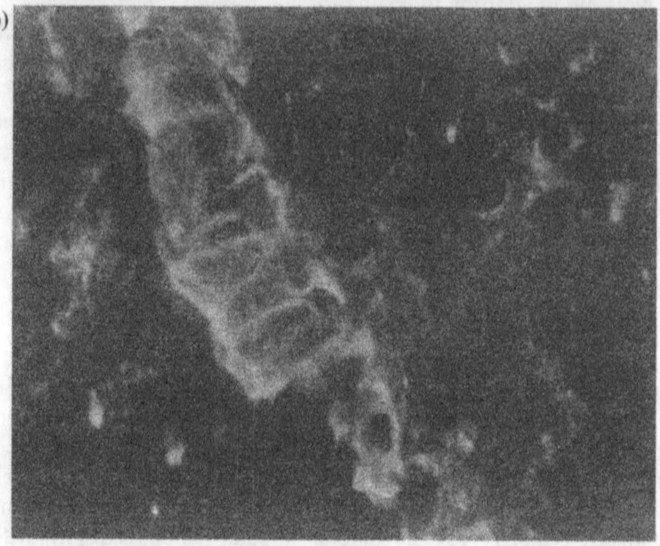

Figure 1 **(a)** Small bowel biopsy from an infant with autoimmune enteropathy reveals subtotal villous atrophy, crypt hyperplasia and moderate infiltration of the lamina propria (HPS × 250). **(b)** Indirect immunofluorescence using the patient's serum on a frozen section of normal human small bowel reveals linear deposition of the patient's IgG antienterocyte antibodies, primarily along the apical border of the villous epithelium

may also be of IgM and IgA isotypes. Serial assays are worthwhile, as antienterocyte antibodies may appear late, exceptionally after onset of disease. Titres tend to decrease or even disappear following therapy, and typically recur with clinical and histopathological relapse[25,26]. These antienterocyte antibodies are absent in other chronic, immune-mediated inflammatory bowel disorders, including coeliac, Crohn's disease and ulcerative colitis. Ultrastructural examination of small bowel biopsies reveals swelling and degenerative changes of the surface epithelial cells[1]. Antibodies to goblet cells are also known to occur in some patients; usually in older cases[27]. The duodenal biopsies in such cases reveal milder changes in terms of villous atrophy and inflammation. On the other hand, depletion or frank absence of goblet, Paneth, and enteroendocrine cells is characteristic[1,27].

The differential diagnosis of autoimmune enteropathy can be divided into two main categories, based on the presence or absence of intestinal inflammation (Table 2). In the former category it is essential to exclude a congenital, or more rarely an acquired, immunodeficiency disorder as causal of the enteritis[19]. Although Unsworth and Walker-Smith's definition of autoimmune enteropathy excluded cases with an underlying immunodeficiency[6], this notion has been challenged by clinical experience and by a better understanding of the immunology of autoimmunity and self-tolerance[15]. Interestingly, the case first reported by McCarthy had IgA deficiency[4]. Murch *et al.*[18] reported the case of a child with autoimmune enteropathy in association with a T-cell activation deficiency. Catassi *et al.*[28] reported a case of autoimmune enteropathy with type 1 diabetes in a boy with common variable hypogammaglobulinaemia. Thus, not only are immunodeficiency disorders and autoimmune enteropathy important differential diagnostic considerations among patients with intractable diarrhoea of infancy, they may coexist in the same patient. It must also be pointed out, however, that immunodeficiency disorders are very commonly associated with IBD-like, chronic intestinal inflammation, which may be of an infectious or non-infectious nature[19].

Recently a congenital dysmorphic variant of autoimmune enteropathy was described (Table 2), in association with radial aplasia, poikilodermia, sensorineural deafness and a number of other congenital abnormalities[29].

Aside from immunodeficiency disorders the list of causes of atrophic villi and significant inflammatory infiltrates of the lamina propria is quite extensive (Table 2). Severe food protein allergy generally responds to dietary exclusion, and immune cell infiltrates typically have a predominance of eosinophils. The morphological features of coeliac disease may resemble those of autoimmune

Table 2 Differential diagnosis of autoimmune enteropathy

A. Disorders with histological inflammation

- Autoimmune enteropathy

  Other variants of autoimmune enteropathy: X-linked type (IPEX syndrome); dysmorphic type; predominant goblet cell depletion; thymoma-associated
- Autoimmune polyendocrinopathy–candidiasis–ectodermal dystrophy (APECED) syndrome
- Post-infectious enteritis
- Immunodeficiency disorders
- Food protein allergy or hypersensitivity
- Coeliac disease
- Crohn's disease
- Carbohydrate-deficient glycoprotein (CDG Ib) syndrome, or mannose-sensitive glycosylation defect
- Syndromic diarrhoea
  - Kamouraska syndrome (enterocolitis, ichthyosis, mental retardation, and deafness)

B. Epithelial cell ultrastructural disorders

- Microvillous inclusion disease
- Tufting enteropathy
- Epithelial dysplasia (basement membrane)

enteropathy[1]. However, the resolution of symptoms and histological findings with a gluten-free diet is diagnostic of the former. Nevertheless, it is worth pointing out that two of our six most recent cases of autoimmune enteropathy relapsed clinically and histologically when gluten was finally introduced into the diet, despite adequate control with immunosuppressive drugs. Thus, these conditions may coexist (Table 1). Although Crohn's disease is rare in this age group, we have recently reported a series of infants diagnosed below the age of 2[30]. Crohn's disease will be distinguished by the lack of antienterocyte antibodies, but can resemble autoimmune enteropathy in terms of clinical manifestations, endoscopic and histological findings (with the exception of granulomas, when present). Post-infectious enteropathies are usually less severe, of shorter duration, and resolve spontaneously.

A similar but distinct syndrome is autoimmune polyendocrinopathy–candidiasis–ectodermal dystrophy (APECED), caused by mutations in the autoimmune regulator gene (AIRE). This disorder is associated with mucocutaneous candidiasis, autoimmune tissue destruction that predominantly affects endocrine glands, and ectodermal dystrophy[31]. In our experience[32], patients with this disorder have malabsorption that is unrelated to severe villous atrophy and is not associated with antienterocyte antibodies. Anti-CYP2A6 antibodies are associated with autoimmune hepatitis in patients with APECED[33].

Congenital disorders of glycosylation, or carbohydrate-deficient glycoprotein syndromes (CDG) are a heterogeneous group of disorders which are often undiagnosed[34]. The patients with CDG Ib are important to recognize, as their enteropathy responds to oral mannose. Thus, mannose-sensitive glycosylation defect is an important diagnostic consideration in infants with non-specific enterocolitis. The disorder is typically associated with severe hepatic fibrosis as well as a protein-losing enteropathy. It is caused by deficiency of phosphomannose isomerase, and can be screened for using isoelectric focusing of serum transferrin[35].

The second category of disorders is characterized by the lack of mucosal inflammation, and generally consists of epithelial cell structural disorders (Table 2). Electron microscopy is required to confirm the precise diagnosis. Abnormal deposition of laminin at the basement membrane has been described in certain cases on intractable diarrhoea of infancy[36]. In terms of the relative frequency of the various causes of severe protracted diarrhoea of infancy, a recent Italian survey[37] suggested that autoimmune enteropathy was the most common cause (25%). Ultrastructural anomalies of the enterocyte followed closely behind (21%), with food allergies and post-infectious enteritis less common. Another survey from Korea confirmed that autoimmune enteropathy is the dominant cause of parenteral nutrition-dependent protracted diarrhoea within the first 2 years of life[38].

ASSOCIATED MANIFESTATIONS

Autoimmune enteropathy is a heterogeneous group of disorders with protean clinical findings and numerous potential autoimmune extraintestinal manifestations, the hallmark of these disorders (Table 1). Patients with nephropathy usually have circulating antibodies to renal, as well as intestinal, epithelial cells[26]. Insulin-dependent diabetes and hypothyroidism are relatively common manifestations[39]. Occasional patients may have bullous pemphigoid and chronic autoimmune hepatitis, with characteristic autoantibodies[40]. An X-linked variant (IPEX syn-drome) is associated in males with neonatal diabetes mellitus, thrombocytopenia, severe infections and polyendocrinopathy[41]. Systemic vasculitis[42] or arthritis[43] may dominate the clinical picture.

THERAPY

Autoimmune enteropathy represents a spectrum of disease, ranging from milder cases to those with a high risk of mortality[1]. Immunosuppressive drugs are the mainstay of treating this autoimmune disease, while dietary restrictions, parenteral nutrition (PN) and anti-secretagogues are generally supportive adjuncts (Figure 2). Unfortunately, this disorder was often reported to be resistant to multiple immunosuppressive therapies. Since our first description of its use in 1990[44], cyclosporine remains the most successful treatment overall. During the active phase of the disease, trough blood levels of about 250 ng/ml are required to control symptoms and permit villous regeneration. A trough blood level in the 150 range is generally effective in maintaining prolonged remission and is relatively safe in terms of toxicity. Cyclosporine has also been shown to control the extraintestinal autoimmune manifestations of the disease[38,45]. Renal function, as monitored by serial measurement of glomerular filtration rate, generally reverses to normal when therapy is finally discontinued. This is not the case if nephrotoxic doses were maintained for prolonged periods, or if the kidneys are involved in the underlying autoimmune disorder. On the other hand, relapses may be expected if cyclosporine is stopped prematurely or if the levels fall below the therapeutic threshold in the first 5–10 years of treatment. Tacrolimus has also been successful in weaning patients off PN and inducing clinical and histological remission, even in steroid- and cyclosporine-resistant cases[46]. Unfortunately, however, no therapeutic regimen has proven to be successful

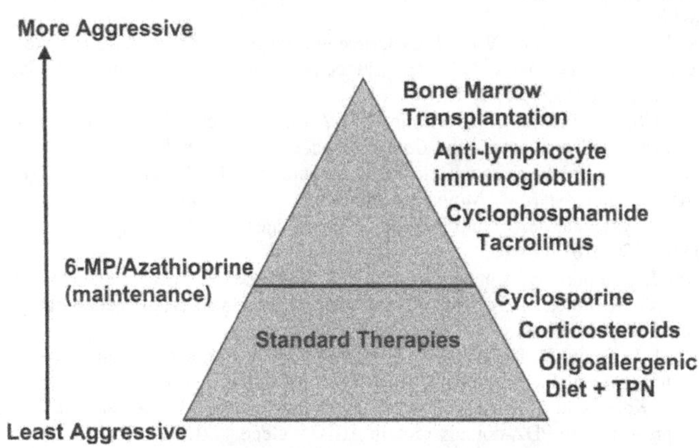

Figure 2 Step-up approach to the management of autoimmune enteropathy

in all cases. Surprisingly, we have observed favourable clinical responses to corticosteroids and azathioprine in cases in which both cyclosporine and tacrolimus failed.

Patients who do not respond to any immunomodulation may be candidates for bone marrow transplantation. Goulet[47] has recently described successful remission of disease post-allogeneic bone marrow transplantation, with a follow-up of 1 year. In a recent study Rabusin and colleagues[48] tested the effectiveness of a non-myeloablative conditioning regimen with cyclophosphamide or fludarabin and antilymphocyte globulin. This was followed by autologous haematopoietic stem cell infusion after preincubation with vincristine and methylprednisolone. Among the 19 patients so treated for severe autoimmune disease, one had an autoimmune enteropathy. Persistent remission was observed in some cases, without mortality or severe morbidity related to the procedure[48]. Bone marrow transplantation would be a particularly relevant consideration in cases of autoimmune enteropathy associated with a severe underlying immunodeficiency.

References

1. Russo PA, Brochu P, Seidman EG, Roy CC. Autoimmune enteropathy. Pediatr Dev Pathol. 1999;2:65–71.
2. Corazza GR, Biagi F, Volta U, Andreani ML, De Franceschi L, Gasbarrini G. Autoimmune enteropathy and villous atrophy in adults. Lancet. 1997;350:106–9.
3. Avery GB, Villavincencio O, Lilly JR. Intractable diarrhea in early infancy. Pediatrics. 1968;41:712–22.
4. McCarty DM, Katz SJ, Gazzel L, Waldmann TA, Nelson DL, Strober W. Selective IgA deficiency associated with total villous atrophy of the small intestine and an organ-specific anti-epithelial cell antibody. J Immunol. 1978;120:932–8.
5. Powell BR, Buist NRM, Stenzel P. An X-linked syndrome of diarrhea, polyendocrinopathy, and fatal infection in infancy. J Pediatr. 1982;100:731–7.
6. Unsworth DJ, Walker-Smith JA. Autoimmunity in diarrhoeal disease. J Pediatr Gastroenterol Nutr. 1985;4:375–80.
7. Peetermans WE, D'haens GR, Ceuppens JL, Rutgeerts P, Geboes K. Mucosal expression by B7-positive cells of the 60-kilodalton heat-shock protein in inflammatory bowel disease. Gastroenterology. 1995;108:75–82.
8. Sukegawa Y, Kamiya S, Yagita A, Sugamata M, Atomi Y. Induction of autoimmune colitis by *Yersinia enterocolitica* 60-kilodalton heat-shock protein. Scand J Gastroenterol. 2000; 35:1188–93.
9. Paeng N, Morikawa A, Kato Y *et al.* Experimental murine model for autoimmune enterocolitis using *Klebsiella pneumoniae* O3 lipopolysaccharide as a potent immunological adjuvant. Microbiol Immunol. 1999;43:45–52.
10. Goodyear CS, O'Hanlon GM, Plomp JJ *et al.* Monoclonal antibodies raised against Guillain–Barré syndrome-associated *Campylobacter jejuni* lipopolysaccharides react with neuronal gangliosides and paralyze muscle–nerve preparations. J Clin Invest. 1999;104:697–708.
11. Moran AP, Prendergast MM. Molecular mimicry in *Campylobacter jejuni* and *Helicobacter pylori* lipopolysaccharides: contribution of gastrointestinal infections to autoimmunity. J Autoimmun. 2001;16:241–56.
12. Kobayashi I, Imamura K, Yamada M *et al.* A 75-kD autoantigen recognized by sera from patients with X-linked autoimmune enteropathy associated with nephropathy. Clin Exp Immunol. 1998;111:527–31.
13. Kobayashi I, Imamura K, Kubota M *et al.* Identification of an autoimmune enteropathy-related 75-kilodalton antigen. Gastroenterology. 1999;117:823–30.
14. Ishikawa S, Kobayashi I, Hamada J *et al.* Interaction of MCC2, a novel homologue of MCC tumor suppressor, with PDZ-domain protein AIE-75. Gene. 2001;267:101–10.
15. Seidman EG, Hollander GA. Autoimmunity with immunodeficiency: A logical paradox. J Pediatr Gastroenterol Nutr. 1999;28:377–9.

16. Mais DD, Mulhall BP, Adolphson KR, Yamamoto K. Thymoma-associated autoimmune enteropathy. A report of two cases. Am J Clin Pathol. 1999;112:810–15.
17. Hill S, Milla PJ, Ciampolillo A, Napolitano G, Bottazzo GF, Mirakian R. LFA-1 and ICAM-1 molecule expression in jejunal mucosa from children with autoimmune enteropathy. Autoimmunity. 1992;13:233–41.
18. Murch SH, Fertleman CR, Rodrigues C *et al.* Autoimmune enteropathy with distinct mucosal features in T-cell activation deficiency: The contribution of T cells to the mucosal lesion. J Pediatr Gastroenterol Nutr. 1999;28:393–9.
19. Seidman E. Gastrointestinal manifestations of primary immunodeficiency disorders. In: Walker WA *et al.*, editors. Pediatric Gastrointestinal Disease – Pathophysiology, Diagnosis, Management, 3rd edn. Hamilton, Ont.: BC Decker. 2000:525–47.
20. Bennett CL, Christie J, Ramsdell F *et al.* The immune dysregulation, polyendocrinopathy, enteropathy, X-linked syndrome (IPEX) is caused by mutations of FOXP3. Nat Genet. 2001; 27:20–1.
21. Wildin RS, Ramsdell F, Peake J *et al.* Nat Genet. 2001;27:18–20.
22. Bennett CL, Ochs HD. IPEX is a unique X-linked syndrome characterized by immune dysfunction, polyendocrinopathy, enteropathy, and a variety of autoimmune phenomena. Curr Opin Pediatr. 2001;13:533–8.
23. Lachaux A. Autoimmune enteropathy. Arch Pediatr. 1996;3:261–6.
24. Hill SM, Milla PJ, Bottazzo GF, Mirakian R. Autoimmune enteropathy and colitis: is there a generalised autoimmune gut disorder? Gut. 1991;32:36–42.
25. Unsworth J, Hutchins P, Mitchell J *et al.* Flat small intestinal mucosa and autoantibodies against the gut epithelium. J Pediatr Gastroenterol Nutr. 1982;1:503–13.
26. Colletti RB, Guillot AP, Rosen S *et al.* Autoimmune enteropathy and nephropathy with circulating anti-epithelial cell antibodies. J Pediatr. 1991;118:858–64.
27. Moore L, Xu X, Davidson G, Moore D, Carli M, Ferrante A. Autoimmune enteropathy with anti-goblet cell antibodies. Hum Pathol. 1995;26:1162–8.
28. Catassi C, Mirakian R, Natalini G *et al.* Unresponsive enteropathy associated with circulating enterocyte autoantibodies in a boy with common variable hypogammaglobulinemia and type I diabetes. J Pediatr Gastroenterol Nutr. 1988;7:608–13.
29. Hilhorst-Hofstee Y, Shah N, Atherton D, Harper JI, Milla P, Winter RM. Radial aplasia, poikiloderma and auto-immune enterocolitis – new syndrome or severe form of Rothmund–Thomson syndrome? Clin Dysmorphol. 2000;9:79–85.
30. Marx G, Seidman EG, Martin SR, Deslandres C. Outcome of Crohn's disease diagnosed before two years of age. J Pediatr. 2002;140:470–3.
31. Heino M, Peterson P, Kudoh J *et al.* APECED mutations in the autoimmune regulator (AIRE) gene. Hum Mutat. 2001;18:205–11.
32. Ward L, Paquette J, Seidman E *et al.* Severe autoimmune polyendocrinopathy–candidiasis–ectodermal dystrophy in an adolescent girl with a novel AIRE mutation: Response to immunosuppressive therapy. J Clin Endocrinol Metab. 1999;84:844–52.
33. Obermayer-Straub P, Perheentupa J, Braun S *et al.* Hepatic autoantigens in patients with autoimmune polyendocrinopathy–candidiasis–ectodermal dystrophy. Gastroenterology. 2001; 121:668–77.
34. de Lonlay P, Seta N, Barrot S *et al.* A broad spectrum of clinical presentations in congenital disorders of glycosylation. I: A series of 26 cases. J Med Genet. 2001;38:14–19.
35. Westphal V, Kjaergaard S, Davis JA, Peterson SM, Skovby F, Freeze HH. Genetic and metabolic analysis of the first adult with congenital disorder of glycosylation type Ib: Long-term outcome and effects of mannose supplementation. Mol Genet Metab. 2001;73:77–85.
36. Goulet O, Kedinger M, Brousse N *et al.* Intractable diarrhea of infancy with epithelial and basement membrane abnormalities. J Pediatr. 1995;127:212–19.
37. Catassi C, Fabiani E, Spagnuolo MI, Barera G, Guarino A. Severe and protracted diarrhoea: results of the 3-year SIGEP multicenter survey. Working group of the Italian Society of Pediatric Gastroenterology and Hepatology (SIGEP). J Pediatr Gastroenterol Nutr. 1999;29:63–8.
38. Beck MN, Kuchler H, Roulet M, Beck D. Prolonged remission induced by cyclosporine in a patient with familial thrombocytopenia and enteropathy. Pediatr Hematol Oncol. 1995;12: 289–93.
39. Yamamoto H, Sugiyama K, Nomura T, Taki M, Okazaki T. A case of intractable diarrhea firmly suspected to have autoimmune enteropathy. Acta Paediatr Jpn. 1994;36:97–103.

40. Lachaux A, Bouvier R, Cozzani E *et al*. Familial autoimmune enteropathy with circulating anti-bullous pemphigoid antibodies and chronic autoimmune hepatitis. J Pediatr. 1994;125:858–62.
41. Levy-Lahad E, Wildin RS. Neonatal diabetes mellitus, enteropathy, thrombocytopenia, and endocrinopathy: Further evidence for an X-linked lethal syndrome. J Pediatr. 2001;138:577–80.
42. Jenkins HR, Jewkes F, Vujanic GM. Systemic vasculitis complicating infantile autoimmune enteropathy. Arch Dis Child. 1994;71:534–5.
43. Pearson RD, Swenson I, Schenk EA, Klish WJ, Brown MR. Fatal multisystem disease with immune enteropathy heralded by juvenile rheumatoid arthritis. J Pediatr Gastroenterol Nutr. 1989;8:259–65.
44. Seidman EG, Lacaille F, Russo P, Galeano N, Murphy G, Roy CC. Successful treatment of autoimmune enteropathy with cyclosporine. J Pediatr. 1990;117:929–32.
45. Satake N, Nakanishi M, Okano M *et al*. A Japanese family of X-linked auto-immune enteropathy with haemolytic anaemia and polyendocrinopathy. Eur J Pediatr. 1993;152:313–15.
46. Bousvaros A, Leichtner AM, Book L *et al*. Treatment of pediatric autoimmune enteropathy with tacrolimus (FK506). Gastroenterology. 1996;111:237–43.
47. Goulet O. Autoimmune enteropathy. In: Delvin EE, Lentze M, editors. Nestlé Nutrition Workshop Series, Pediatric Program. Gastrointestinal Functions. Philadelphia: Lippincott Williams & Wilkins, 2001;46:275–84.
48. Rabusin M, Andolina M, Maximova N *et al*. Immunoablation followed by autologous hematopoietic stem cell infusion for the treatment of severe autoimmune disease. Haematologica. 2000; 85:81–5.

16
Long-term outcome of autoimmune enteropathy (AE)

P. J. MILLA

Enteropathic disorders account for 85% of children with protracted diarrhoea. In about 15%, the protracted diarrhoea is associated with an enterocolitis and circulating autoantibodies, particularly enterocyte antibodies. There may also be antibodies to other epithelial or closely allied cells, such as thyroid, pancreatic islets, hepatocytes or renal tubular cells and non-organ-specific antigens in smooth muscle cells and subcellular organelles, including mitochondria and nuclei. The autoimmune process results in a panenteric inflammatory process causing severe intestinal failure.

We have studied 25 children with AE, aged 1 month to 5 years (median 17 months) at presentation for a period of 1–17 years (median 5 years). All children were initially treated by total parenteral nutrition followed by the introduction of an oligo antigenic diet (OAD) in which cow's milk, egg, wheat and soya were excluded. Eighteen children, Group A, failed to respond and were treated with prednisolone ($n = 4$), prednisolone + azathioprine ($n = 9$), or prednisolone + azathioprine + cyclosporin ($n = 5$). The clinical condition improved in 9 with improvement in enteropathy and loss of ECAb in 5. Only 1 remains on PN but 7 still require immunosuppression; 9 failed to improve; 1 child died; 7 remain on PN; and 1 on enteral nutrition. All remain on immunosuppression. Seven children responded to OAD, Group B: 2 children required enteral nutrition and 5 OAD. Now 3 require OAD and 4 are on a normal diet. Group A had more severe disease with usually subtotal villous atrophy and high titres of ECAbs and other organ-specific auto-antibodies. Fifty per cent responded to immunosuppressive treatment and 38% are PN dependent. Group B had less-severe disease with a milder enteropathy which was ultimately self-limiting.

References

1. Hill SM, Milla PJ, Bottazzo GF, Mirakian R. Autoimmune enteropathy and colitis: is there a generalised autoimmune disorder? Gut. 1991;32:36–42.
2. Mirakian R, Richardson A, Milla PJ *et al.* Protracted diarrhoea of infancy: evidence in support of an autoimmune variant. Br Med J. 1986;293:1132–6.
3. Seidman EG, Lacaille F, Russo P, Galeano N, Murphy G, Roy CC. Successful treatment of autoimmune enteropathy with cyclosporin. J Pediatr. 1990;117:929–32.

Section V
Clinical manifestations and treatment of inflammatory bowel disease

17
Pathology of ulcerative colitis and Crohn's disease

J.-O. GEBBERS

INTRODUCTION

Ulcerative colitis (UC) and Crohn's disease (CD) are the two major forms of chronic relapsing inflammatory bowel disease (IBD). Despite extensive investigations over several decades, a simple explanation for the cause of these disorders has not emerged; moreover, a simple cause-and-effect relationship may not exist. Rather, it is likely that the pathogenesis of IBD, like that of all chronic diseases, is complex and probably represents an interaction between predisposing factors, exogenous and endogenous triggers, and modifying factors (Figure 1). It involves an interaction between three essential factors: genetic susceptibility, the enteric bacterial flora and the intestinal immune system. The outcome of these interactions is a spontaneously relapsing and remitting inflammatory process, in which tissue injury is mediated by the immune system.

Although extraordinary progress has been made in the field of immunology in general (and in relation to IBD), in recent decades, we have to conclude that the major clinical problems of allergy, autoimmunity, and inflammation remain unsolved[1]. Yet, we have reached a point at which the advances in immunology and genetics should explain what causes the immune system to respond at times by damaging normal tissues instead of eliminating an invading microbe. Better knowledge of the regulation of the cells of the immune system will improve medical intervention and the design of rational therapies.

IMMUNOPATHOLOGY

Chronic inflammation is a common, possibly the commonest, cause of tissue injury. With the exception of acute self-limited processes of infectious aetiology, it is invariably mediated by intricate pathways of innate and acquired immunity. This is particularly evident in IBD where tissue destruction occurs in areas heavily infiltrated by leukocytes[1–5].

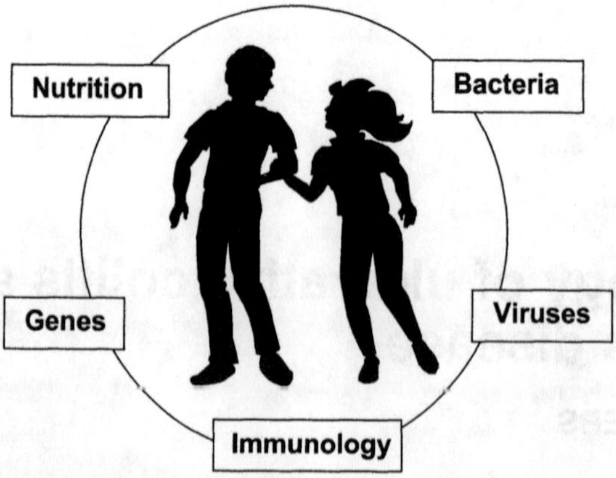

Figure 1 Inflammatory bowel disease: multifactorial aetiology.

Unfortunately, this clear-cut morphological evidence does not have an equally strong functional counterpart because the steps leading from mucosal immune activation to tissue injury are still incompletely understood. There is no paucity of information on the type and function of the immune components involved in intestinal inflammation, but rather on how the various cellular and soluble mediators relate to each other and what distinct sequence of events culminates in tissue destruction or resolution of inflammation.

Perhaps the single most pressing question in studies of chronic intestinal inflammation is the nature of the antigens originally inciting T-cell activation. The answer to this question is still unknown, but, at least in human IBD, bacterial antigens of enteric origin may be involved[6]. If autoantigens were involved, these could result from a chemical modification of normal intestinal proteins, or a specific enzymatic digestion of dietary proteins as in coeliac disease. An abnormality of mucosal immune regulation would be an obvious explanation. However, a primary immunoregulatory defect has not been identified so far[1].

Many of the immunological alterations that have been reported are probably secondary to the inflammatory process and reflect an appropriate response to increased antigenic stimulation in the presence of increased mucosal permeability[2,5]. Instead of an intrinsic mucosal immune defect, it has been proposed that there may be a disturbance in lympho–epithelial communication. Intestinal epithelial cells may take part in the mucosal response, and can present antigen to the responding T cells *in vitro*. Under normal circumstances, the responding T cell is a non-antigen-specific CD8+ suppressor, but, in IBD, the capacity of epithelial cells to induce suppressor T cells is apparently lost, thereby promoting or favouring the persistence of T-cell activation[7]. Since this abnormality occurs in UC and CD, other explanations would have to account for the differences between the two disorders.

Another potential factor that may drive mucosal T-cell activation in IBD is an interaction between host genetic factors and the intestinal microbial flora[8]. Microbial superantigens have been implicated.

In view of these complexities, a pertinent question is whether an antigen-specific T-cell response is *per se* sufficient to induce all the changes we ultimately recognize as IBD, or whether a downstream non-specific amplification process is required to cause full-blown inflammation. Although the number of activated T cells is increased in IBD mucosa, these are not likely to reflect a primary response but one secondary to the local inflammatory milieu. A classical notion teaches that the number of antigen-specific T cells is minuscule in the bulk of immune cells that make up the inflammatory response. Therefore, a global understanding of intestinal inflammatory pathophysiology must also include in-depth studies of immune–non-immune cell interactions, like those of the epithelium and the lymphocyte population.

Whether mucosal immune activation in IBD is due to autosensitization or to non-autoimmune T-cell activation, the final common pathway is the local influx of granulocytes as cells of an acute (active) state of inflammation[9]. Neutrophils are the predominant effector cells within the active lesions and probably mediate most of the tissue damage[5].

Maternal immunity and autoimmune disease

In a stimulating article, R. Zinkernagel[10] broadened a hypothesis, initially developed in relation to allergy, that the increasing incidence of autoimmune diseases and allergies may well be related to recent advances in hygiene, antibiotic use and immunizations. These may deflect a physiological maturation of the immune system in infancy, thus predisposing persons to unwanted immune responses later in life. Particularly, with the advent of the era of increased hygiene, we have entered a dramatic new environment.

The argument is that the antibody repertoire of the mother (her immunological memory reflecting also the protective immunity present in her neighbours – herd immunity) influences not only the susceptibility of her child to infectious agents but also to autoimmune diseases. The period shortly before and after birth may be the key to understanding immunological memory. During this phase of development, the systemic and gut-associated immune system is relatively incompetent[11]. For this reason, transferable maternal immunological memory is essential for the survival of the fetus, newborn and infant. Moreover, the attenuation of infection by transferable maternal immunity (by transferred maternal antibodies) permits microbial agents to immunize the child under optimal conditions.

Maternal protection influences infections with typical pathogens and with pathogens that are usually not life-threatening, like gastrointestinal and respiratory viruses that are not cytopathic or only poorly cytopathic. If the levels of maternal antibodies are insufficient to protect the child against this virus, and such an infection is not noticed clinically, then the immune response it evokes may well be regarded as an autoimmune disease[10].

Inflammatory bowel disease in children

About 2% of all patients with IBD present before the age of 10 years, but 30% develop symptoms between the ages of 10 and 19 years. The classic gastrointestinal symptoms of bloody diarrhoea, abdominal pain and weight loss, as well as distribution of bowel involvement and response to therapy, are similar in children and adults. However, growth failure is a unique feature in paediatric IBD, particularly those with CD. Absolute height deficits are reported in 10–40% of these patients, and height velocities may be reduced in 88%. Growth retardation can be the first sign of IBD and is often already present before other signs become apparent. The inflammatory process, accompanied by an increased caloric requirement, malabsorption, and malnutrition, plays a more important role in the occurrence of growth faltering than steroid treatment. Growth failure is an important marker of disease activity and the success of therapy. Enteral nutrition with an elemental or semi-elemental liquid diet is used as an alternative to corticosteroids in treating paediatric IBD, and energy and protein intake can be increased to 150% of recommended daily allowances for height and age. Depression and delayed puberty are also signs of ongoing IBD in children and adolescents.

ULCERATIVE COLITIS AND CROHN'S DISEASE AS DISTINCT ENTITIES

While UC and CD may share some genetic predisposition factors and immunological mechanisms, the weight of evidence suggests that they are genetically and otherwise fundamentally distinct disease processes[1,12]. There are clear differences in the distribution of inflammation within the gastrointestinal tract, in the depth of involvement of the bowel wall and the macroscopic appearance (Figure 2; Table 1). In addition, one epidemiological factor that indicates a clear dichotomy between UC and CD is the opposing effect of cigarette smoking on the two disorders (reviewed in Reference 1).

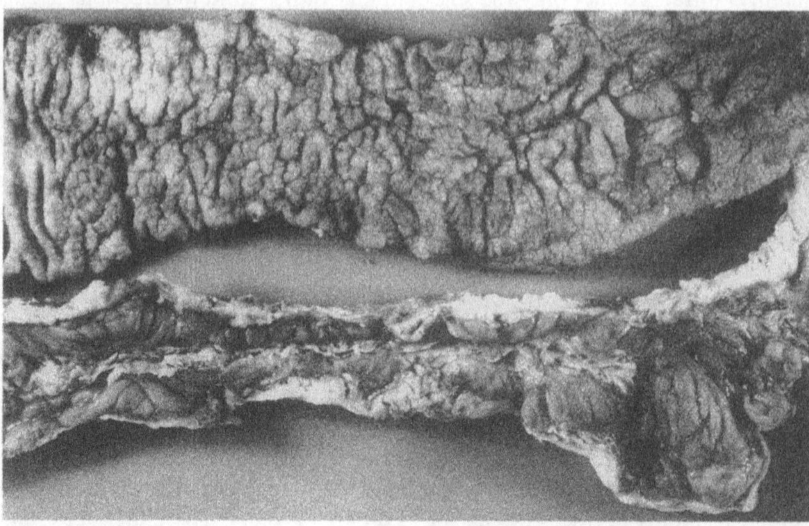

Figure 2 Macroscopic comparison of large bowel resection specimens of ulcerative colitis (top) and Crohn's disease (bottom), the latter with fissural ulcers and narrowed lumen.

Table 1 Differential diagnosis of Crohn's disease vs. ulcerative colitis

Crohn's disease	*Ulcerative colitis*
Inflammation	Inflammation
transmural	mucosal
focal	continuated
disproportional	
Crypts with little changes	Crypts marked altered
Goblet cells preserved	Goblet cells reduced
Granulomas	Cryptitis
Rectum often uninvolved	Rectum always involved

PATHOLOGY OF ULCERATIVE COLITIS

The major clinical features of ulcerative colitis (UC) include diarrhoea and rectal bleeding, which can be modified by the extent and degree of the mucosal inflammation. Essentially, the disease is a chronic relapsing inflammatory process confined to the mucosa involving the large bowel in different extensions.

Generally, the inflammation begins in the rectum and remains limited to this part (ulcerative proctitis) or spreads proximally to involve the sigmoid colon (in about 20% of patients), transverse colon (in about 40% of patients), or the entire large bowel (in about 40% of patients).

One of the major reasons for biopsies in patients with UC is to evaluate the extent and activity of the disease, a task which can only be performed accurately using histological examination. The biopsy is also quite useful in evaluating the severity of the inflammatory process as well as the stage of disease, i.e. is the epithelium regenerating, actively ulcerating or atrophic? The earliest histological changes include dilatation and congestion of the mucosal vasculature, goblet cell depletion, and focal epithelial necrosis. Goblet cell depletion, and reduction in mucin content are important signs of active colitis (Table 1). A very early sign of activity is the presence of microabscesses with polymorphonuclear leukocytes (PML) within the intercryptal (surface) epithelium, and, further, their collections as focal aggregates within the crypts, producing cryptitis with abscesses and empyemas and crypt rupture (Figure 3; reviewed in References 13 and 14).

Lymphocytes and plasma cells accumulate in the lamina propria mucosae and lymphocyte clusters form around activated macrophages, propably representing an early immunological reaction (Figure 4). Yet, the inflammatory changes are non-specific. In severe cases, ulceration may extend to the muscularis propria, and penetration of the outer muscular layer occurs in toxic megacolon. The pattern of inflammation is always diffuse but variations in the intensity of inflammation may give a false impression of discontinuous or skip lesions. In this instance, endoscopic biopsy of apparently grossly involved and uninvolved sites should be performed because, although the apparent intervening mucosa appears to be grossly intact, microscopic examination will demonstrate residual architectural abnormalities characteristic of a resolving or inactive colitis. Perhaps the most reliable sign of a resolving colitis is the restoration of the epithelial goblet cell population, often accompanied by reactive epithelial hyperplasia along the crypt bases. Both the acute and chronic inflammatory components decrease and

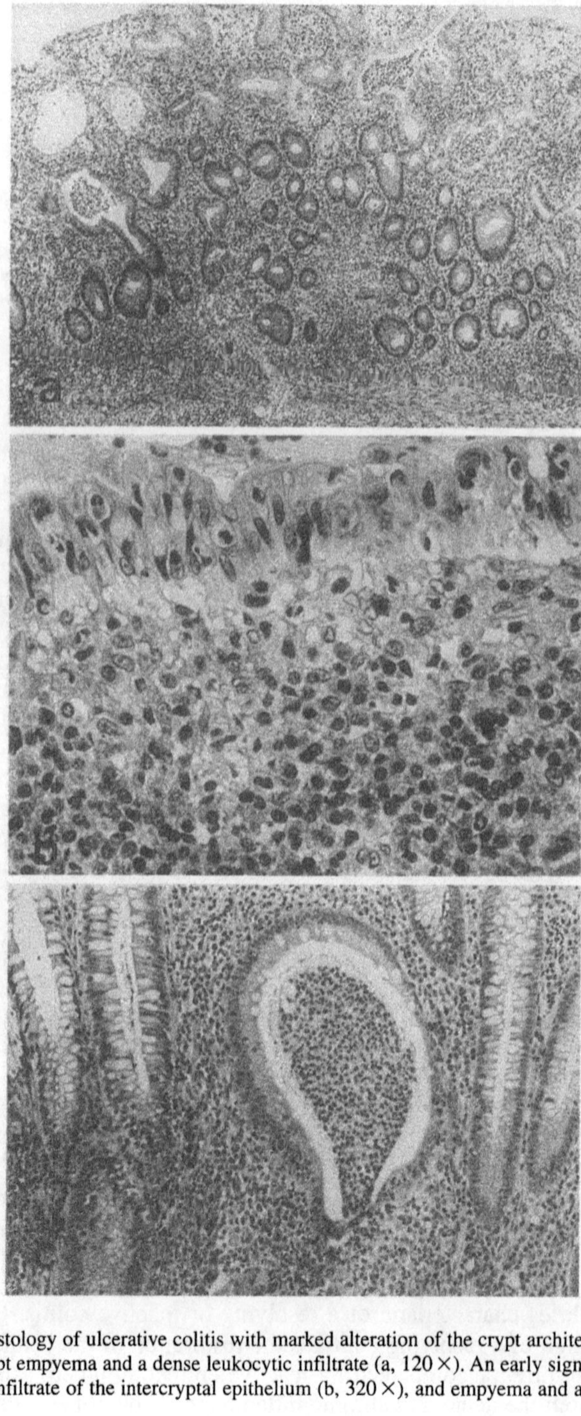

Figure 3 Histology of ulcerative colitis with marked alteration of the crypt architecture, goblet cell depletion, crypt empyema and a dense leukocytic infiltrate (a, 120 ×). An early sign of activity is the granulocytic infiltrate of the intercryptal epithelium (b, 320 ×), and empyema and abscess of a crypt (c, 280 ×).

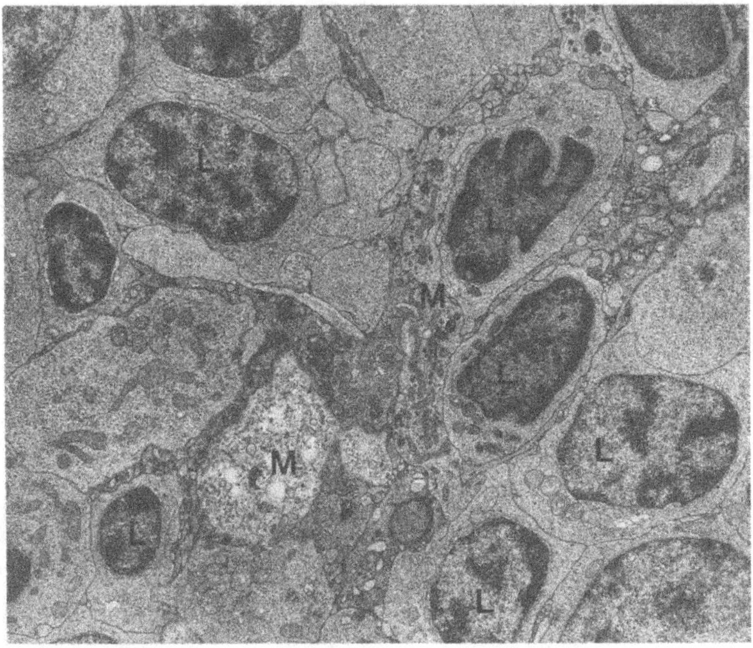

Figure 4 Lamina propria mucosae in ulcerative colitis with a lymphocyte cluster (L) around an activated macrophage (M) indicating a local immune response. Electron microscopy, 3200 ×.

become more focal as active disease subsides spontaneously or in response to therapy. Evidence of regeneration, including prominent crypt branching, enlarged hyperchromatic epithelial cell nuclei, and numerous mitotic figures, may lead to confusion with dysplasia (see below). If the initial mucosal damage is not severe and repair is complete, restoration of the normal mucosal architecture may occur. More commonly, permanent architectural abnormalities provide evidence of formerly active disease and of an ongoing inflammatory process.

Mucosal atrophy in the form of crypt branching, crypt foreshortening, or a reduction in the relative number of crypts per unit mucosa area, in the absence of increased inflammatory cells, characterizes UC in remission. Repeated episodes of ulceration followed by healing can cause glandular entrapment in the submucosa or muscularis propria, posing a diagnostic dilemma when it coexists with marked regenerative atypia or dysplasia. Paneth cells distal to the hepatic flexure, presence of pyloric gastric glands, and endocrine cell hyperplasia may all be seen in long-standing UC.

Occasionally, patients with quiescent colitis have a chronic continuous form of disease without obvious remission and exacerbations. The histological features in these patients often resemble those seen in the resolution phase. Crypts may be distorted or irregularly branched and often separated from the muscularis mucosae. Following deeper ulceration, the muscularis regenerates and becomes markedly thickened. Mucosal inflammation is confined to an

Table 2 Differential diagnosis of ulcerative colitis and Crohn's disease

- Microangiopathy
- Lymphomas
- Behçet's disease
- Solitary rectal ulcer
- NSAID – side-effects
- Ischaemia
- Irradiation enteritis/colitis
- Infections:
  - Mycobacteriae
  - Yersiniae
  - Amoebae
  - Cytomegalo virus

increased lymphocytic and plasmacytic content in the lamina propria and an occasional crypt abscess.

It is important to note that it is not always possible to distinguish histologically clinically active disease from disease in the resolving phase or disease in exacerbation. Yet, the hallmark of an active state is the microabscessing infiltration of granulocytes of the intercryptal epithelium that correlates well with the disease's state of activity[5].

Since the definitive diagnosis of CU is one of exclusion (Table 2), biopsies obtained in an attempt to establish a diagnosis of IBD should always be interpreted as 'consistent with', as opposed to 'diagnosis of', UC. In any case, step biopsies along the whole large bowel, particularly of the rectum, are essential for the evaluation of the diagnosis, the state of activity and the recognition of dysplasia.

PATHOLOGY OF CROHN'S DISEASE

CD is classically a disease of the terminal ileum and proximal colon when it first presents clinically, but any part of the gastrointestinal tract may be involved. Crohn's *colitis* accounts for about 15–20% of all cases, and poses a diagnostic challenge in its differentiation from other inflammatory conditions (Table 2), particularly UC. The differentiation between UC and CD is best accomplished by considering morphological and distributional features (Table 1). The histological diagnosis of CD is likely in the presence of non-caseating epitheloid granulomas with Langhans' giant cells (sarcoid-type granulomas) (Figure 5), fissures or sinuses, transmural inflammation, and a well-segmented colonic involvement is characteristic, but requires histological confirmation that the grossly normal skip areas are indeed normal histologically.

Granulomas occur most commonly in the submucosa (Figure 5) but are also found in the mucosa, muscularis propria, serosa and regional lymph nodes. The presence of granulomas does not indicate disease activity but may be considered a relatively reliable histopathological criterion for differentiating CD from UC in countries where other causes of granulomatous gastrointestinal inflammation are

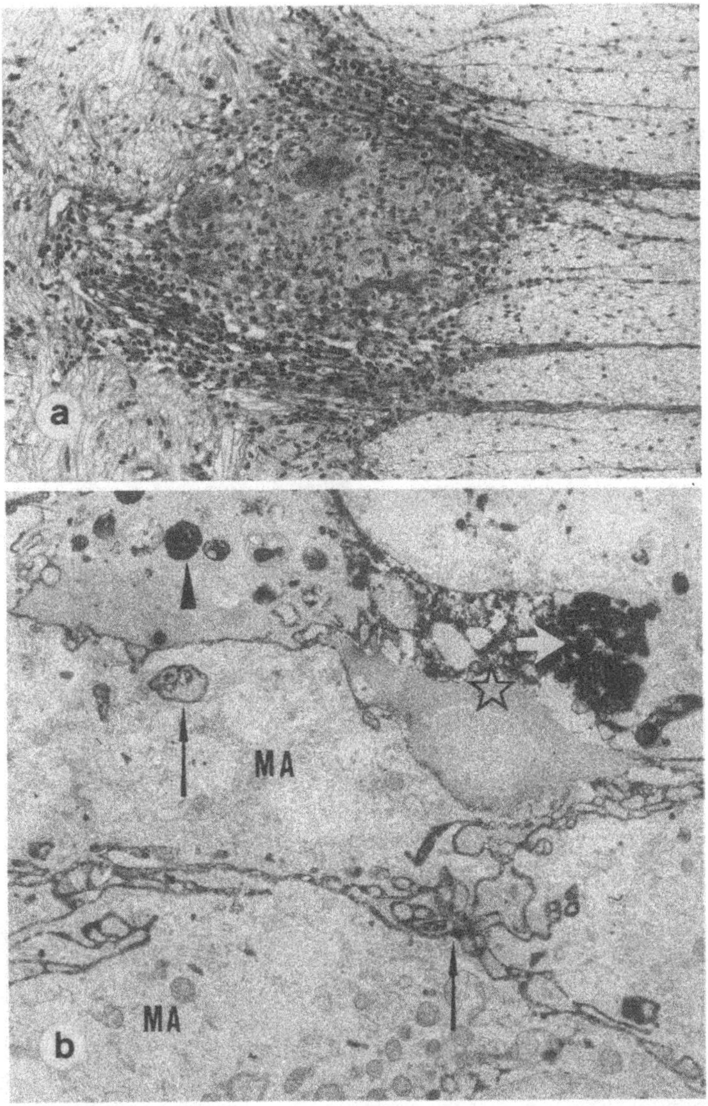

Figure 5 Granulomas in Crohn's disease close to the muscularis propria with epitheloid and multinucleated giant cells. (a) Photomicrograph (340 ×) and (b) ultracytochemistry with acid phosphatase in lysosomes (arrow head) of macrophages (MA), extracellularly (arrows), in necrotic tissue (☆) and with deteriorated collagen fibres (white arrow), 3800 ×.

rare. Again, it should be stressed that granulomas are not specific for CD and can be seen with some forms of bacterial colitis. The reported frequency with which characteristic granulomas may be identified in biopsy specimens varies markedly between studies, but their incidence may be enhanced by obtaining multiple levels of biopsy specimens (reviewed in References 13 and 14).

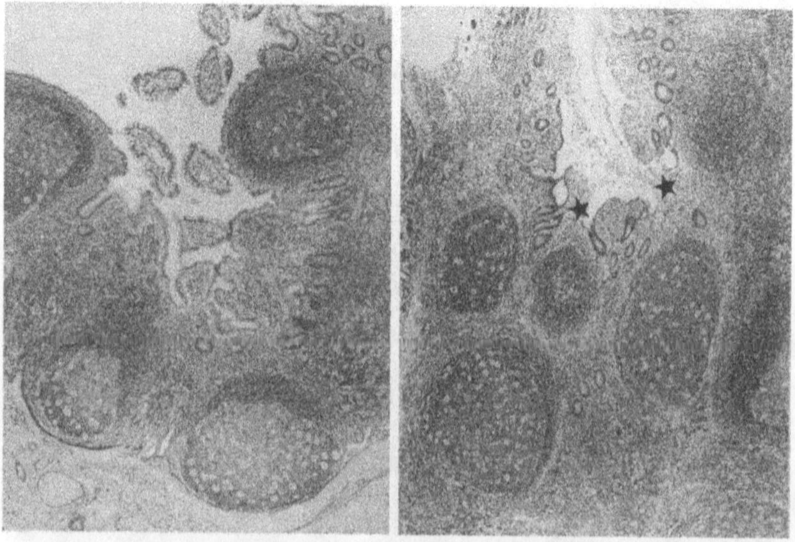

Figure 6 Histology of human Peyer's patches in the normal ileum (left) and in Crohn's disease with eroded lymphoepithelium (★= early lesions), 50 ×

Two relatively distinctive forms of ulceration occur in CD. The first is the histological equivalent of the aphthous ulcer and consists of a central microabscess in the follicle-associated epithelium of solitary lymphatic follicles or of the Peyer's patches (Figure 6). The second type of ulcer is the fissure, which occurs at right angles to the long axis of the bowel wall. The fissure is usually lined by granulation tissue and contains mucopurulent debris. Epitheloid histiocytes may or may not be present.

The diagnostic value of rectal biopsy in CD is proportional to the distance of the disease segment from the anal margin. When disease is distal to the splenic flexure, approximately 50% of all biopsies will yield diagnostic material. In contrast, diagnostic biopsies are obtained in only about 12% of patients with isolated ileal disease.

Thus, in patients in whom the diagnosis of IBD is suspected clinically, biopsies serve several functions: (1) to confirm the clinically suspected diagnosis; (2) to monitor the extent and the severity of the disease; and (3) to distinguish between UC and CD where possible (Table 1). The last feature can be very difficult or impossible in the small percentage of cases where overlap of the two syndromes occurs. Finally, biopsies are performed to detect complications, such as the development of dysplasia or cancer.

COLORECTAL DYSPLASIA AND LARGE BOWEL CANCER IN IBD

Patients with IBD are at increased risk for the development of carcinoma of the large bowel. Factors which increase the cancer risk include disease duration and extent. Actuarial statistical analyses of the high-risk group indicate a cancer rate of 20% per decade (2% per year) after the first 10 years of UC.

An increase in the development of intestinal carcinoma in CD has also been recognized. When the risk of developing carcinoma is compared between UC and CD, it is found that the risk of developing cancer in CD is similar in magnitude to that found in left-sided colitis, but is much less than that found in extensive pan-colitis. Since colitis-associated tumours tend to afflict younger patients and present at an advanced stage, biopsies are now regularly performed to screen for the precursor lesion, dysplasia.

Dysplasia is defined as an unequivocal neoplastic alteration of the intestinal epithelium, and its presence may indicate those patients in whom carcinoma is already present or is likely to develop.

A standardized terminology and grading system for dysplasia was developed by the Inflammatory Bowel Disease Dysplasia Morphology Group. It consists of three major categories: (1) negative for dysplasia; (2) indefinite for dysplasia; and (3) positive for dysplasia. Negative biopsy specimens encompass those that show normal areas or evidence of active or inactive colitis. Cases that are indefinite for dysplasia are further subdivided into those that probably result from inflammation (probably negative); those in which dysplasia is thought to be more likely, but the histology is equivocally dysplastic (probably positive); and those that do not permit a reasonable estimate (unknown). Dysplasia is identified on the basis of a combination of microscopic features, including: (1) architectural alterations exceeding those resulting from usual reparative processes; and (2) cytological abnormalities, including cellular and nuclear pleomorphism, nuclear hyperchromatism, loss of nuclear polarity and marked nuclear stratification. The category 'positive for dysplasia' includes only cases containing unequivocally neoplastic mucosa and these cases are further separated into low- and high-grade subgroups. In low-grade dysplasia, crypt architecture is relatively well preserved, often with increased nuclear stratification, particularly near the crypt base. Mitoses may be present in the upper portion of the crypt and goblet cell mucin is usually moderately depleted. The classification of high-grade dysplasia encompasses all biopsy specimens with more complex glandular architectural derangement. Most cases of high-grade dysplasia also show nuclear stratification that extends into the intercryptal epithelium, prominent hyperchromatism, pleomorphism and loss of nuclear polarity. The category of high-grade dysplasia also includes carcinoma *in situ*.

The biopsy diagnosis of dysplasia creates two types of dilemmas. The first is in making the diagnosis and the second is what to do with the diagnosis once it has been made. There is always a certain degree of interobserver and intraobserver variability in interpreting cellular mucosal abnormalities, particularly in distinguishing these from inflammation and repair. The least controversal biopsies are those that are perfectly normal and those containing areas of high-grade dysplasia, often resembling adenomatous epithelium. If a biopsy exhibits features of dysplasia, a second opinion and/or further biopsy confirmation is suggested before clinical action is taken. The problem related to establishing the diagnosis includes the distinction between reactive versus dysplastic changes, interobserver disagreement about the diagnosis, sampling error, and the fact that dysplasia may not be an obligate precursor of cancer.

Because of the difficulty of reliably establishing a diagnosis of dysplasia, particularly in equivocal cases, a number of approaches have been utilized to try to 'objectify' the diagnosis. These have included the use of special stains for mucin, immunohistochemical analysis of carcinoembryonic antigen (CEA) expression, lectin binding studies, flow cytometry and analysis of oncogenes. Of these, flow cytometric studies to detect aneuploidy in the epithelial cell population is the most valuable approach. However, the difficulty is that, whereas this approach may be useful in analysing a series of patients, in a given patient, the results may not be predictive of the presence or absence of dysplasia. Similarly, the search for oncogenes or their encoded proteins may not be rewarding. In a study of *myc* genes and UC, it was found that *myc* was overexpressed in dysplasia in comparison with normal mucosa. However, it is generally accepted that the expression of this oncogene is related to the cell cycle and one would expect that both normal regenerative as well as dysplastic epithelium would have increased cellular proliferation and, therefore, increased *myc* expression.

The biopsy diagnosis of dysplasia can be extremely difficult or impossible, particularly if the patient is in a period of disease exacerbation. If the diagnosis of dysplasia can be made, it indicates the fact that neoplastic alterations have occurred. However, with current technology it is impossible to provide an exact estimate of the risk of cancer developing in a given patient.

Recent studies suggest that environmental factors related to long-standing inflammation contribute more to this increased cancer risk than inherited susceptibility. Molecular changes that may represent the first steps in the development of neoplasia are being increasingly identified in non-neoplastic colitic mucosa. There is now good evidence suggesting that UC-related colorectal cancer may develop along more than one molecular pathway. Details of the molecular heterogeneity of this kind of UC-related dysplasia and carcinomas may also help to develop reliable tools for diagnosing the former and for predicting the behaviour of the latter[15].

Finally, there is increasing awareness of non-epithelial colorectal malignancies (lymphomas, sarcomas) which are associated with IBD and may potentially increase in incidence with changes in the medical management of the IBD[15]. However, in a recent study, no increased risk for lymphomas was found in patients with IBD compared with the general population[16], but the authors state that they cannot completely rule out a modest increased risk of lymphoma with azathioprine or 6-MP therapy (see also Reference 17).

The development of dysplasia in ileal pouches performed for UC is probably a rare event within 15–20 years after surgery[18].

ALTERATIONS OF THE INTESTINAL MUCOSAL BLOCK IN IBD

The gut is equipped with its own extensive immune apparatus. There are several observations indicating that this local immune system functions fairly independently of the systemic immunity and that the immunobiology of lymphoid cells when resident in the gut may be different from the functional capabilities of lymphocytes in the peripheral blood or spleen[11]. Some of the factors involved in mucosal immunity are produced very close to the surface at which they act (e.g. secretory IgA, lysozyme). The sum of the mechanical, humoral, cellular, immunological and non-immunological defence factors in the intestinal mucosa is called the mucosal block[5,11].

Since the gut has the largest surface (300 m^2) with the heaviest antigenic burden of the body, the intestines can be termed the most important immunological contact organ. The essential barrier against this permanent antigenic burden is the mucosal layer, the actual site of the lesions in IBD.

If there is a relationship between the pathogenesis of IBD and alterations of the mucosal block, three questions arise: (1) Is the local defence system defective? (2) To what extent is the local immune system involved? (3) What is the pathogenesis of the local tissue injury?

In order to answer these questions, some observations are described here on epithelial alterations and on local immune phenomena in relation to the inflammatory process and the tissue injury.

Ulcerative colitis

Epithelial alterations are found by electron microscopy with marked changes of the brush border (microvilli) and its glycocalyx in areas with and without inflammatory changes (Figure 7). The secretory component and IgA is obviously deficient within the intercryptal epithelium (Figure 7). This is found in the active state of the disease, but also in remission and in non-inflamed areas of the bowel. Roediger[19] investigated the metabolic performance of isolated colonic epithelia by assessing the utilization of n-butyrate, the main respiratory fuel of these epithelia. In cells from patients with UC, he found a failure of butyrate oxidation that reflects a variable yet definite metabolic defect of the epithelium. These observations suggest a possible primary epithelial insufficiency that may weaken the mucosal barrier.

During the active state of UC, a marked plasma cell response occurs with quantitative and qualitative deviations from the normal in the sense of a plasma cell dyscrasia. Whereas the IgA-cell number only doubles, the number of IgG cells undergoes a 30-fold increase (Figure 8)[5,9,20]. Plasma cells with Russell bodies and necrobiotic IgG cells are found within the inflammatory infiltrate[21] (Figure 9). These findings indicate an overstimulation of the local B-cell population and could also explain the free extracellular IgG that is found in the lamina propria[5]. IgG is also bound to the basement membrane of the intercryptal epithelium, where the complement fractions, C1q and C3, can be detected simultaneously[5,9,22] (Figure 10). This is evidence for locally bound immune complexes in the active state of the disease[9].

These early findings were confirmed by Brandtzaeg's group 13 years later[23]. The findings prompted Das *et al.* to search for possible autoantibodies to the colonic epithelium in UC which were actually specified[24,25] and finally localized at the intercryptal epithelium[26]. Circulating immune complexes are detectable in UC and correlate well with disease activity[27].

The very early microscopic feature of the onset or relapse of UC is the granulocytic infiltration of the surface epithelium (Figure 11). Ultrastructurally, these intraepithelial granulocytes are often seen in a state of degranulation, indicating enhanced phagocytotic activity. In their neighbourhood, extralysosomal peroxidase and acid phosphatase are present[5] (Figure 12). In homogenates of mucosal

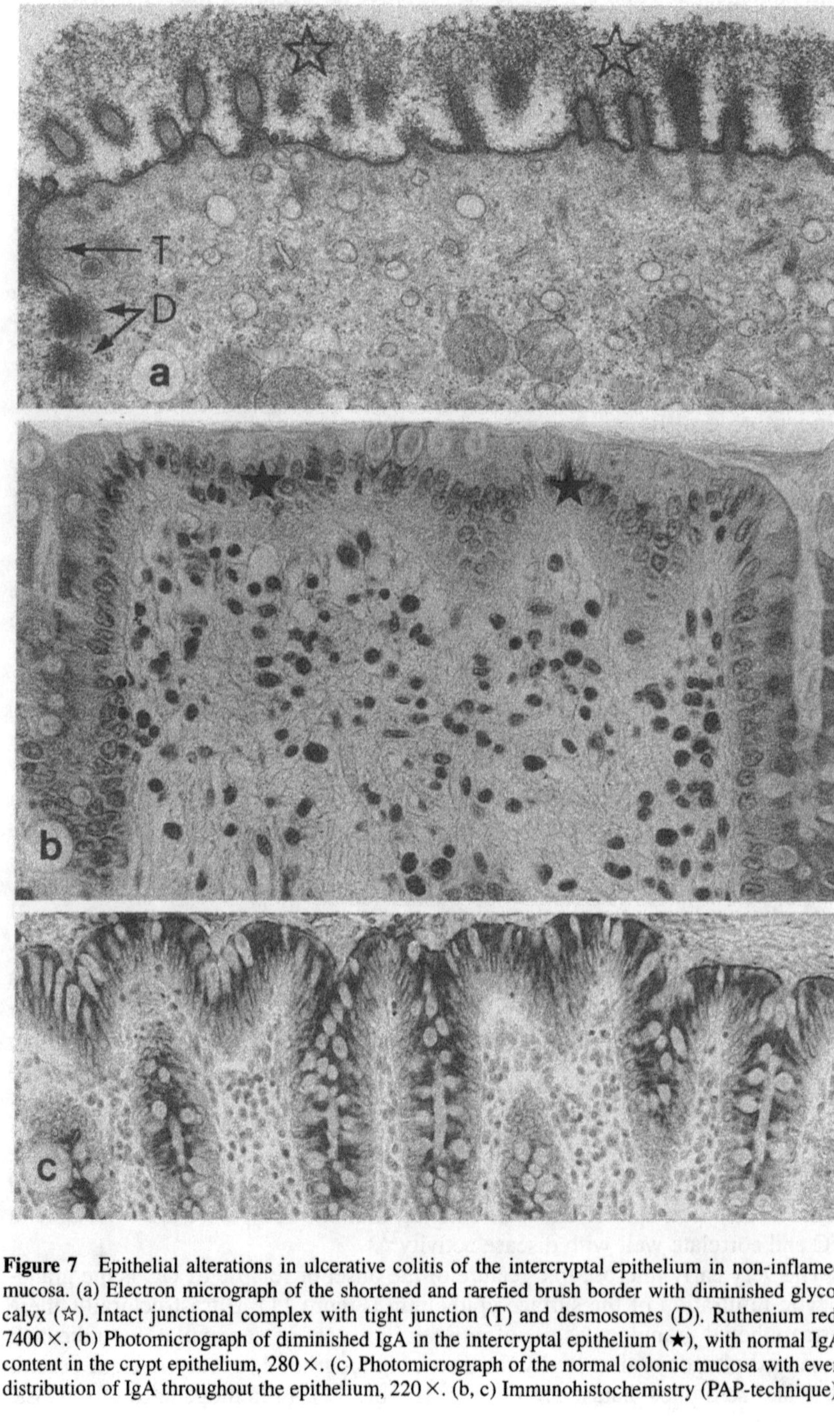

Figure 7 Epithelial alterations in ulcerative colitis of the intercryptal epithelium in non-inflamed mucosa. (a) Electron micrograph of the shortened and rarefied brush border with diminished glycocalyx (☆). Intact junctional complex with tight junction (T) and desmosomes (D). Ruthenium red, 7400 ×. (b) Photomicrograph of diminished IgA in the intercryptal epithelium (★), with normal IgA content in the crypt epithelium, 280 ×. (c) Photomicrograph of the normal colonic mucosa with even distribution of IgA throughout the epithelium, 220 ×. (b, c) Immunohistochemistry (PAP-technique).

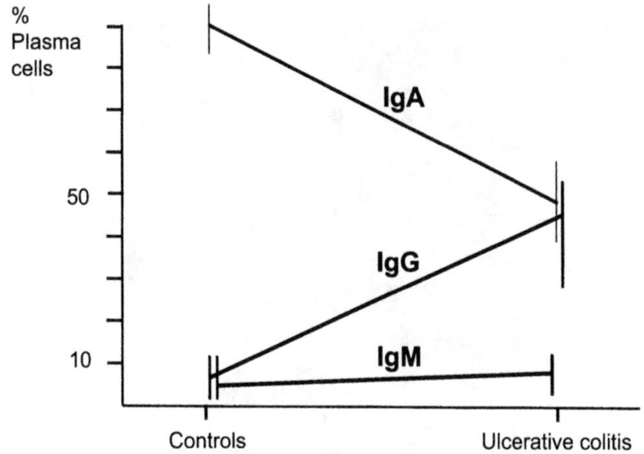

Figure 8 Quantification of the mucosal plasma cell populations in ulcerative colitis and healthy controls with a 30-fold increase of IgG cells in UC.

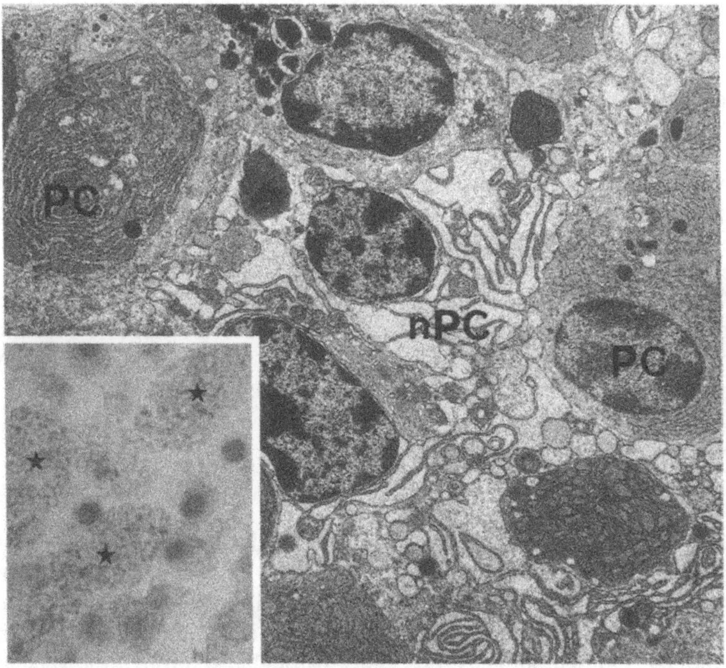

Figure 9 Necrobiotic (nPC) beside normal plasma cells (PC) (electron micrograph, 3200 ×) releasing their IgG (inset demonstrating necrotic IgG-plasma cells. Immunohistochemistry, PAP technique, 600 ×).

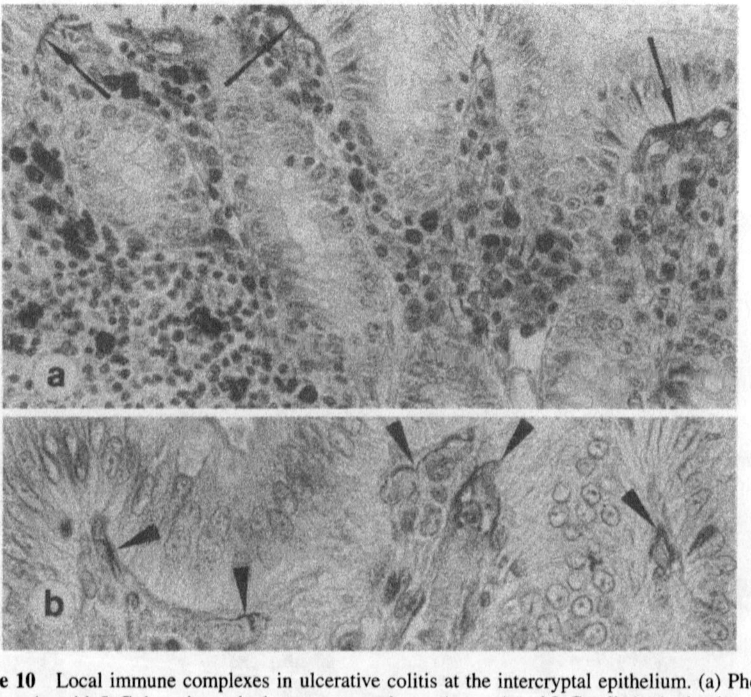

Figure 10 Local immune complexes in ulcerative colitis at the intercryptal epithelium. (a) Photomicrographs with IgG deposits at the basement membrane (arrows) and IgG cells in the lamina propria and (b) at the same site, the C3 fraction of complement (arrow heads). Immunohistochemistry (PAP technique, 320 ×).

specimens from colitic bowels, an abnormally increased activity of acid phosphatase is detectable[28]. This release of lysosomal enzymes is possibly the cause of the tissue injury, as these enzymes are predominantly seen around necrotic epithelial cells and tiny ulcers[5]. The release of lysosomal enzymes could be triggered by the phagocytosis of the immune complexes (Figure 13). In particular, whenever immune complexes are bound to a surface too large to be engulfed (e.g. basement membranes), an advanced secretion of lysosomal enzymes by the phagocytes can be induced[29].

Crohn's disease

Epithelial alterations

Ultrastructurally, we have demonstrated epithelial defects and tiny ulcerations in the (dome) epithelium overlying Peyer's patches in histologically unaffected areas of the small intestine[30] (Figure 14). It is well known that Peyer's patches are key organs of the local immune apparatus, acting as immune contact organs by 'sampling' luminal antigens, especially particulates, through the specialized dome epithelium. This controlled antigen uptake leads to the priming of lymphoid cells of Peyer's patches. These antigen-specific B (and T) cells leave the organ, enter the circulation and populate the lamina propria mucosae along the

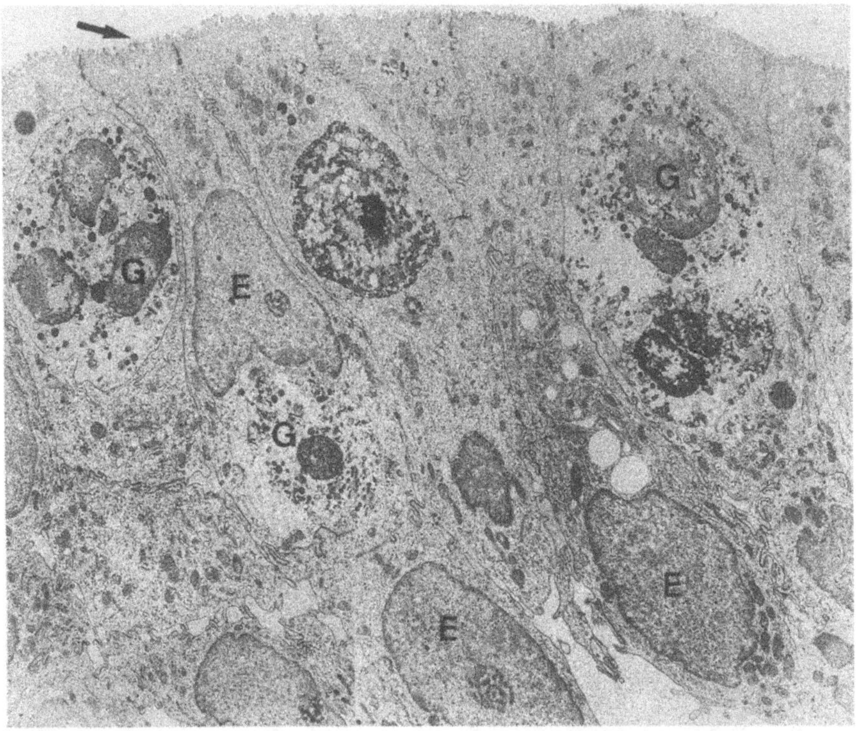

Figure 11 Early lesion in ulcerative colitis with granulocytic infiltrate (G) of the intercryptal epithelium (E). Note the irregular and diminished brush border (arrow). Electron micrograph, 3400 ×.

intestines (and other mucosal sites), where mature B cells produce specific IgA antibodies after a second encounter with the antigen. Additionally, Peyer's patches are regarded as a weak link in the mucosal block in host defence[31], e.g. against invasive pathogenic bacteria.

The microulcerations of the dome epithelium of Peyer's patches could be viewed as an early lesion in CD where luminal antigens gain uncontrolled access to this important immune contact organ. This could lead to an overstimulation of the local immune system, thus causing a disturbed immune homeostasis, which, in fact, is reflected by the local plasma cell response during the course of the disease (Figure 15).

The inflammatory process in the intestine is predominantly an intense B-cell reaction[32,33]. The early B-cell response (in non-ulcerated mucosa) is characterized by a balanced augmentation of the number of plasma cell populations, IgA, IgG, IgM (Figure 16), and corresponds to a typical humoral immune response. During the course of the disease and in relation to the severity of inflammatory changes, there is a progressive increase in IgG cells (Figure 16). The ratio of the two dominating plasma cell classes, IgA/IgG, decreases from the normal value of 14 to 0.7 in severely inflamed mucosa[32]. A marked infiltration of IgE cells is observed around ulcers[30]. This points to local hypersensitivity reactions, which

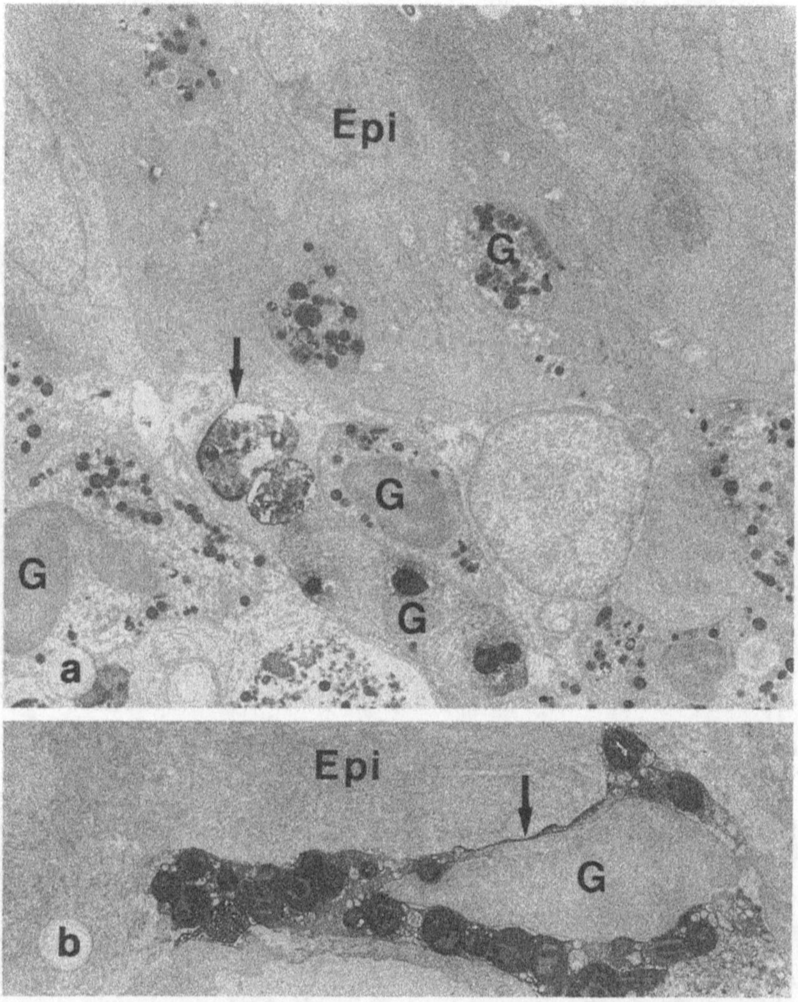

Figure 12 Ulcerative colitis: lysosomal peroxidase in granulocytes (G) within the epithelium (Epi) and released into the interstitial space (arrows). Ultracytochemistry (a: 3100 ×; b: 4200 ×)

could correspond to ultrastructural findings of degranulated mast cells in severely inflamed mucosa. These observations indicate a local plasma cell dyscrasia which has also been shown in the blood of patients with IBD since they express abnormal light-chain distributions according to a monoclonality[34].

Intracellular *E. coli* antigen and IgG is found in granulocytes and macrophages in the inflamed mucosa as evidence for the phagocytosis of immune complexes consisting of *E. coli* antigen and IgG[30]. This corresponds to findings of blood granulocytes in patients with IBD, suggesting also binding or ingestion of immune complexes[35].

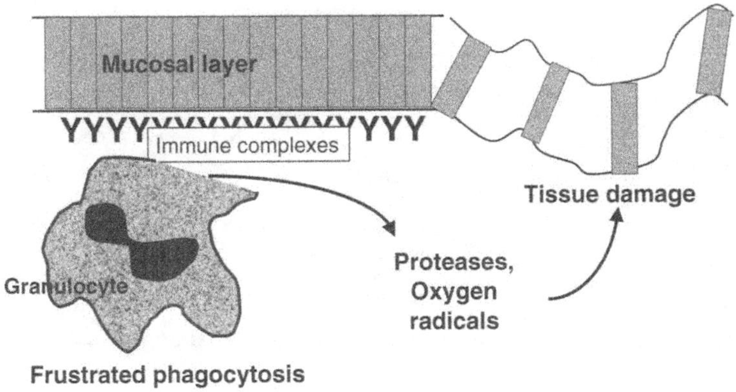

Figure 13 Schematic explanation of local tissue damage in ulcerative colitis. Immune complexes bound to the large surface of the epithelial basement membrane attract granulocytes which undergo frustrated phagocytosis, releasing their lysosomal contents, causing cell and tissue damage.

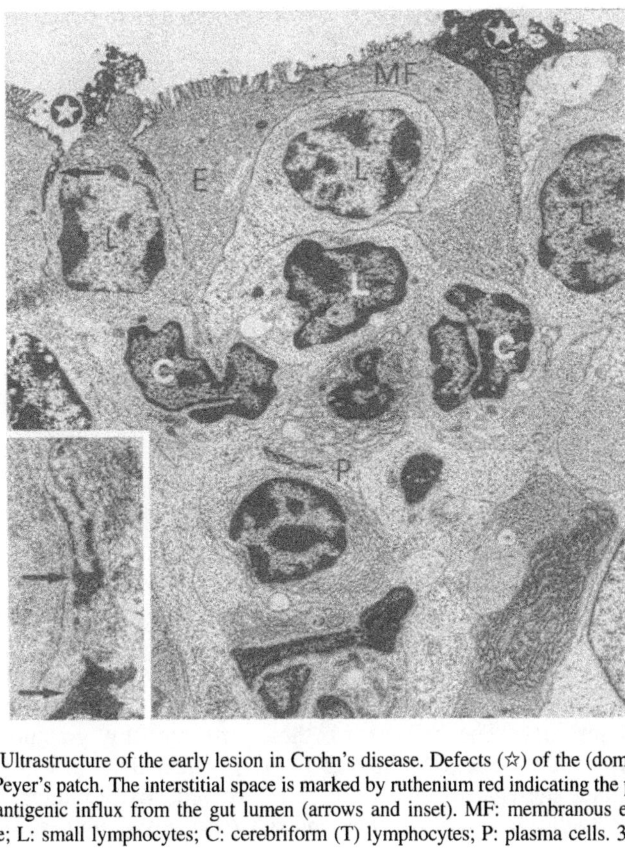

Figure 14 Ultrastructure of the early lesion in Crohn's disease. Defects (☆) of the (dome) epithelium overlying a Peyer's patch. The interstitial space is marked by ruthenium red indicating the possible pathway of the antigenic influx from the gut lumen (arrows and inset). MF: membranous epithelial cell; E: enterocyte; L: small lymphocytes; C: cerebriform (T) lymphocytes; P: plasma cells. 3800 ×; inset: 6100 ×.

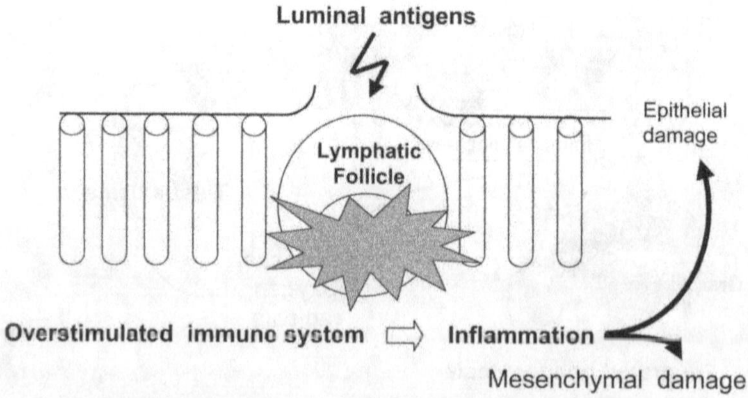

Figure 15 Schematic explanation of the early pathogenesis in Crohn's disease. Defects of the follicle-associated epithelium lead to an uncontrolled influx of luminal antigens causing an overstimulation of the local immune system and an inflammatory process with cell and tissue damage

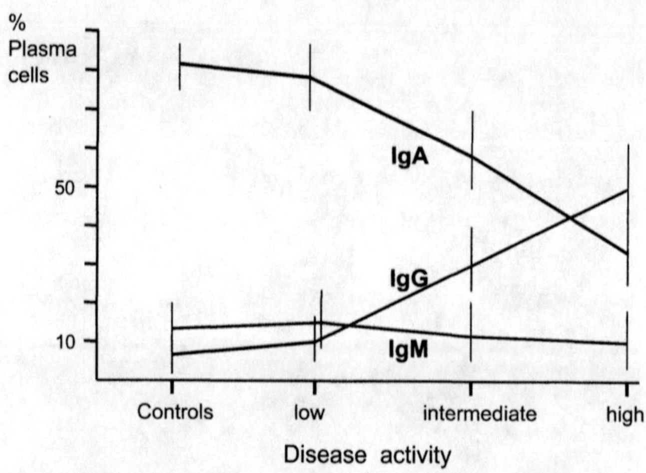

Figure 16 Quantification of the mucosal plasma cell populations in Crohn's disease and healthy controls with a marked IgG response in CD

Granulomas are found around extracellular deposits of IgG. It is of interest in this context that experimental granuloma formation can be dependent on the presence of immune complexes in antibody excess[36].

Extracellular peroxidase and acid phosphatase are conspicuously present within the granulomas (Figure 5)[30]. Both substances are marker enzymes for those of lysosomes. The release of these enzymes by granulocytes and macrophages could be due to an increased phagocytic activity in which immune complexes and aggregated IgG could be involved. Extracellular lysosomal enzymes are found near granulocytes and macrophages as well as in areas of

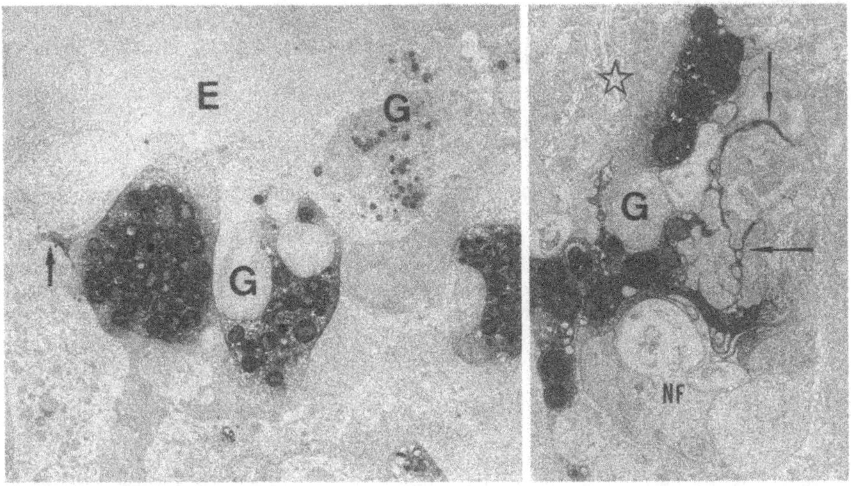

Figure 17 Lysosomal enzymes of granulocytes (G) and their release (arrows) in Crohn's disease. *Left*: Tunica mucosa; *right*: Tunica submucosa with altered collagen (☆). E: epithelium; NF: nerve fibre. Ultracytochemistry, 3000 ×

necrosis and altered collagen fibres (Figure 17). This indicates the mechanism of the ongoing cell and tissue damage in CD.

In this context, Weissmann's concept[37] of the pathogenesis of autoimmune disease is interesting. The release of degenerative enzymes from lysosomes denatures the native constituent of cells and of tissues. Such denatured products might induce the formation of antibodies, which react not only against the breakdown products but also crossreact with antigenetically related normal tissue. Thus, antoimmunity is mounted.

In conclusion and tentative interpretation, there is evidence for an 'early' epithelial defect both in UC and CD. This could cause an undue penetration of luminal antigens with consequent excessive stimulation of the local immune system, leading to a breakdown of the secretory IgA system. The local IgG accumulation, as a 'second line of defence', could have adverse effects in forming complement-activating immune complexes and inducing antibody-dependent cell-mediated cytotoxicity (ADCC). In fact, there is good evidence for the occurrence of local IgG–immune complexes both in UC and in CD.

The observations of IgG deposits and granulocytic and macrophagocytic infiltrates with extracellular lysosomal enzymes at sites of necrosis point to the mechanism of immune phagocytosis leading to release of lysosomal enzymes which cause the ongoing cell and tissue damage[5,30,32].

References

1. Kirsner JB. Origins and Directions of Inflammatory Bowel Disease. Early Studies of the "Nonspecific" Inflammatory Bowel Diseases. Dordrecht, Boston, London: Kluwer Academic Publisher, 2001.

2. Elson CO. The immunology of inflammatory bowel disease. In: Kirsner JB, editor, Inflammatory Bowel Disease. 5th edn. Philadelphia: WB Saunders Co, 1999:208–39.
3. Targan SR, Karp LC, Shanahan F. Immunopathogenesis. In: Gitnick G, editor, Inflammatory Bowel Disease – Diagnosis and Treatment. New York: Igaku-Shoin, 1991:43–52.
4. von Herbay A, Gebbers J-O, Otto HF. Immunopathology of ulcerative colitis: a review. Hepato-gastroenterology. 1990;37:99–107.
5. Gebbers J-O. Immun- und Ultrastrukturpathologie der Colitis ulcerosa. Stuttgart, New York: Thieme, 1981.
6. French N, Petterson S. Microbe-host interactions in the alimentary tract: the gateway to understanding inflammatory bowel disease. Gut. 2000;162:162–3.
7. Mayer L, Eisenhardt D. Lack of induction of suppressor T cells by intestinal epithelial cells from patients with inflammatory bowel disease. J Clin Invest. 1990;86:1255–60.
8. Cong Y, Brandwein SL, McCabe RP *et al.* CD4+ T cells reactivate to enteric bacterial antigens to spontaneously colitic C3/HeijBir mice: Increased T helper cell Type 1 response and ability to transfer disease. J Exp Med. 1998;187:855–64.
9. Gebbers J-O, Otto HF. Evidence for local immune complexes in ulcerative colitis. Acta Gastroent Belg. 1978;41:329–50.
10. Zinkernagel R. Maternal antibodies, childhood infections, and autoimmune diseases. N Engl J Med. 2001;345:1331–5.
11. Gebbers J-O, Laissue JA. Postnatal immunomorphology of the gut. In: Hadziselimovic F, Herzog B, Bürgin-Wolff A, editors, Inflammatory Bowel Disease and Coeliac Disease in Children. Dordrecht, Boston, Lancaster: Kluwer Academic Publisher (MTP Press), 1990: 3–44.
12. Podolsky DK. Inflammatory bowel disease. N Engl J Med. 1991;325:928–37, 1008–16.
13. Riddell RH. Algorithms for the histological diagnosis of IBD: fact, hope and fantasy. In: Tytgat GNJ, Bartelsman JFWM, van Deventer SJH, editors, Falk Symposium 85 - Inflammatory Bowel Diseases. Dordrecht: Kluwer Academic Publisher, 1995:122–32.
14. Jenkins D, Balsitis M, Gallivan S *et al.* Guidelines for the initial biopsy diagnosis of suspected chronic idiopathic inflammatory bowel disease. Br Soc Gastroenterol. 1997:1–20.
15. Wong NACS, Harrison DJ. Colorectal neoplasia in ulcerative colitis – recent advances. Histopathology. 2001;39:221–34.
16. Lewis JD, Bilker WB, Brensinger C *et al.* Inflammatory bowel disease is not associated with an increased risk of lymphoma. Gastroenterology. 2001;121:1080–7.
17. Loftus EV, Sandborn WJ. Lymphoma risk in inflammatory bowel disease: Influences of referral bias and therapy. Gastroenterology. 2001;121:1239–41.
18. Thompson-Fawcett MW, Marcus V, Redston M *et al.* Risk of dysplasia in long-term ileal pouches and pouches with chronic pouchitis. Gastroenterology. 2001;121:275–81.
19. Roediger WEW. The colonic epithelium in ulcerative colitis: An energy-deficiency disease? Lancet. 1980;2:712–5.
20. Brandtzaeg P, Baklien K, Fausa O, Hoel PS. Immunohistochemical characterization of local immunoglobulin formation in ulcerative colitis. Gastroenterology. 1974;66:1123–36.
21. Gebbers J-O, Otto HF. Plasma cell alterations in ulcerative colitis. An electron microscopic study. Path Eur. 1976;11:271–9.
22. Gebbers J-O, Otto HF. Immunohistochemical and electronmicroscopic observations on the local immune response in ulcerative colitis. Virchows Arch A. 1977;374:271–3.
23. Halstensen TS, Mollnes TE, Garred P, Fausa O, Brandtzaeg P. Epithelial deposition of immunoglobulin G1 and activated complement (C3b and terminal complement complex) in ulcerative colitis. Gastroenterology. 1990;98:1264–71.
24. Das KM, Dubin R, Nagai T. Isolation and characterization of colonic tissue-bound antibodies from patients with idiopathic ulcerative colitis. Proc Natl Acad Sci USA. 1978;75:4528–32.
25. Takahashi F, Das KM. Isolation and characterization of a colonic autoantigen specifically recognized by colon tissue-bound immunoglobulin G from idiopathic ulcerative colitis. J Clin Invest. 1985;76:311–8.
26. Halstensen TS, Das KM, Brandtzaeg P. Epithelial deposits of immunoglobulin G1 and activated complement co-localise with M, 40 kD putative autoantigen in ulcerative colitis. Gut. 1993;34:650–7.
27. Nielsen H, Binder V, Daugharty H, Svehag S-E. Circulating immune complexes in ulcerative colitis. I. Correlation to disease activity. Clin Exp Immunol. 1978;31:72–80.
28. Danovitch SH, Gallucci A, Shora W. Colonic mucosal lysosomal enzyme activities in ulcerative colitis. Am J Dig Dis. 1972;17:977–92.

29. Henson PM. Interaction of cells with immune complexes: Adherence, release of constituents, and tissue injury. J Exp Med. 1971;134:114s–35s.
30. Gebbers J-O, Otto HF. Immuno- and ultracytochemical observations in Crohn's disease. In: Peña AS *et al.*, editors, Recent advances in Crohn's disease. The Hague, Boston, London: Martinus Nijhoff, 1981:136–42.
31. Owen RL. And now pathophysiology of M-cells – good news and bad news from Peyer's patches. Gastroenterology. 1983;85:468–70.
32. Otto HF, Gebbers J-O. Electron microscopic, ultracytochemical and immunohistochemical observations in Crohn's disease of the ileum and colon. Virchows Arch A. 1981;391:189–205.
33. Baklien K, Brandtzaeg P. Immunohistochemical characterization of the local immunoglobulin formation in Crohn's disease of the ileum. Scand J Gastroenterol. 1976;11:447–57.
34. Ginsburg CH, Ault KA, Falchuk ZM. Monoclonal B lymphocytes in the peripheral blood of patients with inflammatory bowel disease. Gastroenterology. 1981;81:1111–4.
35. Kirk AP, Cason J, Fordham JN *et al.* Polymorphonuclear leukocyte function in ulcerative colitis and Crohn's disease. Dig Dis Sci. 1983;28:236–48.
36. Spector WG, Heesom N. The production of granuloma by antigen-antibody complexes. J Pathol. 1969;98:31–9.
37. Weissmann HG. Lysosomes, autoimmune phenomena and diseases of connective tissue. Lancet. 1964;2:1373–5.

18
Aetiology of inflammatory bowel disease

A. J. WAKEFIELD

Whilst distinct in many ways, Crohn's disease and ulcerative colitis may be part of a disease continuum, rather than reflecting separate pathologies. This is indicated by the recognition of indeterminate colitis and the apparent transition over time from one phenotype to another. In addition, at the population level, these diseases have exhibited a sequential emergence over time in developed countries with, first, sporadic cases followed by UC as the dominant phenotype and the later emergence of Crohn's disease, with the latter disease ultimately becoming the more common, particularly in children. These two diseases occur together in different family members and within monzygotic and dizygotic twin pairs. At the aetiological level, therefore, it has been proposed that these diseases reflect a different pattern of exposure to a common environmental agent(s) in genetically predisposed individuals. The shared features of sequential emergence and rising incidence throughout the developed world indicate that the aetiological agent(s) may be relatively common, but that it is the *pattern of exposure* to this agent(s) that is an important determinant of risk, as with polio virus and paralytic poliomyelitis.

There is now abundant evidence that IBD has its origins early in life – reflecting a possible aetiological exposure – even though the disease may not emerge until many years later. This evidence includes: birth cohort effects, with shared period and season of birth; a migration effect, such that migrants born into a low-incidence population retain the risk of their population of origin, but that their children born into high-risk developed world populations exhibit a risk for IBD equal to or even in excess of that seen in the indigenous high-risk population; an inverse relationship to infant mortality rates both over time in the same country, and at one time in different countries that have used the same diagnostic criteria; and influences of birth order and family structure, that appear to be distinct in their risk for either Crohn's disease or ulcerative colitis. These features indicate an infectious aetiological exposure in early life.

At the level of morbid pathology, Crohn's disease, in particular, exhibits features of an infection, including multifocal granulomatous and lymphocytic inflammation. In predicting a rational aetiology, therefore, it is surprising that more attention has not been given to the question of the tissue relationship(s) of these key structures. Not only are they a recognized response to antigen that may be causative, but also their tissue relationships may allow prediction of the nature of any antigen. We have identified that many granulomas are part of a vasculitis associated with a $CD8^{+}TIA^{+}perforin^{+}$ cytotoxic T cell–endothelial cell interaction. We hypothesize an enterotropic vasculatropic viral aetiology.

Common infectious exposures that have been implicated include M. Paratuberculosis from infected milk, based upon analogy with Jonne's disease in ruminants. The facts that the original PCR-based detection of M. Para gene sequences in affected tissues has not been reproducible, and that M. Para has been systematically eradicated from Swedish dairy herds while Sweden retains one of the highest incidence rates in the world, are not consistent with this hypothesis. This does not preclude a role for M. Para in Crohn's disease in other settings. We have proposed the measles virus as an aetiological agent for IBD and suggested that the pattern of exposure, including age and dose, may determine both risk and phenotype of disease. While the pattern of exposure issues are complex, measles virus exposure *in utero*, a birth cohort effect with measles epidemics, early measles virus exposure and patterns of measles vaccination have been linked to IBD risk. Measles virus antigens, nucleocapsid-like structure and RNA have been identified in the Crohn's granuloma. RT-PCR-based studies have, until recently, failed to detect measles virus RNA in Crohn's disease. Recent studies from Canada have confirmed the presence of measles virus, including vaccine strain virus, in intestinal tissues affected by IBD and some controls. The implications for an aetiological association with IBD are unknown at this time, although measles virus clearly remains a contender.

19
Medical therapies for inflammatory bowel disease: an overview

G. R. LICHTENSTEIN

ORAL, TOPICAL AND INTRAVENOUS TREATMENT

Aminosalicylates

Sulphasalazine is comprised of an antibacterial, sulphapyridine, bonded to 5-aminosalicylic acid (5-ASA, mesalamine)[1]. 5-ASA serves as the principal therapeutic moiety, while sulphapyridine serves as the inactive carrier until 5-ASA is released in the colon[2]. 5-ASA has been shown to have effects on cyclooxygenase, 5′-lipoxygenase, prostaglandin and thromboxane synthesis, and, additionally, inhibition of platelet activating factor synthase[3]. Furthermore, 5-ASA inhibits the production of oxidants and free radicals[4], decreases the production of interleukin-1 (IL-1) and immunoglobulins, and impairs the function of lymphocytes and monocytes[3,5,6]. Sulphasalazine has been shown to inhibit activation and production of nuclear factor kappa B (NFκB), mitogen-activated protein kinase and tumour necrosis factor-α (TNF-α)[7,8].

In mild-to-moderately active ulcerative colitis, sulphasalazine will induce remission in 35–80% of patients when taken at a dose of 4–6 g/day. The rate of induction of remission is about twice that seen to occur with placebo[9]. Approximately 15% of patients taking sulphasalazine have side-effects significant enough to require discontinuation of the medication. The occurrence of side-effects, including fever, rash, nausea, vomiting, and headaches, precipitated the development of mesalamine products that deliver the 5-ASA moiety without using the sulphapyridine carrier molecule probably responsible for many of these adverse effects (Table 1). Reversible sperm abnormalities may also be seen with use of sulphasalazine. Up to 90% of people who are intolerant to sulphasalazine are tolerant of mesalamine[10]. Side-effects of mesalamine include nausea, vomiting, abdominal pain, hypersensitivity reactions and, occasionally, worsening of colitis. Sulphasalazine may impair folate absorption and contribute to anaemia, thus folate supplementation should be prescribed to patients receiving sulphasalazine[6,11].

Table 1 Oral 5-aminosalicylate derivatives

Drug	*Constituents*	*Site of release*	*Formulation*
Sulphasalazine	Sulphapyridine, 5-ASA	Colon	Tablets
Olsalazine	5-ASA dimer	Distal ileum, colon	Gelatin capsules
Mesalamine			
Asacol	5-ASA	Distal ileum, colon	pH-sensitive, resin-coated tablet
Pentasa	5-ASA	Duodenum, jejunum ileum, colon	Ethycellulose-coated microgranules in a capsule
Rowasa*	5-ASA	Ileum	pH-sensitive, resin-coated tablet
Salofalk*	5-ASA	Ileum	pH-sensitive, resin-coated tablet
Balsalazide*	5-ASA + 4 amino-benzoyl + β-alanine	Colon	Capsule
Ipsalazide*	5-ASA + 4-amino-benzoylglycine	Colon	Capsule

*Currently not available in the United States; 5-ASA, 5-aminosalicylate

Oral mesalamine compounds have been shown to be superior to placebo for mild-to-moderately active ulcerative colitis[9]. A dose–response trend has also been observed, with the lack of significant effect for doses of mesalamine <2 g/day, and increased response at doses of 4–4.8 g/day[11]. No significant differences in response have been shown between any of the mesalamine preparations, nor between the various mesalamine preparations when compared with sulphasalazine. However, one recent study has shown balsalazide to be more effective and better tolerated than mesalamine in the treatment of active ulcerative colitis[12]. Additional confirmatory studies are appropriate before this conclusion can be generally accepted.

The use of any of the aminosalicylates for severely active ulcerative colitis has not been evaluated in controlled trials, but generally are not thought to provide benefit in these patients. Once remission is achieved, aminosalicylates have been shown to be effective as maintenance therapy, as doses of 1.5–4.8 g/day maintain remission in over half of patients. Furthermore, these agents appear to be safe as longer-term maintenance therapies[11,13].

Sulphasalazine appears to provide benefit in patients with ileocolonic and colonic Crohn's disease but not in those with isolated small bowel disease[14,15]. However, those with jejunal and ileal disease may benefit from newer mesalamine preparations that deliver 5-ASA to the small bowel (Table 1). Several of these agents, including Pentasa and Asacol at doses of up to 4 g/day and 3.2 g/day, respectively, have been shown to be superior to placebo in the treatment of active Crohn's ileocolitis[16,17]. Recent data, from two large unpublished studies coupled with the data from a large previous study[16] suggest that mesalamine at 4 g/day is more effective than placebo to induce remission ($p = 0.04$); however, the difference in the Crohn's disease activity index is not clinically significant (18 point difference)[18]. Recent data also suggest 4 g/day Asacol may be as effective as 40 mg/day of oral methylprednisolone for the treatment of active Crohn's ileitis[19]. Moreover, results of a recently published meta-analysis indicate that oral mesalamine preparations are beneficial in maintaining remission of Crohn's disease, although the benefit was mainly observed in patients with surgically induced remission, ileitis and/or prolonged disease duration[20]. Mesalamine seems to have a somewhat limited role in facilitating withdrawal from steroid therapy once remission has been achieved[21,22]. It has been shown to decrease the rate of steroid dependency in this patient population[21].

Topical aminosalicylates

A recent meta-analysis reviewing 17 randomized double-blind controlled trials concluded that topical mesalamine was useful for both the induction and the maintenance of remission of mild-to-moderate distal ulcerative colitis[23]. In such treatment, mesalamine enemas were as effective as oral sulphasalazine, but were associated with fewer side-effects[24]. Similar efficacy has been demonstrated for 1 g, 2 g and 4 g mesalamine enemas for the induction of remission of patients with mild-to-moderate left-sided ulcerative colitis not requiring concurrent corticosteroids[25]. A combined treatment of rectal and oral mesalamine may also be more effective than oral treatment alone for the induction and maintenance of remission of distal ulcerative colitis, suggesting a dose–response effect[26,27]. In the treatment of acute ulcerative proctitis, mesalamine, administered as a 500-mg suppository twice daily, has been shown to be beneficial[28]. Mesalamine suppositories have also been shown to be effective in preventing relapse[29], and the dose may be titrated to patient response and tolerance[30]. Mesalamine foam, not approved in the United States, has a more uniform distribution and longer persistence in the distal colon compared with mesalamine enemas[31] and, in one trial, provided better patient acceptance than the enema preparation[32].

Corticosteroids

Corticosteroids modify cell-mediated immunity and the production of inflammatory mediators including prostaglandins, leukotrienes, platelet activating factors and cytokines[11]. Corticosteroids are efficacious for the treatment of active ulcerative colitis[33] and active luminal Crohn's disease[14], regardless of disease distribution. In moderate-to-severe flares of inflammatory bowel disease, corticosteroids in doses equivalent to 40–60 mg/day of prednisone, are effective first-line therapy. The use of higher doses is associated with increased side-effects without appreciable clinical benefit[34]. In moderate-to-severely active ulcerative colitis or Crohn's colitis, adding sulphasalazine to corticosteroids does not result in better efficacy compared with corticosteroids alone[35].

Corticosteroids have not been shown to be beneficial for maintenance of remission in either Crohn's disease or ulcerative colitis[14,15,36]. Intravenous adrenocorticotropic hormone (ACTH) may be more effective than methylprednisolone for ulcerative colitis patients who have not received prior corticosteroid treatment[37], although adrenal haemorrhage has been reported as a complication of ACTH therapy.

The beneficial effects of corticosteroids are counterbalanced by side-effects that are frequently seen with their prolonged use. Common side-effects include acne, striae, mood changes, sleep disturbance and cushingoid appearance. One important irreversible side-effect includes osteonecrosis, which has also been reported in Crohn's disease patients prior to initiation of corticosteroid therapy[38]. Other important adverse effects include osteopenia, osteoporosis and posterior subcapsular cataracts. The use of bisphosphonates has not been critically evaluated in inflammatory bowel disease patients requiring corticosteroids, but hormone replacement has been shown to be beneficial for prevention of bone loss[39], and should be considered in appropriate patients. Daily calcium (1200–1500 mg/day) and vitamin D (400–800 IU/day) should also be prescribed to IBD patients receiving corticosteroid therapy.

Newer corticosteroid preparations (e.g. budesonide, fluticasone may provide certain advantages over traditional corticosteroids by achieving clinical efficacy associated with fewer systemic side-effects and less adrenal suppression than prednisone. The improved toxicity profile of these agents relates to their low systemic bioavailability, which is achieved via their extensive first-pass metabolism in the liver and erythrocytes. Oral budesonide is the best studied of these newer corticosteroids. Recent trials comparing oral budesonide with prednisolone demonstrate comparable efficacy for inducing remission in active ulcerative colitis[40] and Crohn's disease[41]. Controlled ileal release (CIR) oral budesonide has also been shown to be effective in treating active ileal and ileocaecal Crohn's disease[42], with a higher rate of remission and fewer adverse events when compared at 9 mg orally to 4 g daily of mesalamine[43]. Overall the use of budesonide is associated with fewer acute side-effects than prednisone[44]. Budesonide appeared to also have maintenance benefit, and a one-year study suggested that budesonide might prolong time to relapse in patients with Crohn's disease[45]. Additional placebo-controlled trials have not demonstrated a benefit of oral budesonide as maintenance therapy in Crohn's disease; however, Greenberg *et al.* found that the effect was not sustained at one year of follow-up[46,47]. Budesonide has also been shown in another short-term study to reduce endoscopic recurrence in patients who had surgery for active disease, but not in those who had fibrostenotic disease as the indication for surgery[48].

Topical corticosteroids

Topical corticosteroids in liquid and foam formulations are effective as short-term therapy for active ulcerative colitis distal to the splenic flexure[49]. Foam preparations are often better tolerated by patients and may be easier to retain[50]. In a meta-analysis, topical corticosteroids were found to be less effective than topical mesalamine for inducing remission of distal ulcerative colitis[51]. However, the combination of topical corticosteroids with topical mesalamine is often more efficacious than either alone in the short-term treatment of distal ulcerative colitis[52]. Although absorption of corticosteroids after topical administration is less than after oral administration, prolonged treatment with topical steroids may still be associated with steroid-related side-effects. Recently, a new generation of topical corticosteroids, (e.g. budesonide), has been developed in an attempt to reduce these side-effects. Danielsson *et al.* compared budesonide enemas at a dose of 2 mg/100 ml with placebo for active distal colitis or proctitis[53]. Budesonide was more effective than placebo without noted systemic side-effects. A separate study showed that doses up to 4 mg/day of budesonide for two weeks had no effect on morning plasma cortisol levels[54]. This and subsequent trials have shown topical budesonide to be as efficacious as prednisolone enemas, mesalamine enemas and even systemic corticosteroids in the treatment of distal ulcerative colitis[54–56]. Additional trials are needed to determine the effect of longer-term topical budesonide use.

Antibiotics

Experimental and clinical evidence suggests that bacterial flora may play a role in the pathogenesis of inflammatory bowel disease[11]. Treatment with metronidazole at doses of 10–20 mg/kg/day as primary therapy for active Crohn's colitis has demonstrated efficacy superior to placebo[57] and equal to sulphasalazine[58]. Metronidazole may be particularly useful in managing perianal complications, such as fistulae. Non-randomized trials have shown that at least half the patients achieve healing of perianal disease with metronidazole use[59]. There is currently a randomized placebo-controlled trial ongoing evaluating ciprofloxacin vs. metronidazole vs. placebo for perineal Crohn's disease. Metronidazole may also be beneficial in preventing postoperative recurrence in Crohn's disease. A preliminary study found that use of metronidazole for three months postoperatively decreased the severity of endoscopic recurrence after ileal resection for Crohn's disease[60]. Nitroimidazole, a compound similar to metronidazole but with less intolerance, has demonstrated similar efficacy in preventing postoperative recurrence[61]. No randomized controlled studies have evaluated the efficacy of metronidazole for the maintenance of remission in non-operative Crohn's disease.

Metronidazole has not been shown to be beneficial as acute therapy for ulcerative colitis in controlled trials[62]. One small trial has demonstrated benefit of metronidazole for maintenance of remission in ulcerative colitis; however the evidence is not compelling[63]. The use of long-term metronidazole may result in the development of peripheral neuropathy, which typically is reversible. Other common side-effects of metronidazole include nausea, vomiting, a disulphuram-like reaction with alcohol, and metallic taste.

Ciprofloxacin may have immunomodulatory properties as well as antimicrobial activity[64], and one preliminary report demonstrated equal efficacy of ciprofloxacin and 5-ASA for the induction of remission of active Crohn's disease[65]. Adding ciprofloxacin to metronidazole has also been shown to decrease Crohn's disease activity in some patients[66]. Ciprofloxacin may be especially helpful in treating fistulae and perianal symptoms in Crohn's disease, and can be used in those intolerant of metronidazole[67]. A recent study suggested that six months of oral ciprofloxacin may be beneficial in the treatment of active ulcerative colitis[68]; however additional confirmatory controlled trials are needed. Other similar quinolones and antibiotics (e.g. clarithromycin) have been studied in uncontrolled trials[11] and are currently being investigated in additional clinical trials.

Immunomodulators

Azathioprine and 6-mercaptopurine

The rationale for the therapeutic use of immunomodulators in patients with ulcerative colitis and Crohn's disease stems from observations implicating immunological mechanisms in the pathogenesis of inflammatory bowel disease. The most widely used immunosuppressant agents are the purine analogues, azathioprine and 6-mercaptopurine (6-MP). It is believed that 6-MP and azathioprine have similar efficacy and toxicity, although their exact mechanisms of action are uncertain. Azathoprine is non-enzymatically converted to 6-MP, which is then metabolized to the active end product, 6-thioguanine nucleotides. 6-Thioguanine nucleotides inhibit purine ribonucleotide synthesis and cell proliferation in the S phase of the cell cycle[6]. Azathioprine and 6-MP also inhibit natural killer cell cytotoxicity, cytotoxic T-cell activity, and reduce suppressor T-cell function and cell-mediated immunity.

Azathioprine and 6-MP have been used primarily for patients with active Crohn's disease and ulcerative colitis who are unresponsive to corticosteroids, or who are steroid dependent. In a meta-analysis of randomized double-blinded studies, azathioprine/6-MP were shown to be more efficacious than placebo in patients with active Crohn's disease[69]. Furthermore, in one of these studies, 73% of patients were able to discontinue or reduce the daily dosage of corticosteroids[70]. In another trial, combined treatment with azathioprine and prednisolone was more efficacious than treatment with prednisolone alone for the induction of remission of Crohn's disease[71]. A limiting factor in the use of these agents in the management of active disease is their delayed onset of action of three to six months[69]. Recently, it was thought that the slow response to azathioprine might be avoided by the administration of an intravenous loading dose[72]; however, a recent controlled trial refuted this claim[73]. There have been seven studies which have similarly demonstrated efficacy of azathioprine/6-MP for maintenance of remission in patients with Crohn's disease[69,74]. A recent study of patients with Crohn's disease in remission showed that the five-year relapse rate of those who stopped azathioprine/6-MP was 75%, compared with 32% for those who continued these medications[75]. Preliminary data suggest that 6-MP is also effective in preventing postoperative relapse of Crohn's disease[76].

There have been several controlled studies demonstrating efficacy of azathioprine for the treatment of active ulcerative colitis[77–80]. In addition, controlled trials have demonstrated efficacy of these agents for the maintenance of remission of ulcerative colitis. In one controlled trial of patients with ulcerative colitis who initially achieved remission on azathioprine, a one-year relapse rate of 36% was seen in those who were continued on azathioprine, compared with a 59% relapse rate for those who were switched to placebo[81]. Another study reported that more than 61% of patients with ulcerative colitis who were originally dependent on steroids were able to stop or reduce the steroid use when they were maintained on 6-MP[82].

Side-effects of azathioprine and 6-MP include nausea, vomiting, bone marrow toxicity, abnormal liver associated chemistry tests, and pancreatitis[6,83]. An increased incidence of lymphoma and leukaemia have been reported in patients with renal transplants taking azathioprine/6MP; however, the risk does not seem to be increased in patients with inflammatory bowel disease who are treated with these agents[84,85]. Typically, the maximal doses for 6-MP and azathioprine are 1.5 mg/kg/day and 2.5 mg/kg/day, respectively; however, at these doses, there may still be non-responders and higher doses may be used. Based upon retrospective analyses, some investigators have suggested that induction of leukopenia (white blood cell count <5000 mm^3) may increase the likelihood of therapeutic response[86]. However, a recent controlled trial suggested no benefit for those who achieved leukopenia[73]. Preliminary data suggest that 6-thioguanine levels >235–250 pmoles/8 × 10^8 RBCs correlate with a clinical response in patients with inflammatory bowel disease[87–89]. Additional prospective trials will be necessary to determine whether an individual patient's azathioprine dose can be adjusted safely to achieve therapeutic metabolite levels. Moreover, recent data has demonstrated that mesalamine derivatives inhibit thiopurine methyltransferase (TPMT) activity *in vitro*[90,91] and may thus serve to augment efficacy of 6-MP or azathioprine at a given dose, while limiting toxicity. Continued investigation of the importance and utility of monitoring TPMT genotype, as well as 6MP metabolite levels in IBD remains under intense investigation.

Methotrexate

Methotrexate is a folic acid antagonist, which has both antimetabolite and anti-inflammatory activities. It inhibits the enzyme dihydrofolate reductase, thymidine synthetase and other enzymes involving DNA synthesis[6]. It also interferes with the production of the proinflammatory cytokines, IL-1 and IL-2. Intramuscular methotrexate (25 mg/week) was shown to be beneficial in patients with active Crohn's disease in a multicentre, double-blind placebo-controlled 16-week trial[92]. In contrast, lower-dose oral methotrexate has demonstrated less-consistent results. A recent study demonstrated efficacy of oral methotrexate (15 mg/week) trending towards (but not achieving) statistical significance[93], whereas another controlled study showed that methotrexate, 12.5 mg orally once a week, was only minimally better than placebo in patients with active Crohn's disease[94]. Another multicentre placebo-controlled study by the same group demonstrated that methotrexate, 12.5 mg orally once a week, was no better than placebo in active ulcerative colitis[95]. A randomized placebo-controlled trial was recently published demonstrating maintenance benefit of methotrexate given intramuscularly at a dose of 15 mg once weekly to patients with quiescent Crohn's disease[96]. No maintenance benefit has been proven in ulcerative colitis by means of controlled clinical trials. Potential toxicities of methotrexate include leukopenia, nausea, vomiting and, rarely, hypersensitivity pneumonitis. Hepatic fibrosis is one of the most serious potential sequelae of long-term therapy with methotrexate. A pretreatment liver biopsy is indicated in patients who have abnormal liver associated laboratory chemistries and in those at potentially increased risk for hepatic toxicity (obsess patients etc.). Follow-up liver biopsy, although recommended by some clinicians for patients who have received a cumulative dose in excess of 1.5 g, has not been critically assessed in controlled clinical trials in IBD.

Cyclosporine A

Cyclosporine A (CyA) is a lipophilic undecapeptide extracted from the soil fungus *Tolypocladium infatum gams*. It acts by binding to an endogenous peptide (cyclophilin) which blocks the entry of activated T lymphocytes into the S phase of the cell cycle, thus inhibiting the production of IL-2. It also alters B-cell function by inhibiting T-helper cells. Furthemore, it decreases recruitment of cytotoxic T cells and blocks other cytokines, including IL-3, IL-4, INF-γ, and TNF-α[6,97–99].

The only randomized double-blind placebo-controlled study evaluating the efficacy of intravenous CyA in severe ulcerative colitis was reported in 1994[100]. In 11 patients who failed to respond to at least seven days of intravenous hydrocortisone, 9 responded favourably to continuous intravenous infusion of CyA (4 mg/kg/day) within a mean of 7.1 days, compared with none of the patients receiving placebo. During a 6-month follow-up period, 44% of those who were successfully treated with intravenous CyA ultimately required colectomy despite being maintained on oral CyA[101]. The addition of azathioprine or 6-MP appears to be beneficial in patients who have responded to intravenous CyA, and may lead to a reduced rate of relapse or colectomy[102–104]. These findings suggest that CyA may be used as a 'bridge' for control of disease until azathioprine or 6-MP becomes efficacious, or until elective surgery is performed. There is preliminary evidence to suggest that CyA used alone without corticosteroids may be effective for treatment of severe ulcerative colitis in some patients[105]. Cyclosporine enemas appear to be ineffective in left-sided ulcerative colitis[106].

Four controlled trials have evaluated the efficacy of oral CyA in active Crohn's disease[107–110]. One study demonstrated efficacy with a mean dose of 7.6 mg/kg[107], whereas the other three did not show any benefit over placebo with a mean dose of 5 mg/kg[108–110]. Uncontrolled data have shown efficacy of intravenous CyA (4 mg/kg/day) in the treatment of fistulous Crohn's disease unresponsive to corticosteroids, antibiotics or antimetobolites[111]. Side-effects of CyA reported during the treatment of IBD include hypertension, seizures, parethesias, tremor, gingival hyperplasia, hypertrichosis, electrolyte abnormalities, opportunistic infections and nephrotoxicity[111,112]. CyA blood levels should be followed regularly while on therapy, and careful monitoring for side-effects is critical for those using CyA[113]. A newer microemulsion formulation of CyA (Neoral) has improved oral absorption and may be as effective as intravenous CyA in the treatment of steroid-resistant ulcerative colitis[114].

Other immunomodulating agents

Tacrolimus (FK506) is a fungus (Streptomyces)-derived immunosuppressant that has a mechanism of action similar to that of CyA[115]. Mycophenolate mofetil, another potent immunosuppressant, inhibits lymphocyte proliferation by selectively blocking the synthesis of guanosine nucleotide in T cells. Both agents have been used successfully to treat steroid-refractory Crohn's disease and ulcerative colitis in preliminary trials[116–123]. Tacrolimus has a toxicity profile similar to that of CyA, while the major limiting adverse effect of mycophenolate mofetil is diarrhoea. Future prospective evaluations need to be performed to determine the efficacy and long-term side-effect profiles of these agents in inflammatory bowel disease.

Biological agents

Cytokines are glycosylated proteins that are synthesized by a variety of cell types in response to tissue injury. Certain cytokines, such as TNF-α, IL-1, IL-6, IL-8 and IL-12, are categorized as 'proinflammatory' owing to their ability to induce inflammation, while others such as IL-4, IL-10, IL-11 and IL-13 are categorized as 'anti-inflammatory' due to their ability to reduce inflammation. There is increasing evidence that a disturbed balance between proinflammatory and anti-inflammatory cytokines is present in inflammatory bowel disease. For example, tissue levels of proinflammatory cytokines are elevated in active inflammatory bowel disease, and correlate with the severity of the inflammation[124]. This has led to the development of treatments directed at blocking the proinflammatory actions of these cytokines.

Antibodies against TNF-α

Infliximab (Remicade) is a chimeric (75% human, 25% murine) IgG_1 monoclonal antibody directed against TNF-α. In the initial open-label study, infusion of a single dose of infliximab resulted in remission of active Crohn's disease in 8 of 10 patients previously unresponsive to steroid therapy[125]. Response was seen within four weeks and was maintained for at least eight weeks in most patients. No side-effects related to infliximab were observed. The efficacy and safety of infliximab was confirmed in a multicentre randomized placebo-controlled trial, showing that a single intravenous dose of infliximab (5, 10 or 20 mg/kg) resulted in clinical response in 65% of patients with resistant moderate-to-severe Crohn's disease, as compared with a response of 17% among patients given placebo within four weeks[126]. The 5 mg/kg dose provided the best results, with 81% of treated patients demonstrating a response. Clinical remission occurred in 33% of all patients compared with 4% of patients receiving placebo. The mean duration of response was 8–12 weeks[127], and preliminary data suggest that repeated doses of 10 mg/kg infliximab are effective in maintaining remission of Crohn's disease for up to 36 weeks[128]. Results of a large controlled trial of maintenance infliximab therapy in Crohn's disease (ACCENT I) have been completed and have confirmed that infliximab is effective for maintenance of remission in patients with Crohn's disease[129].

Infliximab has also proved to be efficacious in the treatment of Crohn's disease-associated enterocutaneous fistulae. In one study, complete closure of more than half of all fistulae occurred in 62% of infliximab-treated patients, and complete closure of all fistulae was observed in 46% of infliximab-treated patients, compared with 13% of patients receiving placebo[130]. The optimal dose of infliximab in this trial was 5 mg/kg given as three infusions at weeks 0, 2 and 6. The beneficial effect of infliximab was rapid (usually within two weeks) and persisted with reinfusion at 2-month intervals. In August 1998, the FDA approved infliximab for the treatment of patients with moderate-to-severe Crohn's disease refractory to conventional medication, and for those with draining enterocutaneous fistulae. Concurrent use of infliximab with 6-MP or azathioprine may be associated with prolonged remission in Crohn's disease[131]. However, the long-term effects of infliximab are not known and are currently under investigation in clinical trials.

Side-effects of infliximab include upper respiratory tract infection, sinus congestion, headache, nausea and myalgias. Some patients may develop antibodies against infliximab (formerly known as human antichimeric antibodies or HACA), although the clinical significance of these antibodies remains unclear. Delayed hypersensitivity-like reactions have been reported when prolonged periods (typically between 2 and 4 years) have elapsed between subsequent infusions[132]. Antineutrophil antibodies and double-stranded DNA antibodies may also occur as a result of therapy; however, the clinical significance of these findings remains under investigation. Two lymphomas have been reported to date (and one other has been observed in the ACCENT I trial) in two patients with long-standing Crohn's disease following infliximab infusions, and additional data will be needed to determine the long-term potential risk of lymphoproliferative disorders following infliximab infusion in Crohn's disease[133,134]. At present, it is believed that the risk for development of lymphoma is not higher in those receiving infliximab than the risk in the general population.

The genetically engineered humanized IgG_4 chimeric antibody to TNF-α, CDP571, has also shown good clinical response when administered to patients with moderately active Crohn's disease, or when given to patients in remission to attempt steroid withdrawal, with response rates similar to those seen with infliximab[135–137]. CDP571 appears to be well tolerated; however, longer-term data are needed to evaluate its efficacy and side-effect profile in this group of patients. Anti-TNF-α antibodies also have been evaluated in patients with ulcerative colitis. Infusion of CDP571 was administered in an open-label trial of 15 patients with mild-to-moderate ulcerative colitis. Twelve patients who completed four weeks of treatment had overall improvement[138]. Similarly, infliximab has shown short-term efficacy in four of eight patients with severe ulcerative colitis in another study where patients received single-dose therapy who had failed corticosteroids[139]. Another open-label pilot study demonstrated that approximately half of patients are induced into remission with therapy and that maintenance of remission can be achieved in these patients. Those patients who were steroid dependent responded well whereas those who were steroid refractory were less likely to respond[140]. Larger controlled studies are now ongoing to help determine the role of anti-TNF-α agents in the management of ulcerative colitis.

In addition to intravenous monoclonal antibody therapy directed at TNF-α, thalidomide, an oral agent known to inhibit TNF-α, has shown preliminary benefit in the treatment of intestinal and fistulizing Crohn's disease unresponsive to standard therapies[141–144]. Besides its known teratogenic properties, thalidomide often causes sedation and may cause peripheral neuropathy. Controlled trials of thalidomide in inflammatory bowel disease are necessary to determine its utility in these patients.

Anti-inflammatory cytokines

IL-10 and IL-11 are two anti-inflammatory cytokines that are being investigated for the treatment of Crohn's disease. IL-10 inhibits class I major histocompatibility complex expression on macrophages, decreases T-cell secretion of IL-2 and IFN-γ, and diminishes activated monocyte production of IL-1, IL-6, IL-8 and TNF-α[145]. In a randomized double-blind placebo-controlled multicentre trial, 45 patients with steroid-resistant Crohn's disease received intravenous boluses of recombinant human IL-10 (rhIL-10) or placebo daily for seven days[145]. Fifty per cent of patients who received IL-10, and 23% of those who received placebo, achieved complete remission. IL-10 was well tolerated by all patients. A subsequent study in patients with chronic active Crohn's disease was not able to demonstrate superiority of IL-10 in inducing remission over placebo[146].

Additionally, a recent study demonstrated that IL-10 does not decrease endoscopic recurrence of Crohn's disease after ileal or ileocolonic resection[147]. Very little information is available on the use of IL-10 in ulcerative colitis, although one small study described three patients who improved after rectal application of IL-10[148]. Additional controlled studies need to be done to evaluate the efficacy and safety of this agent in the management of IBD.

Promising results have also been observed utilizing recombinant human IL-11 (rhIL-11) for the treatment of active IBD. IL-11 is a pleiotropic cytokine that has protective effects on the intestinal cells. It has been shown to decrease colitis in animal models of inflammatory bowel disease[149]. In a randomized placebo-controlled trial involving 76 subjects with active Crohn's disease, twice-weekly administration of rhIL-11 for three weeks reduced disease activity significantly when compared with placebo[150]. The medication was well tolerated. Another similar trial involving 148 patients demonstrated efficacy in patients with Crohn's disease not receiving corticosteroids[151]. Larger controlled trials with rhIL-11 have recently been completed.

Intracellular adhesion molecules

Intracellular adhesion molecules (ICAM) are transmembrane glycoproteins that facilitate the emigration of leukocytes from the intravascular space in response to inflammation. They are upregulated in inflamed mucosa in Crohn's disease. ISIS 2302, an antisense oligonucleotide that downregulates the expression of ICAM-1, demonstrated promising results in a phase II trial in 20 patients with active Crohn's disease despite steroid treatment[152] although published results of a larger controlled trial failed to demonstrate positive results[153].

Interferon

In recent years, it has become apparent that the overproduction of the Th-1 cytokines, IL-12 and IFN-γ is the probable driving force behind murine models of intestinal inflammation resembling Crohn's disease and intestinal inflammation in humans with Crohn's disease. In addition, studies of murine models strongly suggest that this overproduction is associated with inadequate secretion of the counter-regulatory and anti-inflammatory cytokine TGF-β. Thus, mucosal inflammation in models (and possibly in humans) may result from an imbalance between normally occurring positive (immunogenic or inflammatory) responses and negative (tolerogenic or anti-inflammatory) mucosal immune responses. These new findings and the hypotheses that arise from them are being used to construct new approaches to the treatment of Crohn's disease that are based on the administration of anti-inflammatory cytokines and anticytokine antibodies. Additionally, it should be stressed that it has been shown that IFN-γ induces the cell-surface expression of MHC molecules[154] and fragment crystallizable (Fc)-γ receptors[155], enhances the cytolytic activity of NK cells, activates macrophages[156], modulates the immunoglobulin isotype profile of a humoral response[157], and exerts an antiproliferative effect on some cell types[158].

As a result of the effects that IFN-γ has on the body and since levels are elevated in patients with Crohn's disease, a trial has been suggested of anti-IFN-γ antibodies. An initial study has been completed and a larger multicentre trial is now ongoing.

NUTRITIONAL THERAPY AND OTHER AGENTS

Bowel rest and TPN are often effective as primary therapy for the treatment of active Crohn's disease but have not proven effective as primary therapy in ulcerative colitis[159–161]. Oral elemental diets (nutritional supplements comprised primarily of L-amino acids) may also be effective in active Crohn's disease but are not well tolerated for any length of time due to their unpalatability. Neither TPN nor elemental diets have proven efficacy for maintenance of remission in Crohn's disease[161]. Use of short-chain fatty acids, which serve as important nutrients of the colonic epithelium, may be beneficial in some patients with active ulcerative colitis[162], and oral fish oil preparations have shown modest benefit in active and quiescent ulcerative colitis and Crohn's disease[161].

Nicotine has been administered to patients with ulcerative colitis due to the protective effect smoking has in this condition[163]. This is in contrast to the deleterious effect smoking has in Crohn's disease. Transdermal nicotine has shown response in active ulcerative colitis, while maintenance therapy appears to be less efficacious[163]. Preliminary data suggest that heparin may be effective for

Table 2 Adverse effects of drugs commonly used in inflammatory bowel disease

Agent	*Route of administration*	*Adverse effects*
Sulphasalazine	PO	Nausea, headache, rash, fever, hypersensitivity reactions, folate malabsorption, sperm abnormalities
5-ASA	PO, topical	Nausea, dyspepsia, headache, rare hypersensitivity reactions*
Corticosteroids	IV, PO, topical	Acne, weight gain, striae, fat redistribution, mood changes, myopathy, hyperglycemia, cataracts†, osteoporosis, osteonecrosis†, growth failure in children†
Azathioprine/6-MP	PO	Nausea, fever, rash, pancreatitis (3–15%), infection, bone marrow suppression‡
Cyclosporine	IV, PO	Hypertension, headache, electrolyte abnormalities, tremor, paresthesias, ↑ LFTs, gingival hyperplasia, nephrotoxicity, seizure (rare), opportunistic infections (rare)
Methotrexate	PO, IM, SC	Nausea, vomiting, diarrhoea, leukopenia, hepatic fibrosis, pneumonitis
Metronidazole	PO	Nausea, abdominal pain, metallic taste, disulphuram-like reaction with alcohol, peripheral neuropathy
Infliximab	IV	Nausea, abdominal pain, upper respiratory infection, myalgias, infusion reactions, possible delayed hypersensitivity-like reactions

*5-ASA usually well tolerated. 80% of patients intolerant to sulphasalazine are able to tolerate 5-ASA. †Posterior subcapsular cataracts, osteonecrosis and growth failure in children are usually associated with prolonged exposure to corticosteroids. ‡Bone marrow suppression with azathioprine or 6-MP may be delayed. 5-ASA, 5-aminosalicylate; AZA, azathioprine; 6-MP, 6-mercaptopurine; IV, intravenous; IM, intramuscular; SC, subcutaneous; LFTs, liver function tests.

induction of remission in ulcerative colitis[164,165], but further randomized controlled trials are necessary. A trial using low-molecular-weight heparin is now ongoing. Other investigational therapies in inflammatory bowel disease, including lymphocytoplasmapheresis, bismuth preparations, novel aminosalicylates and, most recently, growth hormone[166] require additional evaluation prior to acceptance in the management of the inflammatory bowel diseases.

Table 3 Medical therapy of Crohn's disease

	Intestinal disease			*Active fistulae*
	Active disease		*Maintenance*	
	Mild–moderate	*Severe*		
5-ASA				
Oral	+	−	+	−
Topical	ND*	−	ND*	−
Corticosteroids				
Oral	++	+	−	−
Topical	ND	ND	−	−
IV	++	++	−	−
Antibiotics	+	−	ND*	++
AZA/6-MP	++	ND	++	++
Methotrexate	++	ND	++	ND
Cyclosporine A	+	ND	−	ND
Infliximab	++	++	++	++

5-ASA, 5-aminosalicylic acid; AZA, azathioprine; 6-MP, 6-mercaptopurine; ++, significant benefit; +, benefit; −, no benefit; ND, no controlled data available; ND*, no controlled data, but clinical practice is often to prescribe these agents for active symptoms, and perhaps continue these agents as maintenance therapy.

Table 4 Medical therapy of ulcerative colitis

	Active Disease		*Maintenance*
	Mild–moderate	*Severe*	
5-ASA			
Oral	++	ND	++
Topical	++	ND	++
Corticosteroids			
Oral	++	++	−
Topical	++	ND	−
IV	++	++	−
Antibiotics	+	−	ND
AZA/6-MP	++	ND	++
Methotrexate	−	ND	ND
Cyclosporine A	ND	++	−
Infliximab	ND	+	ND

5-ASA, 5-aminosalicylic acid; AZA, azathioprine; 6-MP, 6-mercaptopurine; ND, no controlled data available; ++, significant benefit; +, benefit; −, no benefit.

CONCLUSIONS

At present, medical management of inflammatory bowel disease is far from ideal. It is hoped that further understanding of the basic inflammatory cascade and the perturbations which are present in inflammatory bowel disease will lead to more specific and potent treatments for these disorders. It is not until the specific aetiologic agent(s) causing IBD are discovered that a cure for these chronic and debilitating disorders is likely to be found.

References

1. Baron JH, Connell AM, Lennard-Jones JE, Jones FA. Sulphasalazine and salicylazosulphadimidine in ulcerative colitis. Lancet. 1962;1:1094–6.
2. Azad Khan AK, Piris J, Truelove SC. An experiment to determine the active therapeutic moiety in sulphasalazine. Lancet. 1977;2:892–5.
3. Greenfield SM, Punchard NA, Teare JP. The mode of action of the aminosalicylates in inflammatory bowel disease. Aliment Pharmacol Ther. 1993;7:369–83.
4. Grisham MB. Oxidants and free radicals in inflammatory bowel disease. Lancet. 1994;344:859–61.
5. Gaginella TS, Walsh RE. Sulphasalazine: multiplicity of action. Dig Dis Sci. 1992;37:801–12.
6. Hanauer SB, Meyers S, Sachar DB. The pharmacology of anti-inflammatory drugs in inflammatory bowel disease. In: Kirsner JB, Shorter RG, eds. Inflammatory Bowel Disease, 4th edn. Baltimore: William and Wilkins, 1995:643–63.
7. Kaiser GC, Yan F, Polk B. Mesalamine blocks tumor necrosis factor growth inhibition and nuclear factor kappa beta activation in mouse colonocytes. Gastroenterology. 1999;116:602–9.
8. Wahl C, Liptay S, Adler G, Schmid RM. Sulphasalazine: A potent and specific inhibitor of nuclear factor kappa beta. J Clin Invest. 1998;101:1163–74.
9. Sutherland LR, May GR, Shaffer EA. Sulphasalazine revisited: a meta-analysis of 5-aminosalicylic acid in the treatment of ulcerative colitis. Ann Intern Med. 1993;118:540–9.
10. Giaffer MH, O'Brien CJ, Holdsworth CD. Clinical tolerance to three 5-aminosalicylic acid releasing preparations in patients with inflammatory bowel disease intolerant or allergic to sulphasalazine. Aliment Pharmacol Ther. 1992;6:51–9.
11. Stein RB, Hanauer SB. Medical therapy for inflammatory bowel disease. Gastroenterol Clin N Am. 1999;28:297–321.
12. Green JRB, Lobo AJ, Holdsworth CD *et al.* and the Abacus Investigator Group. Balsalazide is more effective and better tolerated than mesalamine in the treatment of acute ulcerative colitis. Gastroenterology. 1998;114:15–22.
13. Kornbluth A, Sachar DB. Ulcerative colitis practice guidelines in adults. Am J Gastroenterol. 1997;92:204–11.
14. Summers RW, Switz DM, Sessions JT Jr *et al.* National Cooperative Crohn's Disease Study: results of drug treatment. Gastroenterology. 1979;77:847–69.
15. Malchow H, Ewe K, Brandes JW *et al.* European Cooperative Crohn's Disease Study (ECCDS): results of drug treatment. Gastroenterology. 1984;86:249–66.
16. Singleton JW, Hanauer SB, Gitnick GL *et al.* and the Pentasa Crohn's Disease Study Group. Mesalamine capsules for the treatment of active Crohn's disease: results of a 16-week trial. Gastroenterology. 1993;104:1293–301.
17. Tremaine WJ, Schroeder KW, Harrison JM, Zinsmeister AR. A randomized, double-blind, placebo-controlled trial of the oral mesalamine (5-ASA) preparation, Asacol, in the treatment of symptomatic Crohn's colitis and ileocolitis. J Clin Gastroenterol. 1994;19:278–82.
18. Hanauer SB, Stromber U. Efficacy of oral pentasa 4 g/day in treatment of active Crohn's disease: A meta analysis double-blind placebo-controlled trial. Gastroenterology. 2001; [Abstract]120(5), Suppl 1:A 453.
19. Prantera C, Cottone M, Pallone F *et al.* Mesalamine in the treatment of mild to moderate active Crohn's ileitis: Results of a randomized, multicenter trial. Gastroenterology. 1999;116:521–6.
20. Camma C, Giunta M, Rosselli M, Cottone M. Mesalamine in the maintenance treatment of Crohn's disease: a meta-analysis adjusted for confounding variables. Gastroenterology. 1997; 113:1465–73.

21. Modigliani R, Colombel JF, Dupas J-L *et al.* Mesalamine in Crohn's disease with steroid-induced remission: effect on steroid withdrawal and remission maintenance. Gastroenterology. 1996;110:688–93.
22. Hanauer SB, Krawitt EL, Robinson M, Rick GG, Safti MA. Long term management of Crohn's disease with mesalamine capsules (Pentasa). Pentasa Crohn's Disease Compassionate Use Study Group. Am J Gastroenterol. 1993;88:1343–51.
23. Marshall JK, Irvine EJ. Rectal aminosalicylate therapy for distal ulcerative colitis: a meta-analysis. Aliment Pharmacol Ther. 1995;9:293–300.
24. Kam L, Cohen H, Dooley C, Rubin P, Orchard J. A comparison of mesalamine suspension enema and oral sulphasalazine for treatment of active distal ulcerative colitis in adults. Am J Gastroenterol. 1996;91:1338–42.
25. Hanauer SB. Dose-ranging study of mesalamine (Pentasa) enemas of acute ulcerative proctosigmoiditis: Results of a multicentered placebo-controlled trial. Inflamm Bowel Dis. 1998;4:79–83.
26. Safdi M, DeMiccom, Sninsky C *et al.* A double-blind comparison of oral versus rectal mesalamine versus combination therapy in the treatment of distal ulcerative colitis. Am J Gastroenterol. 1997;92:1867–71.
27. D'Albasio G, Pacini F, Camarri E *et al.* Combined therapy with 5-aminosalicylic acid tablets and enemas for maintaining remission in ulcerative colitis: a randomized double-blind study. Am J Gastroenterol. 1997;92:1143–7.
28. Danish 5-ASA Group. Topical 5-aminosalicylate versus prednisolone in ulcerative proctosigmoiditis: a randomized, double-blind multicenter trial. Dig Dis Sci. 1987;32:598–602.
29. D'Ariennzo A, Panarese A, D'Armiento FP *et al.* 5-Aminosalicylic acid suppositories in the maintenance of remission in idiopathic proctitis or proctosigmoiditis: a double-blind placebo-controlled clinical trial. Am J Gastroenterol. 1990;85:1079–82.
30. Marteau P, Crand J, Foucxault M, Rambaud JC. Use of mesalazine slow release suppositories 1 g three times per week to maintain remission of ulcerative proctitis: a randomised double-blind placebo controlled multicentre study. Gut. 1998;42:195–9.
31. Campieri M, Corbelli C, Gionchetti P *et al.* Spread and distribution of 5-ASA colonic foam and 5-ASA enema in patients with ulcerative colitis. Dig Dis Sci. 1992;37:1890–7.
32. Campieri M, Paoluzi P, D'Albasio G *et al.* Better quality of therapy with 5-ASA colonic foam in inactive ulcerative colitis: a multicenter comparative trial with 5-ASA enema. Dig Dis Sci. 1993; 38:1843–50.
33. Truelove SC, Witts LJ. Cortisone in ulcerative colitis: a final report on a therapeutic trial. Br Med J. 1955;2:1041–5.
34. Rosenberg W, Ireland A, Jewell D. High-dose methylprednisone in the treatment of active ulcerative colitis. J Clin Gastroenterol. 1990;12:40–1.
35. Van Hees PAM, Van Lier HJJ, Van Elteren PH *et al.* Effects of sulphasalazine in patients with active Crohn's disease: a controlled double-blind study. Gut. 1981;22:404–9.
36. Lennard-Jones JE. Corticosteroids and immunosuppressive drugs. In: Allan RN, Keighley MRB, Alexander-Williams J, eds. Inflammatory Bowel Disease. London: Churchill Livingstone, 1990: 373–89.
37. Meyers S, Sachar DB, Goldberg JD, Janowitz HD. Corticotropin versus hydrocortisone in intravenous treatment of ulcerative colitis. Gastroenterology. 1983;85:351–7.
38. Freeman HJ, Kwan WCP. Brief report: Non-corticosteroid-associated osteonecrosis of the femoral head in two patients with inflammatory bowel disease. N Engl J Med. 1993;329: 1314–16.
39. Clements D, Compton JE, Evand WD, Rhodes J. Hormone replacement therapy prevents bone loss in patients with inflammatory bowel disease. Gut. 1993;34:1543–6.
40. Lofberg R, Dannielsson A, Suhr O *et al.* Oral budesonide versus prednisolone in patients with active extensive and left-sided colitis. Gastroenterology. 1996;110:1713–18.
41. Rutgeerts P, Lofberg R, Malchow H *et al.* A comparison of budesonide with prednisolone for active Crohn's disease. N Engl J Med. 1994;331:842–5.
42. Greenberg G, Feagan B, Martin F *et al.* Oral budesonide for the treatment of active Crohn's disease. N Engl J Med. 1994;331:836–41.
43. Thomsen OO, Cortot A, Jewell D *et al.* A comparison of budesonide and mesalamine for active Crohn's disease. N Engl J Med. 1998;339:370–4.
44. Yang YX, Lichtenstein GR. Corticosteroids in Crohn's disease. Am J Gastroenterol. 2002; (in press).

45. Lofberg R, Rutgeerts P, Malchow H *et al.* Budesonide prolongs time to relapse in ileal and ileocaecal Crohn's disease: a placebo controlled one year study. Gut. 1996;39:82–6.
46. Cortot A, Colombel JF, Rutgeerts P *et al.* Budesonide controlled ileal release (CIR) capsules in prednisolone-dependent patients with Crohn's disease. Gastroenterology. 1999;116:A692.
47. Greenberg GR, Feagan BG, Martin F *et al.* Oral budesonide as maintenance treatment for Crohn's disease: A placebo-controlled, dose-ranging study. Gastroenterology. 1996;110:45–51.
48. Hellers G, Cortot A, Jewell D *et al.* Oral budesonide for prevention of postsurgical recurrence in Crohn's disease. The IOIBD Budesonide Study Group. Gastroenterology. 1999;116:294–300.
49. Ardizzone S, Bianchi Porro G. The topical treatment of distal ulcerative colitis. Eur J Gastroenterol Hepatol. 1996;8:599–602.
50. Somerville KW, Langman MS, Kane SP *et al.* Effects of treatment on symptoms and quality of life in patients with ulcerative colitis: comparative trial of hydrocortisone acetate foam and prednisolone-21–phosphate enemas. Br Med J. 1985;291:866.
51. Marshall JK, Irvine EJ. Rectal corticosteroids versus alternative treatment in ulcerative colitis: a meta-analysis. Gut. 1997;40:775–81.
52. Mulder CJJ, Fockens P, Meijer JW, Van der Heider H, Wiltink EH, Tytgat GN. Beclomethasone dipropionate (3 mg) versus 5-amonisalicylic acid (2 g) versus the combination of both (3 mg/2 g) as retention enemas in active ulcerative proctitis. Eur J Gastroenterol Hepatol. 1996;8:549–53.
53. Danielsson A, Lofberg R, Persson T *et al.* A steroid enema, budesonide, lacking systemic effects for the treatment of distal ulcerative colitis or proctitis. Scand J Gastroenterol. 1992;27:9–12.
54. The Danish Budesonide Study Group. Budesonide enema in distal ulcerative colitis. A randomized dose-response trial with prednisolone enema as positive control. Scand J Gastroenterol. 1991;26:1225–30.
55. Lemann M, Galian A, Rutgeerts *et al.* Comparison of budesonide and 5-aminosalicylic acid enemas in distal ulcerative colitis. Aliment Pharmacol Ther. 1995;9:557–62.
56. Bianchi Porro G, Prantera C, Campieri M *et al.* Comparative trial of methylprednisolone and budesonide enemas in inactive distal ulcerative colitis. Eur J Gastroenterol Hepatol. 1994;6: 125–30.
57. Sutherland LR, Singleton J, Sessions J *et al.* Double blind, placebo controlled trial of metronidazole in Crohn's disease. Gut. 1991;32:1071–5.
58. Ursing B, Aim T, Barany F *et al.* A comparative study of metronidazole and sulphasalazine for active Crohn's disease: the Cooperative Crohn's Disease Study in Sweden. Gastroenterology. 1982;83:550–62.
59. Bernstein LH, Frank MS, Brandt LJ, Boley SJ. Healing of perineal Crohn's disease with metronidazole. Gastroenterology. 1980;79:357–65.
60. Rutgeerts P, Hieele M, Geboes K *et al.* Controlled trial of metronidazole treatment for prevention of Crohn's recurrence after ileal resection. Gastroenterology. 1995;108:1617–21.
61. Rutgeerts PJ, D'Haens G, Baert F *et al.* Nitroimidazole antibiotics are efficacious for prophylaxis of postoperative recurrence of Crohn's disease: A placebo controlled trial [Abstract]. Gastroenterology. 1999;116:A 808.
62. Chapman RW, Selby WS, Jewell DP. Controlled trial of intravenous metronidazole as an adjunct to corticosteroids in severe ulcerative colitis. Gut. 1986;27:1210–12.
63. Gilat T, Leichtman G, Delphre G *et al.* A comparison of metronidazole and sulphasalazine in the maintenance of remission in patients with ulcerative colitis. J Clin Gastroenterol. 1989; 11:392–5.
64. Tawfik AF, Shoeb HA, Bishop SJ, al-Shammary FJ, Shibl AM. Influence of new quinolones on normal immune capabilities. J Chemother. 1990;2:300–5.
65. Colombel JF, Lemann M, Cassagnou M *et al* and the GETAID. A controlled trial comparing ciprofloxacin with mesalazine for the treatment of active Crohn's disease. Am J Gastroenterol. 1999;94:674–8.
66. Prantera C, Zannoni F, Scribano ML *et al.* An antibiotic regimen for the treatment of active Crohn's disease: a randomized, controlled clinical trial of metronidazole plus ciprofloxacin. Am J Gastroenterol. 1996;91:328–32.
67. Turunen U, Farkkila M, Valtonen V, Seppala K. Long-term outcome of ciprofloxacin treatment in severe perianal or fistulous Crohn's disease [Abstract]. Gastroenterology. 1993;104:A793.
68. Turunen UM, Farkkila MA, Hakala K *et al.* Long-term treatment of ulcerative colitis with ciprofloxacin: a prospective, double-blind, placebo-controlled study. Gastroenterology. 1998; 115:1072–8.

69. Pearson DC, May GR, Fick GH, Sutherland LR. Azathioprine and 6-mercaptopurine in Crohn's disease. A meta-analysis. Ann Intern Med. 1995;122:132–42.
70. Present DH, Korelitz BI, Wisch N, Glass JL, Sachar DB, Pasternack BS. Treatment of Crohn's disease with 6-mercaptopurine: a long-term, randomized, double-blind study. N Engl J Med. 1980;302:981–7.
71. Ewe K, Press AG, Singe CC *et al.* Azathioprine combined with prednisolone or monotherapy with prednisolone in active Crohn's disease. Gastroenterology. 1993;105:367–72.
72. Sandborn WJ, Van Os EC, Zins BJ, Tremaine WJ, Mays DC, Lipsky JJ. An intravenous loading dose of azathioprine decreases the time to response in patients with Crohn's disease. Gastroenterology. 1995;109:1808–17.
73. Sandborn WJ, Tremain WJ, Wolf DC *et al.* Lack of effect of intravenous azathioprine on time to respond to azathioprine for steroid treated Crohn's disease. Gastroenterology. 1999;117: 527–35.
74. Su CG, Stein RB, Lewis JD, Lichtenstein GR. Azathioprine or 6-mercaptopurine for inflammatory bowel disease: Do risks outweigh benefits? Digest Liver Dis. 2000;32:518–31.
75. Bouhnik Y, Lemann M, Mary JY *et al.* Long-term follow-up of patients with Crohn's disease treated with azathioprine or 6-mercaptopurine. Lancet. 1996;347:215–19.
76. Korelitz B, Hanauer S, Rutgeerts P, Present D, Peppercorn M. Post-operative prophylaxis with 6-MP, 5-ASA or placebo in Crohn's disease: a 2 year multicenter trial [Abstract]. Gastroenterology. 1998;114:A1011.
77. Jewell DP, Truelove SC. Azathioprine in ulcerative colitis: final report on controlled therapeutic trial. Br Med J. 1974;4:627–30.
78. Caprilli R, Carratu R, Babbini M. A double-blind comparison of the effectiveness of azathioprine and sulphasalazine in idiopathic proctocolitis. Am J Dig Dis. 1975;20:115–20.
79. Kirk AP, Lennard-Jones JE. A controlled trial of azathioprine in chronic ulcerative colitis. Br Med J. 1982;284:1291–2.
80. Rosenberg JL, Wall AJ, Levin B, Binder HJ, Kirsner JB. A controlled trial of azathioprine in the management of chronic ulcerative colitis. Gastroenterology. 1975;69:96–9.
81. Hawthorne AB, Logan RFA, Hawkey CJ *et al.* Randomised controlled trial of azathioprine withdrawal in ulcerative colitis. Br Med J. 1992;305:20–2.
82. Alder DJ, Korelitz BI. The therapeutic efficacy of 6-mercaptopurine in refractory ulcerative colitis. Am J Gastroenterol. 1990;85:717–22.
83. Present DH, Meltzer SJ, Krumholz MP, Wolke A, Korelitz BI. 6-Mercaptopurine in the management of inflammatory bowel disease: short and long term toxicity. Ann Intern Med. 1989;111: 641–9.
84. Lewis JD, Schwartz JS, Lichtenstein GR. Azathioprine for maintenance of remission in Crohn's disease: Benefits outweigh the risk of lymphoma. Gastroenterology. 2000;118:1018–24.
85. Connell WR, Kamm MA, Dickson M, Balkwill AM, Ritchie JK, Lennard-Jones JE. Long-term neoplastic risk after azathioprine treatment in inflammatory bowel disease. Lancet. 1994;343: 1249–52.
86. Colonna T, Korelitz BI. The role of leucopenia in the 6-mercaptopurine-induced remission of refractory Crohn's disease. Am J Gastroenterol. 1994;89:362–6.
87. Dubinsky MC, Lamothe S, Yang HY *et al.* Pharmacogenomics and metabolite measurement for 6-mercaptopurine therapy in inflammatory bowel disease. Gastroenterology. 2000;118: 705–13.
88. Cuffari C, Sharma S. 6-Mercaptopurine metabolite levels tailored to achieve clinical responsiveness in pediatric Crohn's disease [Abstract]. Gastroenterology. 1999;116:A694.
89. Cuffari C, Picco M, Hunt S, Bayless T. Azathioprine metabolite levels predict clinical responsiveness to therapy in IBD [Abstract]. Gastroenterology. 1999;116:A694.
90. Szumlanski CL, Weinshilboum RM. Sulphasalazine inhibition of thiopurine methyltransferase: possible mechanism for interaction with 6-mercaptopurine and azathioprine. Br J Clin Pharmacol. 1995;39:456–9.
91. Lewis LD, Benin A, Szumlanski CL *et al.* Olsalazine and 6-mercaptopurine-related bone marrow suppression: a possible drug–drug interaction. Clin Pharmacol Ther. 1997;62:464–75.
92. Feagan BG, Rochon J, Fedorak RN *et al.* Methotrexate for the treatment of Crohn's disease. N Engl J Med. 1995;332:292–7.
93. Arora S, Katkov W, Cooley J *et al.* Methotrexate in Crohn's disease: results of a double-blind, randomized, placebo-controlled trial. Hepatogastroenterology 1999;46:1724–9.
94. Oren R, Moshkowitz M, Odes S *et al.* Methotrexate in chronic active Crohn's disease: a double-blind, randomized, Israeli multi-center trial. Am J Gastroenterol. 1997;92:2203–9.

95. Oren R, Arber N, Odes S *et al.* Methotrexate in chronic active ulcerative colitis: a double-blind, randomized, Israeli multi-center trial. Gastroenterology. 1996;110:1416–21.
96. Feagan BG, Fedorak RN, Irvine JE *et al.* A comparison of methotrexate with placebo for the maintenance of remission in Crohn's disease. N Engl J Med. 2000;342:1627–32.
97. Langford CA, Klippel JH, Balow JE, James SP, Sneller MC. Use of cytotoxic agents and cyclosporine in the treatment of autoimmune disease. Part 2: Inflammatory bowel disease, systemic vasculitis, and therapeutic toxicity. Ann Intern Med. 1998;129:49–58.
98. Sandborn WJ. A critical review of cyclosporine therapy in inflammatory bowel disease. Inflamm Bowel Dis. 1995;1:48–63.
99. Sandborn WJ. A review of immune modifier therapy for inflammatory bowel disease: Azathioprine, 6-mrcaptopurine, cyclosporine, and methotrexate. Am J Gastroenterol. 1996;91: 423–3.
100. Lichtiger S, Present DH, Kornbluth A *et al.* Cyclosporin in severe ulcerative colitis refractory to steroid therapy. N Engl J Med. 1994;330:841–5.
101. Kornbluth A, Lichtiger S, Present D, Hanauer S. Long-term results of oral cyclosporin in patients with severe ulcerative colitis: a double-blind randomized multicenter trial [Abstract]. Gastroenterology. 1994;106:A714.
102. Cohen RD, Stein R, Hanauer SB. Intravenous cyclosporin in ulcerative colitis: A five-year experience. Am J Gastroenterol. 1999; 94:1587–92.
103. Fernandez-Banares F, Bertran X, Esteve-Comas M *et al.* Azathioprine is useful in maintaining long-term remission induced by intravenous cyclosporine in steroid-refractory severe ulcerative colitis. Am J Gastroenterol. 1996;91:2498–9.
104. Marion JF, Present DH. 6-Mercaptopurine maintains cyclosporine induced response in patients with ulcerative colitis [Abstract]. Am J Gastroenterol. 1996;91:A1975.
105. D'Haens G, Lemmens L, Hiele M, Aerden I, Rutgeerts P. Remission of severe ulcerative colitis with cyclosporine monotherapy is effectively maintained with further immunosuppression [Abstract]. Gastroenterology. 1999;116:A722.
106. Sandborn WJ, Tremaine WJ, Schroeder KW *et al.* A placebo-controlled trial of cyclosporine enemas for mildly to moderately active left-sided ulcerative colitis. Gastroenterology. 1994; 106:1429–35.
107. Brynskov J, Freund L, Rasmussen SN *et al.* A placebo-controlled, double blind, randomized trial of cyclosporine therapy in active chronic Crohn's disease. N Engl J Med. 1989; 321: 845–50.
108. Stange EF, Modigliani R, Penna AS, Wood AJ, Feutren G, Smith PR and the European Study Group. European trial of cyclosporine in chronic active Crohn's disease: a 12–month study. Gastroenterology. 1993;109:774–82.
109. Feagan BG, McDonald JWD, Rochon J *et al.* and the Canadian Crohn's Relapse Prevention Trial Investigators. Low dose cyclosporine in the treatment of Crohn's disease. N Engl J Med. 1994;330:1846–51.
110. Jewell DP, Lennard-Jones JE and the Cyclosporine Study Group of Great Britain and Ireland. Oral cyclosporine for chronic active Crohn's disease: a multicenter controlled trial. Eur J Gastroenterol Hepatol. 1994;6:499–505.
111. Hanauer SB, Smith MB. Rapid closure of Crohn's disease fistulas with continuous intravenous cyclosporin A. Am J Gastroenterol. 1993;88:646–9.
112. Stein R, Cohen RD, Hanauer SB. Complications during cyclosporine therapy for inflammatory bowel disease. Gastroenterology. 1997;112:A1096.
113. Kornbluth A, Present DH, Lichtiger S *et al.* Cyclosporin for severe ulcerative colitis: A user's guide. Am J Gastroenterol. 1997;92:1424–8.
114. Oppong K, Record CO. Neoral may be as effective as intravenous cyclosporine in the treatment of steroid-resistant ulcerative colitis. Am J Gastroenterol. 1998;93:1188–9.
115. Thomson AW, Starzl TE. FK506 and autoimmune disease: Prospective and prospects. Autoimmunity. 1992;12:303.
116. Fellermann K, Ludwig D, Stahl M, David-Walek T, Stange EF. Steroid-unresponsive acute attacks of inflammatory bowel disease: Immunomodulation by Tacrolimus (FK506). Am J Gastroenterol. 1998;93:1860–6.
117. Sandborn WJ. Preliminary report on the use of oral Tacrolimus (FK 506) in the treatment of complicated proximal small bowel and fistulizing Crohn's disease. Am J Gastroenterol. 1997; 92:876–9.

118. Bousvaros A, Wang A, Leichtner AM. Tacrolimus (FK 506) treatment of fulminant colitis in a child. J Pediatr Gastroenterol Nutr. 1996;23:329–33.
119. Lowry PW, Weaver AL, Tremaine WJ, Sandborn WJ. Combination therapy with oral Tacrolimus (FK 506) and azathioprine (AZA) or 6-mercaptopurine (6MP) for refractory perianal Crohn's disease (CD) [Abstract]. Gastroenterology. 1999;116:A810.
120. Neurath MF, Wanitschke R, Peters M *et al.* Mycophenolate mofetil for treatment of active inflammatory bowel disease. Clinical and immunological studies. Ann NY Acad Sci. 1998; 859:315–18.
121. Florin TH, Roberts RK, Watson MR, Radford-Smith GL. Treatment of steroid refractory inflammatory bowel disease (IBD) with mycophenolate mofetil (MMF) [Letter]. Aust NZ J Med. 1998;28:344–5.
122. Fickert P, Hinterleitner TA, Wenzl HH, Aichbichler BW, Petritsch W. Mycophenolate mofetil in patients with Crohn's disease. Am J Gastroenterol. 1998;93:2529–32.
123. Hassard P, Vasilauskas E, Kam L, Targan S, Abreu-Martin MT. Limited benefit of mycophenolate mofetil (MMF) for the treatment of severe refractory Crohn's disease (CD) [Abstract]. Gastroenterology. 1999;116(4):A733.
124. Reimund JM, Witterheim C, Dumont S *et al.* Mucosal inflammatory cytokine production by intestinal biopsies in patients with ulcerative colitis and Crohn's disease. J Clin Immunol. 1996;16:144–50.
125. van Dullemen HM, van Deventer SJ, Hommes DW *et al.* Treatment of Crohn's disease with anti-tumor necrosis factor chimeric monoclonal antibody (cA2). Gastroenterology. 1995;109: 129–35.
126. Targan SR, Hanauer SB, van Deventer SJH *et al.* A short-term study of chimeric monoclonal antibody cA2 to tumor necrosis factor (alpha) for Crohn's disease. N Engl J Med. 1997;337: 1029–35.
127. Stein RB, Lichtenstein GR. Medical therapy for Crohn's disease: State of the art. Surg Clin N Am. (in press).
128. Rutgeerts P, D'Haens G, Targan S *et al.* Efficacy and safety of retreatment with anti-tumor necrosis factor antibody (Infliximab) to maintain remission in Crohn's disease. Gastroenterology. 1999; 117:761–9.
129. Hanauer SB, Lichtenstein GR, Colombel JF *et al.* Maintenance infliximab (Remicade) is safe, effective and steroid-sparing in Crohn's disease: Preliminary results from the ACCENT I trial. Gastroenterology. 2001;120(5) Suppl 1:A-21.
130. Present DH, Rutgeerts P, Targan S *et al.* Infliximab for the treatment of fistulas in patients with Crohn's disease. N Engl J Med. 1999;340:1398–405.
131. Pittman R, Toy LS, Kornbluth A, Present DH. Pretreatment with 6-mercaptopurine/azathioprine prolongs clinical response time in Crohn's disease patients with fistulizing disease treated with infliximab. Gastroenterology. 2000;118:A4206.
132. Hanauer SB, Rutgeerts PJ, D'Haens G *et al.* Delayed hypersensitivity to infliximab (Remicade) re-infusion after 2–4 year interval without treatment. Gastroenterology. 1999;116:A813.
133. Bickston SJ, Lichtenstein GR, Arseneau KO *et al.* The relationship between infliximab treatment and lymphoma in Crohn's disease. Gastroenterology. 1999;117:1433–7.
134. Lichtenstein GR, MacDermott RP. The future has arrived: Biological therapy for Crohn's disease. Gastroenterology.medscape.com. DDW May, 1999:1–7.
135. Stack WA, Mann SD, Roy AJ *et al.* Randomised controlled trial of CDP571 antibody to tumour necrosis factor-alpha in Crohn's disease. Lancet. 1997;349:521–4.
136. Feagan BG, Sandborn WJ, Baker JP *et al.* A randomized, double-blind, placebo-controlled, multicenter trial of the engineered human antibody to TNF (CDP571) for steroid sparing and maintenance of remission in patients with steroid-dependent Crohn's disease. Gastroententerology. 2000;118:A3599.
137. Sandborn WJ, Targan SR, Hanauer SB *et al.* A randomized controlled trial of CDP571, a humanized antibody to TNFalpha, in moderately to severly active Crohn's disease. Gastroenterology. 2000;118:A3598.
138. Evans RC, Clark L, Heath P, Rhodes JM. Treatment of ulcerative colitis with an engineered human anti-TNFα antibody CDP571 [Abstract]. Gastroenterology. 1996;110:A905.
139. Sands BE, Podolsky DK, Tremaine WJ *et al.* Chimeric monoclonal anti-tumor necrosis factor antibody (cA2) in the treatment of severe steroid-refractory ulcerative colitis (UC) [Abstract]. Gastroenterology. 1996;110:A1008.

140. Su CG, Salzberg B, Lewis J *et al.* Efficacy of anti-tumor necrosis factor therapy in patients with ulcerative colitis. Am J Gastroenterol. 2002;(in press).
141. Vasiliauskas EA, Kam LY, Abreu-Martin MT *et al.* An open-label, stepwise dose-escalating pilot study to evaluate the safety, tolerance, & efficacy of low-dose thalidomide in the treatment of chronically-active, steroid-dependent Crohn's disease [Abstract]. Gastroenterology. 1999; 116:A837.
142. Macumber C, Wettstein AP, Vickers CR *et al.* Thalidomide: effective therapy in chronic resistant inflammatory bowel disease [Abstract]. Gastroenterology. 1999;116:A767.
143. Kane SV, Ehrenpreis ED, Cohen LB, Hanauer SB, Cohen RD. Therapeutic efficacy of thalidomide for patients with refractory Crohn's disease [Abstract]. Gastroenterology. 1999; 116:A745.
144. Wedel S, Bauditz J, Suk A, Lochs H. Efficacy of thalidomide in Crohn's disease [Abstract]. Gastroenterology. 1999;116:A843.
145. van Deventer SJ, Elson CO, Fedorak RN and the Crohn's Disease Study Group. Multiple doses of intravenous interleukin 10 in steroid-refractory Crohn's disease. Gastroenteology. 1997;113:383–9.
146. Schreiber S, Fedorak RN, Nielson OH *et al.* A safety and efficacy study of recombinant human interleukin-10 (rhuIL-10) treatment in 329 patients with chronic active Crohn's disease [Abstract]. Gastroenterology. 1998;114:A1080.
147. Colombel J, Lille C, Rutgeerts P *et al.* Safety and tolerance of subcutaneous recombinant human interleukin-10 (IL-10) in subjects with Crohn's disease after first ileal or ileocolonic resection [Abstract]. Gastroenterology. 1999;116:A689.
148. Schreiber S, Heinig T, Thiele HG, Raedler A. Immunoregulatory role of interleukin 10 in patients with inflammatory bowel disease. Gastroenterology. 1995;108:1434–4.
149. Keith JC, Albert LM, Ferranti TJ *et al.* Recombinant human interleukin-11 (HIL-11) decreases inflammatory bowel disease in HLA-B27 transgenic rats [Abstract]. Gastroenterology. 1995; 108:A846.
150. Bank S, Snisky C, Robinson M *et al.* Safety and activity evaluation of rh-IL-11 in subjects with active Crohn's disease [Abstract]. Gastroenterology. 1997;112:A927.
151. Sands BE, Bank S, Sninsky CA *et al.* Preliminary evaluation of safety and activity of recombinant human interleukin eleven (rhIL-11) in patients with active Crohn's disease. Gastroenterology. 1999; 117:58–64.
152. Yacyshyn BR, Bowen-Yacyshyn MB, Jewell L *et al.* A placebo-controlled trial of ICAM-1 antisense oligonucleotide in the treatment of Crohn's disease. Gastroenterology. 1998;114: 1133–42.
153. Schreiber S, Malchow H, Kruis W *et al.* And the German ICAM-1 Study Group. Anti-sense ICAM-1 (ISIS-2302) for subcutaneous treatment of chronic active Crohn's disease (CACD): Lack of efficacy in a prospective, double-blind, multicenter trial. Gastroenterology. 2000;118:A2971.
154. Manyak CL, Tse H, Fischer P *et al.* Regulation of class II MHC molecules on human endothelial cells. J Immunol. 1988;150:3817–21.
155. Fridman WH, Gresser I, Bandu MT *et al.* Interferon enhances the expression of Fc gamma receptors. J Immunol. 1980;124:2436–41.
156. Young HA, Hardy KJ. Role of interferon gamma in immune cell regulation. J Leuk Biol. 1996;58:373–81.
157. Snapper CM, Paul WE. Interferon-gamma and B cell stimulatory factor-1 reciprocally regulate Ig isotype production. Science. 1987;236:944–7.
158. Lengyl P. Tumor-suppressor genes: News about the interferon connection. Proc Nat Acad Sci. 1993;93:5893–5.
159. Hanauer SB. Drug therapy: Inflammatory bowel disease. N Engl J Med. 1996;334:841–8.
160. Burke A, Lichtenstein GR, Rombeau JL. Nutrition and ulcerative colitis. In: Baillere's Textbook of Clinical Gastroenterology. 1997:153–74.
161. Han PD, Burke A, Baldassano RN, Rombeau JL, Lichtenstein GR. Nutrition and inflammatory bowel disease. Gastroenterol Clin N Am. 1999;28:423–44.
162. Steinhart AH, Brzezinski A, Baker JP. Treatment of refractory ulcerative proctosigmoiditis with butyrate enemas. Am J Gastroenterol. 1994;89:179–84.
163. Sandborn WJ. Nicotine therapy for ulcerative colitis: A review of rationale, mechanisms, pharmacology, and clinical results. Am J Gastroenterol. 1999;94:1161–71.
164. Korzenik JR, Robert ME, Bitton A *et al.* A multi-center, randomized, controlled trial of heparin for the treatment of ulcerative colitis [Abstract]. Gastroenterology. 1999;116:A752.

165. Vrij AA, Schoon EJ, Hemker HC, Stockbrugger RW. Low molecular weight heparin (LMWH) treatment in steroid refractory ulcerative colitis (UC) [Abstract]. Gastroenterology. 1999;116: A841.
166. Slonim AE, Bulone L, Damore MB, Goldberg T, Wingertzahn MA, McKinley MJ. A preliminary study of growth hormone therapy for Crohn's disease. N Engl J Med. 2000;342:1633–7.

EDITORIAL COMMENT

Interferon alpha [IFN-α] was introduced for the first time for treating inflammatory bowel disease [IBD] in 1990 [1,2]. Between 1990 and 1997, 75% (111 patients) of IBD patients treated with IFN-α achieved remission [3–5]. More recently, in an open labelled randomized study, Madsen *et al.* reported that IFN-α depressed the disease activity significantly as well as the histological disease activity of patients with IBD. Their results also suggest that IFN-α may be effective in treating active left-sided ulcerative colitis [6].

1. Hadziselimovic F, Emmons, LR. Letter to the Editor. J Am Med Assoc. 1990; 264:2741.
2. Hadziselimovic F, Emmons LR, Schaub U. Natural killer cell and large granular lymphocytes deficiency in the gut of children with inflammatory bowel disease. Can J Gastroenterol. 1990; 4:303–8.
3. Sümer N. Interferon -α treatment in inflammatory bowel disease (follow-up between 1991 and 1995). In: F. Hadziselimovic, B. Herzog, editors. Inflammatory bowel disease and chronic recurrent abdominal pain. Kluwer Academic Publishers, Dordrecht/Boston/London; 1997:168–78.
4. Hanauer SB, Baert FJ, Robinson M. Interferon treatment in mild to moderate active Crohn's disease: preliminary results of an open label pilot study. Gastroenterology, 1994; 106:A696.
5. Hadziselimovic F, Emmons LR. Long-term follow-up of a treatment with interferon-α-2a for inflammatory bowel disease. In: F. Hadziselimovic, B. Herzog, editors. Inflammatory bowel disease and chronic recurrent abdominal pain. Kluwer Academic Publishers, Dordrecht/Boston/London; 1997:150–167
6. Madsen SM, Schlichting P, Davidsen B, *et al.* An open-labelled, randomized study comparing systemic interferon–α-2A and prednisolone enemas in the treatment of left-sided ulcerative colitis. 2001; 96:1807–15.

20
Azathioprine in the treatment of paediatric ulcerative colitis

H. K. HARMS, M. KAPPLER and R. M. BERTELE-HARMS

Ulcerative colitis (UC) usually starts in childhood when the final growth spurt is expected. The disease threatens normal growth development not only by itself, but, even more, by the frequently unreflected long-term use of growth-suppressing steroids. The latter is probably the main reason for the large number (up to 50%) of paediatric colectomies reported in the literature[1–4].

The unacceptably large number of side-effects of long-term glucocorticoid therapy led to the search for more suitable systemic anti-inflammatory drugs.

In the 1960s, first experiences with the antimetabolites, 6-MP and azathioprine (Aza), as steroid-saving immunosuppressive drugs emerged, and, in 1971, Schäfer *et al.* from Hamburg[5] published the first encouraging results on Aza in the treatment of 15 children with UC. Unfortunately, this concept did not find general acceptance. Possible reasons were the fear of bone marrow depression and the induction of malignancies. An additional factor may have been the long time interval before the full effectiveness of Aza could be expected.

During the past 20 years, we have tried to avoid long-term steroid therapy by using Aza combined with local anti-inflammatory drugs, mainly sulphasalazine.

Between 1978 and 1998, we have cared for 65 patients with UC, including nearly equal numbers of males and females. Their mean age at diagnosis was 11 years; the mean period of observation 7.6 years. Forty-five per cent of the patients suffered from pancolitis and 12% from subtotal colitis; 26% showed a left-sided colitis and 17% a proctosigmoiditis only. Fifteen patients, mostly those with pancolitis, needed initial blood transfusions. The pharmaco therapy was started with 50–75 $mg\,kg^{-1}\,d^{-1}$ sulphasalazine in all patients. Twenty per cent with clinically severe disease, mostly those patients with pancolitis, were also given steroids (2 mg prednisone $kg^{-1}\,d^{-1}$).

After one year of treatment, about half the patients remained in remission with sulphasalazine alone, whereas the others, in particular those with extended colitis, experienced one or more relapses. In general, the relapses could be well controlled by treating them with steroids again, but, because of their well-known side-effects, we switched to an immunosuppressive therapy with Aza (3 $mg\,kg^{-1}\,d^{-1}$).

The increasingly good experience with Aza in maintaining a remission and the small number of side-effects, led to its earlier introduction during the past ten years. Today, in severe colitis when frequent relapses are expected, Aza is given initially in addition to sulphasalazine and prednisone in order to obtain a seamless immunosuppression after tapering and stopping steroid therapy.

In our patients, the mean daily prednisone dose could be significantly reduced 7 months after the introduction of Aza, from $0.64\,mg\,kg^{-1}\,d^{-1}$ to $0.1\,mg\,kg^{-1}\,d^{-1}$. In parallel, the frequency of relapses went down by factor 10, from 3.4/year before the introduction of Aza to 0.3/year on Aza. This significant reduction exceeds by far the natural course of the disease.

Concerning the growth development of our patients with UC, we compared the mean height percentiles at the time of diagnosis and at the age of 18 years in all those patients, who completed their 18th year of life and who were treated at least for five years. The height percentiles of these 38 patients increased significantly from a mean of 37% at time of diagnosis to a mean final height percentile of 52%.

This normal growth was achieved by avoiding long-term steroids and replacing them by Aza in 40% of patients. A further 50% could be well controlled by sulphasalazine only.

We also attribute the small number of colectomies to our therapeutic regimen, since most colectomized young patients reported in the literature, were colectomized because they were steroid dependent or refractory and growth retarded.

Among our patients, only one patient with giant polyposis of the whole colon needed to have a colectomy.

In general, the diagnosis of fulminant colitis, which can only be treated by colectomy, should be established with caution. Most patients may achieve a milder degree of the disease by patient conservative treatment over several weeks.

Concerning the side-effects of Aza therapy, we observed reversible leucopenia, which did not recur after a short interruption, in only one patient. Elevations of liver enzymes, observed by other groups in up to 25% of patients[4], were never seen in our patients although regularly looked for. Since most of our patients received a combination of sulphasalazine with Aza, and sulphasalazine inhibits *in vitro* the activity of thiopurine methyltansferase[6], which is the key enzyme for the toxic liver metabolite, methylmercaptopurine, this could be an explanation for the missing liver toxicity in our patients.

Slightly elevated pancreatic enzymes without any symptoms were seen rarely in our patients and are no justification for interruption of Aza therapy.

From our 20 years experience with Aza in the treatment of ulcerative colitis, we have come to the following conclusions:

- Aza may nearly completely replace steroids in the long-term treatment and maintenance of remission of paediatric UC. It seems similar to the treatment of Crohn's disease.
- Aza allows normal growth and helps to avoid colectomies.
- Aza is safe and the number of side-effects is small and usually reversible.

References

1. Hyams JS, Davis P, Grancher K, Lerer T, Justinich CJ, Markowitz J. Clinical outcome of ulcerative colitis in children. J Pediatr. 1996;129:81–8.
2. Durno C, Sherman P, Harris K *et al.* Outcome after ileoanal anastomosis in pediatric patients with ulcerative colitis. JPGN. 1998;27:501–7.
3. Kirschner BS. Safety of azathioprine and 6-mercaptopurine in pediatric patients with inflammatory bowel disease. Gastroenterology. 1998;115:813–21.
4. Falcone RA, Lewis LG, Warner BW. Predicting the need for colectomy in pediatric patients with ulcerative colitis. J Gastrointest Surg. 2000;4(2):201–6.
5. Schäfer KH, Bläker F. Experiences with immunosuppressive therapy in childhood ulcerative colitis. Z Kinderheilk. 1971;110:317–23.
6. Dubinsky MC, Lamothe St, Yang HY *et al.* Pharmacogenomics and metabolite measurement for 6-mercaptopurine therapy in inflammatory bowel disease. Gastroenterology. 2000;118:705–13.

21 Molecular mechanisms of steroid resistance in chronic inflammatory bowel disease

H. BANTEL and K. SCHULZE-OSTHOFF

Glucocorticoid resistance represents a serious clinical problem in various chronic inflammatory diseases, especially in chronic inflammatory bowel disease (IBD), asthma and rheumatoid arthritis. However, the molecular mechanisms underlying this steroid unresponsiveness are completely unknown. The effects of steroids result largely from the inhibition of pro-inflammatory transcription factors, such as NF-κB. Recently, increased activation of NF-κB in macrophages of the lamina propria from IBD patients has been reported[1]. Moreover, steroid treatment was associated with disappearance of active NF-κB in tissue from IBD patients[2].

NF-κB normally resides in the cytoplasm as an inactive complex bound to inhibitory IκB proteins. Upon stimulation, IκB is proteolytically degraded which exposes the NLS (nuclear localization signal) sequence of NF-κB, allowing it to initiate gene transcription of pro-inflammatory cytokines, adhesion molecules or enzymes. Two mechanisms have been proposed to explain glucocorticoid-receptor (GR)-mediated inhibition of NF-κB. *In-vitro* studies indicated that the GR upregulates IκB synthesis, which, however, may be cell-type specific[3,4]. There is growing evidence that a direct physical interaction between GR and NF-κB plays an important role in repressing each other's activity[5,6]. At present, however, the contribution of each mechanism in GR repression has not been defined under physiological conditions.

In a recent study, we investigated the activation of the pro-inflammatory transcription factors NF-κB and AP-1 as well as of the upstream stress-activated protein kinases, p38 and JNK, in 22 steroid-resistant and 14 steroid-sensitive patients with IBD (Reference 7 and unpublished data). The activity of the mediators was investigated in biopsies from various regions of the affected mucosa using activation-specific antibodies. In steroid-sensitive patients, activation of NF-κB was mainly found in macrophages of the lamina propria. Most surprisingly, in more than 50% of steroid-resistant patients, excessive NF-κB activation was predominantly found in epithelial cells.

Since previous studies have shown that a mutual interaction between the pro-inflammatory transcription factor AP-1 and the GR might be part of the anti-inflammatory effect of steroids[8], we next investigated the activation of AP-1 as well as of the upstream MAP-kinases, p38 and JNK, in tissue biopsies from steroid-sensitive and steroid-resistant patients. Similarly to NF-κB activity, in steroid-sensitive patients, activation of p38, JNK and AP1 was mainly found in macrophages of the lamina propria. In contrast, steroid-resistant patients revealed a remarkably different staining pattern, as extensively activated p38, JNK and AP-1 were predominantly localized in epithelial cells. We therefore suggest that this increased epithelial activation of NF-κB and the other mediators might be involved in the unresponsiveness to steroids. In such a scenario, excessively activated NF-κB and AP-1 may inhibit the anti-inflammatory action of a limited number of GR molecules and prevent their DNA binding. Moreover, detection of their activation state may serve as a diagnostic tool for the early recognition of steroid resistance, sparing these patients the undesired side-effects of prolonged and ineffective steroid treatment.

References

1. Rogler G, Brand K, Vogl D *et al.* Nuclear factor κB is activated in macrophages and epithelial cells of inflamed intestinal mucosa. Gastroenterology. 1998;15:357–69.
2. Thiele K, Bierhaus A, Autschbach F *et al.* Cell specific effects of glucocorticoid treatment on the NF-κB/IκBα system in patients with Crohn's disease. Gut. 1999;45:693–704.
3. Scheinmann RI, Cogswell PC, Lofquist AK, Baldwin AS Jr. Role of transcriptional activation of IκBα in mediation of immunosuppression by glucocorticoids. Science. 1995;270:283–6.
4. Auphan N, DiDonato JA, Rosette C, Helmberg A, Karin M. Immunosuppression by glucocorticoids: inhibition of NF-κB activity through induction of IκB synthesis. Science. 1995;270: 286–90.
5. Heck S, Bender K, Kullmann M, Gottlicher M, Herrlich P, Cato ABC. IκBα-independent down-regulation of NF-κB activity by glucocorticoid receptor. EMBO J. 1997;16:4698–707.
6. De Bosscher K, Schmitz ML, Vanden Berghe W, Plaisance S, Fiers W, Hageman G. Glucocorticoid-mediated repression of nuclear factor-κB-dependent transcription involves direct interference with transactivation. Proc Natl Acad Sci USA. 1997;94:13504–9.
7. Bantel H, Domscke W, Schulze-Osthoff K, Kaskas B, Gregor M. Abnormal activation of transcription factor NF-kappaB involved in steroid resistance in chronic inflammatory bowel disease. Am J Gastroenterol. 2000;95:1845–6.
8. Karin M, Chang L. AP-1-glucocorticoid receptor crosstalk taken to a higher level. J Endocrinol. 2001;169:447–51.

22 Treatment with budesonide in inflammatory bowel disease

R. BEHRENS

The treatment of IBD depends on the extent and activity of the disease. It is well known that both are greater in affected children than in adults. These conditions result in a higher dependency on steroids. However, the adverse effects of steroids are severe and appear in about 70% of patients. Additionally steroids may decrease growth velocity. The pathophysiology is multifactorial and includes inhibition of: the activity of the osteoblasts; calcium absorption; and the expression of growth hormone receptor. Furthermore, they increase renal excretion of calcium and bone metabolism due to secondary hyperparathyroidism[1].

Growth failure is one of the main problems in young patients with inflammatory bowel disease. Therefore, there is a need for drugs other than steroids, with similar efficacy but without the mentioned side-effects.

In the last decade, budesonide has been developed as a new substance which seemed to fullfill these criteria. It has a high first-pass effect in the liver (90%) which guarantees significantly less adverse events than in steroids. The affinity to the glucocorticoid receptor and the local intraluminal concentration are high. In endocrinological tests, the suppression of the adrenal function is much less than in steroids. Unfortunately, release of the substance is dependent on an intraluminal pH > 6. This means that the effect is possible only in the terminal ileum and ascending colon. Therefore, it seems that treatment can be offered only to patients with Crohn's disease. The efficacy has to be assessed from evidence-based medicine. Unfortunately, there are only studies of adult patients published yet.

In acute Crohn's disease, budesonide works better than placebo but not as well as steroids[2–5]. There is only one paediatric study in which remission was achieved in 60% but the group was small (only 32 patients) and the study design was retrospective[6]. A randomized controlled study in paediatric patients with Crohn's disease has been completed but not published yet. In summary, in acute Crohn's disease, steroids are the treatment of choice as mentioned in various guide lines[7,8]. Only when there are severe side-effects due to steroids and ileocaecal extension of the disease should budesonide be considered.

In mild or moderate Crohn's disease, budesonide is one of the preferred drugs if there is ileocaecal involvement[8].

In maintenance therapy, there are several controlled studies with different results[9–13]. A dosage of 3 mg budesonide did not prevent relapse more effectively than placebo[13] but a dosage of 6 mg daily seemed to prolong remission. But, after one year, there were no differences between the treatment and placebo groups[10]. Paediatric studies are not available. In conclusion, the results differ and further studies are necessary to show whether budesonide is significant in preventing relapses.

The same situation exists in the postoperative course where neither 3 nor 6 mg budesonide daily prevented relapse significantly[14,15].

Up to now, it has not been investigated whether paediatric patients need a daily dosage different from that of adults. Therefore, the same dosage (9 mg daily) is recommended.

The adverse effects of budesonide are similar to those of placebo and much less than those of steroids.

On the other hand it is not known yet whether budesonide has a positive effect on growth velocity. There is one retrospective study with only 6 patients and a follow-up of 6 months, which is too short for a good evaluation of growth velocity[6]. There was no increase in growth velocity found.

CONCLUSIONS

In active Crohn's disease, budesonide is less effective than steroids and indicated only for cases with steroid intolerance and ileocaecal involvement. In moderate or mild Crohn's disease, there is a good indication for budesonide. In maintenance therapy, budesonide does not seem to be effctive. Further studies are needed to examine both this situation and also the effect on growth velocity.

References

1. Allen DB. Glucocorticoid-associated growth failure: mechanisms and potential reversal. Endocrinologist. 1998;8:21–30.
2. Greenberg GR, Feagan BG, Martin F *et al.* Oral budesonide for active Crohn's disease. N Engl J Med. 1994;331:886–41.
3. Rutgeerts P, Löfberg R, Malchow H *et al.* A comparison of budesonide with prednisolone for active Crohn's disease. N Engl J Med. 1994;331:842–5.
4. Gross V, Andus T, Caesar I *et al.* Oral pH-modified release budesonide versus 6-methylprednisolone in active Crohn's disease. Eur J Gastroenterol Hepatol. 1996;8:905–9.
5. Campieri M, Ferguson A, Doe W *et al.* Oral budesonide is as effective as oral prednisolone in active Crohn's disease. Gut. 1997;41:209–14.
6. Kundhal P, Zachos M, Holmes JL *et al.* Controlled ileal release budesonide in pediatric Crohn's disease: efficacy and effect on growth. J Pediatr Gastroenterol Nutr. 2001;33:75–80.
7. Schlömerich J. Gibst es Neues in der Standardtherapie der CED? Internist. 1999;40:1288–99.
8. Hanauer SB, Sandborn W. Management of Crohn's disease in adults. Am J Gastroenterol. 2001;96:635–43.
9. Löfberg R, Rutgeerts P, Malchow H *et al.* Budesonide prolongs time to relapse in ileal and ileocaecal Crohn's disease. A placebo controlled one year study. Gut. 1996;39:82–6.
10. Greenberg GR, Feagan BG, Martin F *et al.* Oral budesonide as maintenance treatment for Crohn's disease: A placebo-controlled, dose-ranging study. Gastroenterology. 1996;110:45–51.

11. Cortot A, Colombel JF, Rutgeerts P *et al.* Switch from systemic steroids to budesonide in steroid dependent patients with inactive Crohn's disease. Gut. 2001;48:186–90.
12. Ferguson A, Campieri M, Doe W *et al.* Oral budesonide as maintenance therapy in Crohn's disease – results of a 12-month study. Aliment Pharmacol Ther. 1998;12:175–83.
13. Gross V, Andus T, Ecker KW *et al.* Low dose oral pH modified release budesonide for maintenance of steroid induced remission in Crohn's disease. Gut. 1998;42:493–6.
14. Ewe K, Bottger T, Buhr HJ *et al.* Low-dose budesonide treatment for prevention of postoperative recurrence of Crohn's disease: a multicentre randomized placebo-controlled trial. German Budesonide Study Group. Eur J Gastroenterol Hepatol. 1999;11:277–82.
15. Hellers G, Cortot A, Jewell D *et al.* Oral budesonide for prevention of postsurgical recurrence in Crohn's disease. Gastroenterology. 1999;116:294–300.

23 Anti-TNF strategies in paediatric Crohn's disease

C. P. BRAEGGER

INTRODUCTION

As the treatment of Crohn's disease (CD) cannot be directed against a known aetiological agent, it must focus on the pathogenic mechanisms of the disease leading to chronic intestinal inflammation. Traditionally, non-specific anti-inflammatory and immunosuppressive drugs (aminosalicylates, corticosteroids, azathioprine, 6-mercaptopurine) are used to reduce the inflammatory process. Often, these drugs are not sufficiently effective and induce side-effects.

However, recent advances in the understanding of the pathogenesis of this disease have led to the development of new and more-focused therapeutic strategies in the management of patients with CD. Evidence has been provided from clinical studies as well as from animal models suggesting that one important pathogenic mechanism in CD is the breakdown of tolerance of the intestinal immune system to the resident enteric bacterial flora[1,2]. The resulting mucosal inflammation caused by an upregulated intestinal immune response is largely mediated by Th-1 lymphocytes[3]. Several proinflammatory and immunoregulatory cytokines have been shown to be produced in increased amounts[3–6]. One of them, tumour necrosis factor-α (TNF), has become a key target for many of the new therapeutic agents. TNF is elevated in the blood, the gut mucosa and in the stool of patients with CD[4,7]. Its production correlates well with disease activity[4]. Its wide range of proinflammatory actions, as well as its key role in mediating the mucosal damage and some of the systemic sequelae (cachexia, growth retardation), makes it an ideal candidate for therapeutic intervention. Several pharmacological and biological approaches have been tested in order to reduce TNF production and secretion as well as to neutralize TNF efficacy. This review focuses on the current status of therapeutic agents with anti-TNF activity with special respect to paediatric CD.

MOLECULES BLOCKING TNF PRODUCTION/SECRETION

Pentoxyfylline/oxpentfylline

Pentoxyfylline is a methylxanthine-derivative drug acting as a specific type-4 phosphodiesterase (PDE4) inhibitor. It increases intracellular cAMP which blocks TNF production by modulation of transcription.

In-vitro, pentoxyfylline has been shown to reduce TNF production of lymphocytes of patients with active CD[8]. However, a clinical open-label trial with pentoxyfylline in 16 patients with corticosteroid-dependent chronic active CD showed no improvement in disease activity, endoscopic degree of inflammation or laboratory parameters[9]. Pentoxyfylline has not been tested in children with CD.

Thalidomide

Thalidomide is a hypnotic and sedative agent that was first released to treat insomnia in Germany in 1956 and soon after in many other countries. In the US, FDA approval was delayed because of suspected peripheral neuropathy. After a few years and more than 10 000 babies affected with birth defects (phocomelia), it was realised that thalidomide causes teratogenicity. In recent years, thalidomide has regained some attention[10] due to its ability to suppress TNF production by degrading TNF mRNA, which was first observed in patients with erythema nodosum associated with leprosy (erythema nodosum leprosum).

Two recent open-labelled studies suggested a benefit of thalidomide treatment in adult patients with refractory CD[11,12]. Thalidomide has also been tested successfully in small trials in paediatric CD[13,14].

The toxicity of thalidomide includes teratogenicity and peripheral neuropathy, the latter probably being more frequent than previously suspected[10]. Rare side-effects are dermatitis, constipation and pruritus. In 2001, there have been some case reports on deep vein thrombosis associated with thalidomide in patients with multiple myeloma[15,16]. As thalidomide is administered in one daily dose at bedtime, sedation is usually not a limiting factor.

TNF-BINDING NEUTRALIZING FUSION PROTEINS

Etanercept

Etanercept is a recombinant human TNF-receptor p75-Fc fusion protein. It is produced in a Chinese hamster ovary system by linking DNA encoding the human TNF-receptor 2 to DNA encoding the Fc portion of human imunoglobulin lgG_1. The resulting dimer molecule acts as a competitive inhibitor of TNF. It prevents binding of TNF to cell-membrane TNF receptor. Etanercept does not fix complement nor does it induce antibody-dependent cytotoxicity.

In rheumatoid arthritis, etanercept has been shown to induce a rapid and sustained benefit in patients with severe, treatment-resistant disease[17]. Human anti-human antibodies (HAHA) have been detected in 16% of patients with rheumatoid arthritis receiving treatment with etanercept for up to 18 months. Other autoantibodies have been observed: ANA in 11% (placebo 5%) and anti-DNA antibodies in 15% (placebo 4%) of patients. However, there was no report on delayed hypersensitivity reaction or drug-induced lupus. Injection site reactions were common (37%).

In patients with CD, an open-label, as well as a randomized double-blind placebo-controlled, trial showed that subcutaneous etanercept at a dose of 25 mg twice weekly is not an effective therapy[18,19]. Etanercept has not been tested in children with CD.

MONOCLONAL ANTIBODIES AGAINST TNF

CDP571

CDP571 is a humanized monoclonal antibody to TNF. It is produced by linking the antigen-binding regions (complementarity-determining regions, CDRs) of the variable domain of mouse anti-human TNF antibody to a human immunoglobulin IgG_4. The resulting molecule contains 95% human and 5% mouse protein. CDP571 has a high affinity for circulating TNF. It does not activate complement nor does it induce cytotoxicity.

A first small randomized controlled trial of a single dose of CDP571 antibody to TNF in 30 patients with active Crohn's disease showed some limited beneficial effects[20]. Recently, a larger randomized double-blind placebo-controlled trial with CDP571 in 169 patients with active Crohn's disease has been published[21]. It showed a significant effect on the clinical response at week 2 (45% of CDP571-treated patients compared with 27% in the placebo group; $p = 0.0023$). However, other results for secondary endpoints were statistically not significant.

CDP571 was well tolerated with infusion reactions in 12% of patients (placebo 7%). Delayed hypersensitivity reactions, drug-induced lupus and non-Hodgkin lymphoma (NHL) were not reported. Anti-idiotype antibodies were observed in 7%, and anti-DNA antibodies in 2%, of treated patients. CDP571 has not been tested in children.

Infliximab

Infliximab is a chimeric monoclonal antibody to TNF. It is produced by linking the variable domain of a mouse anti-human TNF antibody to human immunoglobulin IgG_1. It contains 75% human and 25% mouse protein. Infliximab binds to soluble and membrane-bound TNF, activates complement and has been shown to be cytotoxic to TNF-secreting cells. The latter effect may account for the sustained duration of action of infliximab.

Infliximab was first tested in a 14-year-old girl with steroid-resistant CD. After two infusions with infliximab 10 mg/kg at weeks 0 and 2, clinical and endoscopic remission lasting 3 months was achieved[22]. An open-label study with infliximab treatment of 12 patients with active steroid-resistant CD showed beneficial effects[23]. A multicentre double-blind placebo-controlled study of infliximab showed that one single dose can induce a clinical response in 64% and clinical remission in 33% of 108 patients with moderate to severe CD at week 4[24]. Infliximab induces endoscopic and histological healing in CD[24,25]. One study addressed efficacy and safety of retreatment with infliximab to maintain remission in CD[26]. It showed that retreatment with infliximab every 8 weeks maintained the clinical benefit in most patients and was well tolerated. Treatment with infliximab can also lead to closure of fistulas, as demonstrated in a randomized placebo-controlled multicentre trial[27]. Sixty-eight per cent of patients receiving three doses of 5 mg/kg of infliximab had closure of at least half of their fistulas compared with 26% in the placebo group ($p = 0.0002$). Fifty-five per cent of patients receiving 5 mg/kg of infliximab had all their fistulas closed compared with 13% in the placebo group ($p = 0.001$).

Infliximab is well tolerated[28]. Adverse events are usually mild and include abdominal pain, vomiting, nausea, fever and upper respiratory tract infections. Infusion reactions were reported in 16% of treated patients. Most of them occurred after the second infusion and were more common in patients with human anti-chimeric antibodies (HACAs). HACAs have been observed in 13%. Both infusion reactions and development of HACAs appeared to occur less often in patients on concomitant corticosteroid or immunosuppressive treatment (10% vs. 23%). Delayed hypersensitivity reactions may occur in up to 25% of patients after prolonged treatment intervals of 2–4 years. ANA have been reported in 24–36%, and anti-DNA in 9%. Drug-induced lupus and NHL have only rarely been associated with infliximab. Recently, there was a publication on 70 cases of tuberculosis among 147 000 patients treated with infliximab, according to the MedWatch reporting system of the FDA[29]. In most patients, tuberculosis was diagnosed after one to three infusions. Forty out of 70 patients had extrapulmonary disease. The authors conclude that most cases are therefore probably re-activated tuberculosis rather than new infections.

Open questions concerning the routine use of infliximab in patients with CD include the choice of the optimum concomitant immunosuppressive treatment and pretreatment, the optimum treatment interval, and the safety of long-term treatment.

Infliximab has been tested in children. One publication reported a chart review of 19 children and adolescents successfully treated with infliximab[30]. There has been one multicentre double-blind randomized trial of 21 children, between 8 and 17 years old, treated with a single dose of infliximab with a follow-up period of 20 weeks[31]. The study showed that infliximab pharmacokinetics in paediatric patients were similar to those of adults. Ninety-five per cent of patients had a clinical response and 50% achieved remission after the 20-week evaluation. Endoscopic improvement was also observed. Infliximab was well tolerated with no antibodies to infliximab or anti-DNA antibodies detected and no serious infusion reactions. The observed benefit suggests that infliximab is also an option in the treatment of active refractory CD in children and adolescents.

CONCLUSIONS

- The chimeric monoclonal antibody to TNF, infliximab, is very effective in the treatment of moderate to severe refractory CD. It is also effective for the closure of Crohn's fistula. A recent review of cumulative data on infliximab toxicity showed that the use of infliximab is safe. However, safety data on children are unfortunately still insufficient.

- The humanized monoclonal antibody to TNF, CDP571, is presumably also safe, but less effective for the treatment of CD. There are no data on children available.
- Published data show that the TNF-binding neutralizing fusion protein etanercept is not effective in CD.
- There are no data of controlled trials with thalidomide in CD. Open-label pilot studies in adults and in children suggest a beneficial effect. However, there are great safety problems with thalidomide (teratogenicity, neuropathy).

References

1. Duchmann R, Kaiser I, Hermann E *et al.* Tolerance exists towards resident intestinal flora but is broken in active inflammatory bowel disease. Clin Exp Immunol. 1995;102:448–55.
2. Duchmann R, Schmitt E, Knolle P *et al.* Tolerance towards resident intestinal flora in mice is abrogated in experimental colitis and restored by treatment with interleukin-10 or antibodies to interleukin-12. Eur J Immunol. 1996;26:934–8.
3. Breese E, Braegger CP, Corrigan CJ *et al.* Interleukin-2- and interferon-gamma-secreting T cells in normal and diseased human intestinal mucosa. Immunology. 1993;78:127–31.
4. Braegger CP, Nicholls S, Murch SH *et al.* Tumour necrosis factor alpha in stool as a marker of intestinal inflammation. Lancet. 1992;339:89–91.
5. Braegger CP. Immunopathogenesis of chronic inflammatory bowel disease. Acta Paediatr. 1994; Suppl 395:18–21.
6. Murch SH, Braegger CP, Walker-Smith JA, MacDonald TT. Location of tumour necrosis factor alpha by immunohistochemistry in chronic inflammatory bowel disease. Gut. 1993;34:1705–9.
7. Nicholls S, Stephens S, Braegger CP *et al.* Cytokines in stools of children with inflammatory bowel disease or infective diarrhoea. J Clin Pathol. 1993;46:757–60.
8. Reimund JM, Dumont S, Muller CD *et al.* In vitro effects of oxpentifylline on inflammatory cytokine release in patients with inflammatory bowel disease. Gut. 1997;40:475–80.
9. Bauditz J, Haemling J, Ortner M *et al.* Treatment with tumour necrosis factor inhibitor oxpentifylline does not improve corticosteroid dependent chronic active Crohn's disease. Gut. 1997;40: 470–4.
10. Sands BE, Podolsky DK. New life in a sleeper: thalidomide and Crohn's disease. Gastroenterology. 1999;117:1485–8.
11. Ehrenpreis ED, Kane SV, Cohen LB *et al.* Thalidomide therapy for patients with refractory Crohn's disease: an open-label trial. Gastroenterology. 1999;117:1271–7.
12. Vasiliauskas EA, Kam LY, Abreu-Martin MT *et al.* An open-label pilot study of low-dose thalidomide in chronically active, steroid-dependent Crohn's disease. Gastroenterology. 1999; 117:1278–87.
13. Facchini S, Candusso M, Martelossi S *et al.* Efficacy of long-term treatment with thalidomide in children and young adults with Crohn disease: preliminary results. J Pediatr Gastroenterol Nutr. 2001;32:178–81.
14. Weinstein TA, Sciubba JJ, Levine J. Thalidomide for the treatment of oral aphthous ulcers in Crohn's disease. J Pediatr Gastroenterol Nutr. 1999;28:214–16.
15. Osman K, Comenzo R, Rajkumar SV. Deep venous thrombosis and thalidomide therapy for multiple myeloma. N Engl J Med. 2001;344:1951–2.
16. Zangari M, Anaissie E, Barlogie B *et al.* Increased risk of deep-vein thrombosis in patients with multiple myeloma receiving thalidomide and chemotherapy. Blood. 2001;98:1614–15.
17. Moreland LW, Schiff MH, Baumgartner SW *et al.* Etanercept therapy in rheumatoid arthritis. A randomized, controlled trial. Ann Intern Med. 1999;130:478–86.
18. D'Haens G, Swijsen C, Noman M *et al.* Etanercept in the treatment of active refractory Crohn's disease: a single-center pilot trial. Am J Gastroenterol. 2001;96:2564–8.
19. Sandborn WJ, Hanauer SB, Katz S *et al.* A randomized, double-blind, placebo-controlled trial of subcutaneous etanercept in the treatment of moderate to severe Crohn's disease. Gastroenterology. 2001;121:1088–94.
20. Stack WA, Mann SD, Roy AJ *et al.* Randomised controlled trial of CDP571 antibody to tumour necrosis factor-alpha in Crohn's disease. Lancet. 1997;349:521–4.

21. Sandborn WJ, Feagan BG, Hanauer SB *et al.* An engineered human antibody to TNF (CDP571) for active Crohn's disease: a randomized double-blind placebo-controlled trial. Gastroenterology. 2001;120:1330–8.
22. Derkx B, Taminiau J, Radema S *et al.* Tumour-necrosis-factor antibody treatment in Crohn's disease. Lancet. 1993;342:173–4.
23. van Dullemen HM, van Deventer SJ, Hommes DW *et al.* Treatment of Crohn's disease with anti-tumor necrosis factor chimeric monoclonal antibody (cA2). Gastroenterology. 1995;109:129–35.
24. Targan ST, Hanauer SB, VanDeventer SJH *et al.* A short-term study of chimeric monoclonal antibody cA2 to tumor necrosis factor for Crohn's disease. N Engl J Med. 1997;337:1029–35.
25. D'Haens G, Van Deventer S, Van Hogezand R *et al.* Endoscopic and histologic healing with infliximab anti-tumor necrosis factor antibodies in Crohn's disease: a European multicenter trial. Gastroenterology. 1999;116:1029–34.
26. Rutgeerts P, D'Haens G, Targan S *et al.* Efficacy and safety of retreatment with anti-tumor necrosis factor antibody (infliximab) to maintain remission in Crohn's disease. Gastroenterology. 1999;117:761–9.
27. Present DH, Rutgeerts P, Targan S *et al.* Infliximab for the treatment of fistulas in patients with Crohn's disease. N Engl J Med. 1999;340:1398–405.
28. Hanauer SB. Review article: safety of infliximab in clinical trials. Aliment Pharmacol Ther. 1999;13:16–22.
29. Keane J, Gershon S, Wise RP *et al.* Tuberculosis associated with infliximab, a tumor necrosis factor-neutralizing agent. N Engl J Med. 2001;345:1098–104.
30. Hyams JS, Markowitz J, Wyllie R. Use of infliximab in the treatment of Crohn's disease in children and adolescents. J Pediatr. 2000;137:192–6.
31. Baldassano R, Vasiliauskis E, Braegger CP *et al.* A multicenter study of anti-TNF chimeric monoclonal antibody (Infliximab) in the treatment of pediatric patients with active Crohn's disease. Gastroenterology. 1999;116:A665.

24
Long-term 5-ASA treatment and gender-related differences in children with IBD

F. HADZISELIMOVIC, J. O. WIDAUER and L. R. EMMONS

INTRODUCTION

Roughly 25% of those suffering from either Crohn's disease or ulcerative colitis were diagnosed during childhood or early adolescence. Crohn's disease is incurable while ulcerative colitis can be cured by total colectomy. Several medical treatments are effective in achieving remission in both Crohn's disease and ulcerative colitis[1–4]. Drugs, such as sulphasalazine, mesalamine, glucocorticoid, azathioprine and 6-mercaptopurine, are used as standard treatments for inflammatory bowel disease (IBD). 5-ASA (mesalamine) is the treatment of choice for both the acute and remission stages of the disease[5]. 5-ASA is superior to sulphasalazine and it causes fewer side-effects[5]. There are, however, controversial data concerning the influence of 5-ASA on male fertility. Unfortunately, nothing is known about its effect on the fertility of those who have been treated throughout their entire pubertal development. In our study, we have analysed the effects of long-term treatment with 5-ASA in children, with particular emphasis on male sexual development. Furthermore, we investigated the gender-related differences that occur during the course of IBD that may be influenced by long-term treatment with 5-ASA.

PATIENTS AND METHODS

The clinical data of twenty-two patients who were treated with 5-ASA for 258 patient-years were analysed. Seven males and 5 females had Crohn's disease; 5 males and 5 females had ulcerative pancolitis. All but one of the patients with Crohn's disease had ileocolonic involvement. This male patient had isolated small bowel Crohn's disease. All patients at the time of diagnosis were pre- or early pubertal in their development. They were treated with 30 mg of 5-ASA/kg for the entire time. The total observation time for 5-ASA treatment was

258 patient-years, ranging from 10 to 16 years. Only one patient was forced to stop 5-ASA treatment after 6 years because of severe headaches. During the acute stage and at relapse of the disease, patients received other drugs in addition to 5-ASA; these included: prednisolone (22/22), azathioprine (6/22), and, in some cases, Roferon, interferon alpha (IFN-α) (12/22). Growth progress, incidence of surgery, pubertal development, and haematological, as well as liver and kidney parameters, were recorded at regular intervals. All adverse side-effects of the treatment were noted.

The final growth of the patients was compared with their genetically targeted height utilizing the following formula for males: father's height (cm) + mother's height (cm) *plus* 13 cm divided by two ± 8.4 cm (SD); for females: mother's height (cm) + father's height (cm) *minus* 13 cm divided by two ± 8.4 (SD). Educational achievement and socioeconomic status were included. Disease activity was evaluated with Crohn's disease activity index (CDAI) for Crohn's disease and colitis activity index (CAI, Rachmilewitz) for ulcerative colitis. In addition, soluble tumour necrosis factor receptors 55 and 75 (sTNF-R 55/75) levels in urine were assessed at regular intervals.

Semen samples were obtained by masturbation after at least 5 days of abstinence. The ejaculate was delivered in a standard polypropylene container within 3 h of emission (6/8); the ejaculate from two of them was sent by express mail. Eight patients, now young adults, have had their semen analysed; it was compared with World Health Organization standards: sperm density (Mio/ejaculate), motility, morphology and volume (ml)[6]. Motility was expressed as percentage of sperm with forward progression – sum of the fast linear progression and slow progression. Morphology was expressed as the percentage of sperm with normal forms. In addition, the presence of sperm autoantibodies was noted and MAR-penetration test was performed. Serum levels of LH, FSH and testosterone were determined accordingly.

RESULTS

According to clinical data, twenty out of twenty-two patients were in remission at the time of examination. sTNF-R55 and 75 were also within the normal range in 20/22 patients. All patients had normal liver and kidney function. Twenty-one of the patients had normal serum albumin. Two male (2/12) patients had colon-diversion while 70% of the females had colon-diversion (7/10; $p < 0.001$ Fisher test).

All patients were unmarried, the oldest of being 30 years of age. They had completed puberty, achieving the Tanner V stage of development. The female patients had had normal menstrual cycles and the males had normal sexual functional responses (erections and ejaculations); their hormonal levels for LH, FSH and testosterone were within the normal range.

Sperm density per ejaculate in all eight patients was in the normal range; 248 ± 276.3 (Mio/ejaculate); one patient had 899 Mio/ejaculate! The lowest value was 68.8 Mio/ejaculate. Ejaculate volume mean was: 3.8 ± 1.9 ml. Two patients had lower than normal volume (1.9 and 1.2 ml). All patients had normal pH values of the ejaculate; mean: 8.0 ± 0.1 as well as normal motility;

Table 1 Volume, pH, motility and sperm density per ejaculate were quantified and compared with WHO standards (reference values in brackets)

	Patient								
	1	*2*	*3*	*4*	*5*	*6*	*7*	*8*	Mean ± SD
Volume (>2.0 ml)	4.1	5.2	3.6	4.5	1.9	1.2	7.5	2.7	3.8 ± 1.9
pH (7.3–8.0)	7.9	8.2	8.1	7.8	8.2	8.1	8.1	8.0	8.0 ± 0.14
Sperm motility (⩾50%)	75	50	56	56	39	73	*	*	58.1 ± 13.7
Sperm density/ ejaculate ($\geqslant 90 \times 10^6$)	68.8	201.5	257.4	72.9	98.4	111	277.5	899	248.3 ± 275.3
Normal sperm forms (⩾25%)	5	8	4	7	7	27	13	24	11.8 ± 8.8
Pathological sperm head (*% abnormal*)	91	90	90	89	89	69	77	64	82.3 ± 10.8

*Semen ejaculate specimen was sent by express post; consequently, sperm motility was unable to be assessed because of the time delay.

mean: 56.1 ± 13.7 (Table 1). In contrast, sperm morphology was very abnormal in 7 of the 8 patients; mean: 11.8 ± 8.8% of normal sperm forms (Table 1). The most significant pathological finding was that 82.3 ± 10.3% of sperm heads in the ejaculate were abnormal (Table 1). Two males had pathological MAR penetration test results and the same two had sperm IgG autoantibodies in their serum. All patients had completed their elementary school education and had reached a similar educational level to the general Swiss population. Two male patients were drug addicts.

DISCUSSION

We have found that gender-related differences exist in the clinical course of IBD in paediatric patients. The mean time lag between onset of symptoms and the diagnosis was similar in males and females, and there were no differences in presenting symptoms and initial localization of the lesions. However, female patients in our group with inflammatory bowel disease had a significantly higher rate of ileocaecal resection or colectomy than the males. This agrees with data published on adult patients with Crohn's disease[7]. Continuous treatment with 5-ASA did not reduce the number of indications for the necessity for surgery. We did *not* find more extraintestinal manifestations in our paediatric female population. This differed from the findings of Wegtmans *et al.* in their adult patients with Crohn's disease, namely, that extraintestinal manifestations occur much more often in females[7].

This is the first long-term study to consider the effect of 5-ASA on sexual development of prepubertal and pubertal males. Semen analysis of patients with IBD over this long-term treatment with 5-ASA starting in childhood has confirmed that 5-ASA has no deleterious effect on semen quality and thus, on developing testes[8–10]. Some have suggested that impaired sperm density in adults with IBD is associated with disease activity and the nutritional status of the patient[10]. Furthermore, seminal abnormalities, such as oligospermia, reduced sperm motility, and the increased incidence of abnormal sperm forms, was related to treatment with sulphasalazine[10–15]. Following termination of sulphasalazine treatment, or switching to mesalamine, the abnormalities described above were ameliorated[16–18].

The high incidence of necrospermia of the sperm head in our patients was unrelated to disease activity. The normal basal serum LH, FSH and testosterone values in our patients coincide with a normal function of the hypothalamo–pituitary–gonadal axis. Therefore, there is no conclusive evidence that testicular damage causes necrospermia, either due to disease activity or to 5-ASA treatment. Moreover, it is probable that an abnormal epididymal function is responsible for this high incidence of necrospermia. This has never been discussed heretofore.

Adverse drug reactions to mesalamine were reported mainly as haematological reactions such as agranulocytosis and pancytopenia (60% of all mesalamine side-effects) followed by a skin reaction[19]. The same group reported that two fatalities were linked to mesalamine during the observational period from 1988–1997 in Sweden[19]. We have had no such adverse reactions in our cohort during treatment with 5-ASA. Perhaps most of these adverse reactions to mesalamine are related to dose rather than to the drug itself. Our experience has been limited to paediatrics, and the dose regimen of mesalamine is significantly lower than that prescribed for adults.

In conclusion, our long-term study suggests that 5-ASA is a safe and well-tolerated medication that is particularly suited for a long-term treatment in children and adolescents.

References

1. Stein RB, Hanauer SB. Medical treatment for IBD. Gastroenterol Clin N Am. 1999;28(2):297–321.
2. Klotz S. Update in medical therapy in inflammatory bowel disease: a clinician's view. Diagn Dis. 1999;17(3):163–71.
3. Hoffmann JC, Zeitz M. Treatment of Crohn's disease. Hepato-Gastroenterology. 2000;47(31): 90–100.
4. Ludwig D, Stange E. Treatment of ulcerative colitis. Hepato-Gastroenterology. 2000;47(31):83–9.
5. Klotz U. The role of aminosalycilates at the beginning of the new millennium in treatment of chronic inflammatory bowel disease. Eur J Clin Pharmacol. 2000;56(5):353–62.
6. World Health Organization. Semen examination – laboratory manuals. In: WHO Laboratory Manuals for Examination of Human Semen and Semen–Cervical Mucus Interaction, 3rd Edn. Cambridge, England: Cambridge University Press, 1992.
7. Wegtmans MJ, Verspaget HW, Lemers CBHW, van Hogezand RA. Gender-related differences in the clinical course of Crohn's disease. Am J Gastroenterol. 2001;96(5):1541–6.
8. Hrudka F, Singh A. Sperm nucleomalacia in man with IBD. Arch Androl. 1984;13:37–57.
9. Karbach U, Ewe K, Schramm P. Quality of semen in patients with Crohn's disease. Z Gastroenterol. 1982;20:314–20.

10. Farthing MJ, Dawson AM. Impaired sperm quality in Crohn's disease. Ill health or under nutrition. Scand J Gastroenterol. 1983;18:57–60.
11. Levi AJ, Fischer AM, Hughes L, Hendry WF. Male infertility due to sulfasalazine. Lancet. 1979;2:276–8.
12. Birni GG, McLeod TI, Watkinson G. Incidence of sulfasalazine induced male infertility. Gut. 1981;22:452–5.
13. Toovey S, Hudson E, Hendry WF, Levi AJ. sulfasalazine and male infertility: reversibility and possible mechanism. Gut. 1982;22:445–51.
14. Freeman JG, Reece VA, Vanables CV. Sulfasalazine and spermatogenesis. Digestion. 1982;23: 68–71.
15. O'Morain C, Smethurst P, Dore CJ, Levi AJ. Reversible male infertility due to sulfasalazine: studies in man and rat. Gut. 1984;25:1078–84.
16. Riley SA, Lecarpanter J, Mani V, Goodman MJ, Mandal BK, Tumberg LA. Sulfasalazine induced seminal abnormalities in ulcerative colitis: results of mesalazine substitution. Gut. 1987;28:1008–12.
17. Chatzinoff M, Guarino JM, Corson SL, Batzer FR, Friedman LS. Sulfasalazine-induced abnormal sperm penetration assay reversed on changing to 5-aminosalicylic acid enemas. Dig Dis Sci. 1988;33:108–10.
18. Zelissen PM, van Hattum J, Poen H, Scholten P, Geritse R, Velde ER. Influence of salazosulfapyridine and 5-aminosalicylic acid on seminal qualities and male sexual hormones. Scand J Gastroenterol. 1988;23:1100–04.
19. Blomqvist P, Feltelius N, Loefberg R, Ekbom A. A 10-year survey of inflammatory bowel disease drug therapy, costs and adverse reactions. Aliment Pharmacol Ther. 2001;15(4):475–81.

25
Side-effects associated with use of oral budesonide in children and adolescents

A. LEVINE

Successful treatment of inflammatory bowel disease requires medications that will achieve and maintain remission of the disease. However, those medications with the greatest potential to achieve remission also carry the highest risks of side-effects. Oral corticosteroids are highly effective for the treatment of active Crohn's disease. They induce clinical remission fairly rapidly, and lead to weight gain and improved appetitie. However, first-generation systemic corticosteroids induce a variety of side-effects. The most common are cosmetic side-effects such as moon face, acne, hirsuitism, striae and central adiposity. Numerous significant side-effects with greater morbidity have been associated with this therapy.

Budesonide is a potent steroid that undergoes extensive first-pass metabolism to nearly inactive metabolites 6-hydroxy budesonide and 16-hydroxy prednisolone[1]. Its systemic bioavailability is about 10% and it has a significantly higher affinity for the glucocorticoid receptor, 15 times that of prednisolone and 9 times that of dexamethasone. Its lipophilic properties enhance tissue penetration. High local penetration of a potent steroid in inflamed intestinal tissues, with low systemic concentrations should theoretically attain a better therapeutic margin with enhanced efficacy and decreased systemic side-effects.

Oral budesonide has been evaluated and compared with prednisone in mild to moderate Crohn's disease in adults. Multiple studies have shown a significantly lower incidence of side-effects in patients treated with budesonide when compared with patients treated with prednisone. Data from some of these studies are presented in Table 1.

The incidence of side-effects in budesonide-treated patients, while lower, still ranged from 28–78% compared with 55–90% for prednisone or prednisolone[2–5]. In a study comparing budesonide with mesalamine, side-effects in patients treated with budesonide 9 mg/day were similar to those associated with placebo[6].

Examination of the published data shows that the significant decrease in side-effects seen in patients treated with budesonide was mostly due to a decrease in

Table 1 Comparison of side-effects in adults treated with budesonide and conventional corticosteroids

Study	*Number of patients*	*Budesonide side-effects (%)*	*Prednisone side-effects (%)*	*Cosmetic side-effects decreased*	*Other comments*
Campieri *et al.*[3]	178	78*	90	Yes	Moon face more common ×3 with prednisone
Bar-Meir *et al.*[2]	201	44*	67	Yes	No difference in headache, muscle or oedema
Rutgeerts *et al.*[4]	176	33*	55	Yes	Less oedema with budesonide
Gross *et al.*[5]	67	28*	67	Yes	

* = Significantly different from prednisone side-effects at $p < 0.5$.

cosmetic side-effects associated with steroids. Other important side-effects, such as psychiatric effects, insomnia and myopathy, were not decreased or not evaluated independently. Data regarding the use of oral budesonide in children and adolescents are scarce. Published or reported incidents of significant side-effects in children have all come from Israel. These reports disclosed 5 significant adverse events worth reporting, thought to be related to oral budesonide. These include 1 case of severe hypokalaemia with hyperaldosteronism[7], 3 cases of benign intracranial hypertension[8], and 1 case of severe myopathy associated with treatment of autoimmune hepatitis (Shamir *et al.*, personal communication). The cases of benign intracranial hypertension occurred during the first 6 weeks of full-dose therapy, and not during tapering. We tried to identify possible risk factors for adverse events among these five patients. Two of these events occurred in patients with liver disease, and 4/5 patients were in a poor nutritional state. Possible mechanisms of budesonide-related toxicity include increased bioavailability due to decreased metabolism in the face of liver disease and decreased adipose tissue in Crohn's disease, leading to decreased volume of distribution. The patients who developed benign intracranial hypertension were all significantly malnourished with a low BMI. The brain has a high concentration of steroid receptors, and, if budesonide becomes more bioavailable, the higher receptor affinity and lipophilic structure may increase the risk for CNS complications, such as benign intracranial hypertension or headache.

Data from 2 as-yet-unpublished studies in children performed in Israel shed further light on the topic of side-effects related to oral budesonide use. The first study was a retrospective analysis performed in 12 centres, reviewing all children treated with oral budesonide for mild to moderately active Crohn's disease. Inclusion criteria for this study included a paediatric Crohn's disease activity index between 12.5 and 40, use of budesonide (9 mg/day) or oral prednisone

(40 mg/day) as a single therapy. Significant adverse events were evaluated in both groups. This study included 120 children (62 budesonide and 58 prednisone) who met inclusion and exclusion criteria. In the budesonide group, only 1/62 children developed a severe adverse event, in comparison with 8/58 in the prednisone-treated group; this was statistically significant[9]. A concommitant clinical trial (Israeli Pediatric Gastroenterology Society Budesonide Study Group, in press) used similar criteria for disease activity. We prospectively followed 33 children randomly assigned to either budesonide 9 mg/day or prednisone 40 mg/day initial dose, tapered and evaluated at 12 weeks. These children were prospectively monitored for type, frequency and severity of side-effects. Patients treated with oral budesonide had significantly fewer side-effects, and cosmetic side-effects, when compared with children treated with prednisone. There was also a trend towards decreased muscular-associated side-effects. Furthermore, a cosmetic severity score was analysed in both groups. Children treated with oral budesonide had significantly fewer severe cosmetic effects ($p < 0.05$) in comparison with those treated with prednisone.

Both these studies also evaluated weight gain with budesonide or prednisone in patients responding to therapy. Patients treated with prednisone gained approximately twice as much weight during the study period. Use of budesonide led to a significantly lower weight gain than did the use of prednisone. While this may be attributed to less fluid retention, it might also reflect decreased steroid-mediated hyperphagia, a positive side-effect associated with steroid use in IBD.

In conclusion, it is clear that oral budesonide does have the potential to cause significant and cosmetic side-effects associated with corticosteroids. However, budesonide appears to cause fewer overall side-effects, fewer cosmetic side-effects, less-significant side-effects, and less-severe cosmetic disfiguration.

Liver disease and very poor nutritional status may increase the potential for side-effects with oral budesonide. Though it appears to cause fewer side-effects when compared with equivalent-dosed prednisone or prednisolone, it should be used with more caution in patients with previously cited risk factors. The benefit/risk ratio with higher doses and colonic location still need to be evaluated. At the present time, its favorable side-effect profile may warrant an initial trial of budesonide in children and adolescents requiring steroids with appropriately located mild to moderately active Crohn's disease.

References

1. Spencer CM, McTavish D. Budesonide. A review of its pharmocalogical properties and therapeutic efficacy in inflammatory bowel disease. Drugs. 1995;50:854–72.
2. Bar-Meir S, Chowers Y, Lavy A *et al.* Budesonide versus prednisone in the treatment of active Crohn's disease. Gastroenterology. 1998;115:835–40.
3. Campieri M, Ferguson A, Doe W, Persson T, Nilsson LG. Oral budesonide is as effective as oral prednisolone in active Crohn's disease. Gut. 1997;41:209–14.
4. Rutgeerts P, Lofberg R, Malchow H *et al.* A comparison of budesonide with prednisolone for active Crohn's disease. N Engl J Med. 1994;331;842–5.
5. Gross V, Andus T, Caesar I *et al.* Oral pH modified release budesonide versus 6-methylprednisolone in active Crohn's disease. Eur J Gastroenterol Hepatol. 1996;8:905–9.
6. Thomsen OO, Cortot A, Jewell D *et al.* A comparison of budesonide and mesalamine for active Crohn's disease. International Budesonide–Mesalamine Study Group. N Engl J Med. 1998;339: 370–4.

7. Rosenbach Y, Zahavi I, Rachmal A, Dinari G. Severe hypokalemia after budesonide treatment for Crohn's disease. J Pediatr Gastroenterol Nutr. 1997;24:352–5.
8. Levine A, Watemberg N, Hager H, Bujanover Y, Ballin A, Lerman-Sagie T. Benign intracranial hypertension associated with budesonide treatment in children with Crohn's disease. J Child Neurol. 2001;16:458–61.
9. Levine A, Broide E, Stein M *et al.* Evaluation of oral budesonide for treatment of mild and moderate exacerbations of Crohn's disease in children. J Pediatr Gastroenterol Nutr. 2001;32:363A.

Section VI
Short presentations of selected topics

S1
Definition of immunodominant B cell epitopes on soluble liver antigen (SLA) and their implication for molecular mimicry

D.-P. BOGDANOS[1], F. RODRIGUES[2], U. C. SHARMA[1], Y. MA[1], G. MIELI-VERGANI[2] and D. VERGANI[1]

[1]Institute of Hepatology, UCL; [2]Child Health, King's College Hospital, London, UK

Soluble liver antigen (SLA)/UGA suppressor tRNA associated antigenic protein, a major target antigen in autoimmune hepatitis, the sequence of which has been recently established. To define the B cell epitopes on SLA and to investigate whether they are targets of crossreactivity, we tested ab binding to 54 icosameric peptides, spanning the entire sequence of SLA, in 5 anti-SLA seropositive AIH patients tested by radioligand assay, ELISA and immunoblot. Three antigenic regions were defined located towards the SLA C-terminus, 2 of them novel (281–308, 321–348) and one previously described (aa 385–441). This latter was found to contain 2 antigenic subregions separated by an invariably non-reactive sequence (393–412), a discontinuity probably reflecting the conformational nature of this epitopic region. The fine specificity of SLA 385–441 was investigated with 15-mer peptides overlapping by 3 aa and the focus of reactivity was localized to aa 412–441. Since this region was found to share >70% similarity with 9 microbial antigens, the relevant microbial peptides were tested for reactivity. Only the urease alpha subunit (aa 225–239) of *Helicobacter pylori* was crossreactive as confirmed by competition ELISAs. SLA/*H. pylori* peptide crossreactive patients had serological evidence of *H. pylori* infection. Our results provide for the first time a complete linear B cell epitope map of SLA, a major antigen in AIH, and implicate *H. pylori* in the generation of autoimmunity through a mechanism of molecular mimicry.

S2
Serological and histopathological features of children with autoimmune hepatitis – overlapping syndrome

J. CIELECKA-KUSZYK, M. WOZNIAK, J. PAWLOWSKA and W. DURA

Department of Pathology and Gastroenterology, The Children's Memorial Health Institute, Warsaw, Poland

---

Introduction: Autoimmune hepatitis in children is a chronic progressive disease which can coexist with hepatotropic viral infection and primary sclerosing cholangitis.

Aim of the study: This was to compare the antibody profile and histopathological changes in autoimmune hepatitis, coexisting other diseases.

Materials and methods: 100 children with autoimmune hepatitis type I and 21 children with autoimmune hepatitis type II have been scored (IAHP Report 1999) according to the histological criteria (interface hepatitis, bridging necrosis, biliary lesions, granuloma formations, Pearl's stain for iron), serum biochemistry (ALT level, alkaline phosphatase), γ-globulin concentration, including IgG, serum autoantibodies (ANA, AMA, LKM, AMA, pANCA) and viral markers (antibodies against HCV, antiHbs, Hbe, Hbc, PCR for HCV).

Results: At the time of diagnosis, the histology of the liver was characterized by necroinflammatory changes accompanied by fibrosis and/or cirrhosis. Viral infection occurred in 8 children (2 children were infected by HCV, 6 children by HBV), 6 children demonstrated features of primary sclerosing cholangitis, including 3 children with ulcerous colitis. Necroinflammatory changes in autoimmune and viral hepatitis were severe (according to Batts & Ludwig 1995); in HBV: predominantly lobular changes, lymph follicle formations; in HCV: steatosis and Fe accumulation in the hepatocytes and Kupffer cells. Histological features of biliary changes and mild cholestasis were seen in all cases of primary sclerosing cholangitis; granuloma formation in the portal tracts in 2 cases. All children were treated with azathioprine and prednisolone (without interferon in 8 cases of viral hepatitis).

Conclusion: Variable autoantibody levels with false positivity for anti-HCV occurs in autoimmune hepatitis (7 children with PCR negative for HCV) and overlapping syndrome (2 children with PCR positive for HCV). Histopathological changes in overlapping syndrome are not diagnostic, but are suggestive, for the aetiology. Overlapping syndrome in children responded poorly to classical treatment of autoimmune hepatitis.

S3
Liver histopathology in children with autoimmune hepatitis

M. WOZNIAK, M. WOYNAROWSKI, J. KUSZYK and J. SOCHA

Department of Gastroenterology, Hepatology and Nutrition, Child's Health Memorial Institute, Warsaw, Poland

Autoimmune hepatitis (AIH) is an infrequent disease in childhood but it may rapidly progress to liver cirrhosis. The aim of our study was to correlate the initial liver biopsy and outcome of AIH treatment and to compare results of initial and control liver biopsies. All biopsies were evaluated by a single observer who was using a modified Scheuer's classification for grading and staging.

The correlation of the initial liver biopsy and the treatment outcome at the end of the observation period (mean 6 years) was done in 118 children (M 36, F 82; mean age 10.5 ± 3.5 years) treated in our institution from 1989 till 1999. Table 1 shows the mean scores in different outcome groups.

The control liver biopsy was taken in 111 children after 2 years of prednisone or prednisone + azathioprine treatment. We compared the results by subtracting the initial biopsy score from the control score for grading and staging separately. The results of the calculation are shown in Table 2.

Table 1

Treatment outcome	$n = 118$	*Mean grading*	*Mean staging*
Permanent remission	30	2.6 ± 0.9	1.8 ± 0.9
Continued treatment	63	2.7 ± 1.0	2.2 ± 0.9
Relapse after treatment discontinuation	15	2.6 ± 0.8	1.9 ± 0.7
LTX	4	2.9 ± 1.2	2.5 ± 0.6
Death	6	2.8 ± 0.8	2.4 ± 0.8

Table 2

	Improvement				*No change*	*Deterioration*		
	−4	*−3*	*−2*	*−1*	*0*	*1*	2	*3*
Grading	4 (3.6%)	14 (12.7%)	32 (29.1%)	28 (25.5%)	23 (20.0%)	9 (8.2%)	1 (0.9%)	0
Staging	0	2 (1.8%)	7 (6.4%)	29 (26.4%)	60 (54.0%)	9 (8.2%)	3 (2.7%)	1 (0.9%)

Neither the method of AIH treatment nor the AIH type influenced the changes in the histopathology picture.

Conclusions:

1. The initial liver biopsy in children with AIH shows high-grade inflammation and fibrosis, especially in those with poor outcome.
2. Control biopsy shows grading improvement in the majority of children while staging remains unchanged or deteriorates in over 65% of children.

S4
Childhood autoimmune hepatitis (AIH) type I: analysis of 14 cases

H. ÖZEN, N. KOÇAK, I. N. SALTIK, A. YÜCE and F. GÜRAKAN

Hacettepe University School of Medicine, Department of Pediatric Gastroenterology, Ankara, Turkey

AIH is a chronic inflammatory progressive liver disease. Here we report the analysis of 14 children diagnosed at our hospital.

The mean age at diagnosis was 10.9 + 2.6 years and the female/male ratio was 1.3. The median time of diagnosis since the onset of symptoms was 8 months. All patients had high transaminase and γ-globulin values. Hepatomegaly was found in 71.4%, splenomegaly in 64.3% and ascites in 14.3%. Seven patients had only SMA, two ANA, and two AMA. While two children had ANA+SMA, one had ANA+ SMA+AMA positivity. Seven children were positive for ANCA. Liver biopsies revealed severe active hepatitis in addition to cirrhosis in four. The follow-up period was 30.7±15.6 months. Drug therapy consisted of prednisone 2 mg kg^{-1} day^{-1} po initially with the addition of azathioprine 1.5 mg kg^{-1} day^{-1} po at the third–sixth month and slow tapering of prednisone in 12 patients. Both drugs were started together in two children. Prednisone was discontinued in three patients with sustained normal ALTs. All patients' ALTs normalized or decreased significantly with therapy. Biochemical remission did not correlate with disappearance of autoantibodies. None of the patients showed decompensation of liver disease.

Prednisone and azathioprine therapy seems to be adequate in the majority of the patients with AIH. Different drugs, such as ursodeoxycholic acid, may be tried in resistant patients or decreasing the doses of prednisone and azathioprine.

S5
Efficiency of the scoring system for diagnosis of autoimmune hepatitis in children

A. POTAPOV, O. GUNDOBINA, O. BUKANOVICH, Z. ZAINUDINOV and B. KAGANOV

Department of Gastroenterology and Hepatology, Research Center of Children's Health, Moscow, Russia

Background: The International Autoimmune Hepatitis Group have proposed a scoring system for diagnosis of autoimmune hepatitis (AIH) in adults.

Aims: To evaluate the efficiency of the scoring system in children.

Patients and methods: We observed 30 children (26 girls, 4 boys) age 7–15 years with AIH. The average follow-up period was 35 ± 3 months. Blood serum of all the patients was tested for ANA, SMA, anti-LKM 1, routine biochemical parameters, HBV, HCV, HAV markers, and morphological examination of liver specimens was performed. The scoring system was used in all children.

Results: All the patients were found to have ANA and/or SMA in serum: ANA in 21 patients, SMA in 24 (titre range 1 : 20–1 : 1280). Fifteen patients were positive for both ANA and SMA. Anti-LKM 1 was not found in any of the tested patients. ALT/AST serum levels in all children exceeded 2–20 times normal values. γ-Globulin level was elevated by 22–40% in 20 and 41–55% in 10 patients. IgG level was 1.5–2.5 times higher than normal in all children. All patients were negative for hepatitis B and C virus markers. Applying the AIH scoring system, 17 of 30 (58%) children had 'definite' and the other 13 'probable' AIH before treatment. Repeating the counting score 1 year after the introduction of immunosuppressive therapy which was effective, 21 (70%) children fulfilled the criteria for 'definite' and 9 children remained in the category of 'probable' AIH.

Conclusions: The scoring system proved its efficiency in paediatric practice by confirming the diagnosis of AIH in all observed children and facilitates the diagnosis of AIH.

S6
Progression of autoimmune hepatitis type 1 in children

O. GUNDOBINA[1], A. POTAPOV[1], Z. ZAINUDINOV[1], M. RATNIKOVA[2] and B. KAGANOV[1]

[1]Department of Gastroenterology and Hepatology, Research Center of Children's Health; [2]Clinic of Children's Diseases, Moscow Medical Academy, Moscow, Russia

---

Background: Autoimmune hepatitis (AIH) is a necroinflammatory liver disorder of unknown cause, characterized by positive response to immunosuppressive therapy.

Aims: To study the course of autoimmune hepatitis (AIH) in children.

Patients and methods: During the period from 1993 to 2001, we observed 30 children (26 girls and 4 boys) aged from 7 to 15 years with AIH type 1. All children received immunosuppressive therapy consisting of prednisolone and azathioprine. Morphological examination of liver biopsy specimens with definition histological activity index Knodell was done in 24 patients.

Results: In 7 children, histological examination of liver tissue revealed chronic hepatitis (2 severe, 3 moderate and 2 mild) and, in 17 children, cirrhosis (8 severe, 5 moderate and 4 mild). In 5 patients, cirrhosis was found before therapy, in 12 patients it was established during therapy. In 6 children, liver biopsy was not possible and cirrhosis was diagnosed on clinical and laboratory evidence (varicose veins of the anterior abdominal surface, ankle oedema, ascitis, oesophageal varicosis, hypersplenism, prothrombin index <50%, serum albumin level <40%). Ultrasound examination revealed, in all patients with cirrhosis, dilatation of portal and lienal veins with reduction of the blood flow rate and porto-systemic shunt formation.

Thus, liver cirrhosis was found in 23 of 30 (77%) children with AIH. The diagnosis of cirrhosis was established 19 ± 4 months after the first manifestation of the disease.

Conclusions: AIH in children has a progressive course with formation of liver cirrhosis in 77% patients within two years of initial manifestation, not related to the introduction of immunosuppressive therapy.

S7
Autoimmune hepatitis as the first manifestation of systemic lupus erythematosus (SLE)

A. HINSBERGER, U. NEUDORF and A. BALLAUFF

Universitäts-Kinderklinik, Essen, Germany

In about 20% of patients with SLE, the liver is affected but autoimmune hepatitis as the initial main manifestation of SLE is rare. We report on two girls presenting with acute hepatitis with jaundice, elevated transaminases and impaired liver function.

Patient 1, a $14\frac{1}{2}$-year-old girl, became jaundiced after two weeks of fever, abdominal pain, vomitting and malaise. At admission she had hepatomegaly, AST 432 U/L, ALT 221 U/L, bilirubin 8.1 mg/dl, TPZ 78%, protein 6.2 g/dl, IgG normal but ANA 1 : 65536 (<1 : 256). Virology and metabolic screening was negative. There was suspicion of Wilson's disease due to 10-fold elevated urinary copper excretion and 5-fold elevated copper concentration in liver tissue. After a few days, there was development of neurological and psychiatric symptoms as well as haemolytic anaemia, malar rush, photosensitivity and renal impairment in the course of the disease. Liver histology included: cholestasis, hepatocellular single-cell necrosis and signs of hepatocellular regeneration, no inflammatory infiltrations. Clinical symptoms and anti-ds-DNA 64 U/L (0.1–40) led to the diagnosis of SLE.

Patient 2, a $15\frac{1}{2}$-year-old girl, was admitted with jaundice as the only clinical symptom, with AST 673 U/L, ALT 451 U/L, bilirubin 8.5 mg/dl, protein 10.1 g/dl, TPZ 45%, IgG 5080 mg/dl, ANA 1 : 1000000, non-haemolytic anaemia. There was only slightly elevated copper excretion in the urine. Liver histology showed: sectal fibrosis, large infiltrations with lymphocytes, plasma cells and eosinophilic granulocytes, leading to the histological diagnosis of autoimmune hepatitis. In this patient too, anti-ds-DNA 978 U/ml led to the diagnosis of SLE.

In girls with ANA-positive autoimmune hepatitis, SLE has to be considered and anti-ds-DNA should be measured.

S8
Autoimmune hepatitis – clinical findings of Wilson's disease in early childhood

M. GEORGIEVA-SHAKOLA[1], D. KONSTANTINOVA[1], V. TZANEVA[1], P. TZANKOVA[2], A. SAVOV[3] and M. POPOVA[1]

[1]Department of Pediatrics, [2]Department of Nephrology, Medical University, Varna; [3]Genetic Centre, Medical Academy, Sofia, Bulgaria

---

Wilson's disease (WD) is an uncommon autosomal recessive condition of impared hepatic copper excretion, resulting in excessive amounts of body copper. Clinical findings are very different in the different age groups. This study's aim was to reveal some unusual clinical findings of this pathology in early childhood and its treatment. In 1997–1999, a diagnosis of WD was proved in 2 girls (3 years and 3.7 years) by clinical, laboratory (+specific), ultrasonographic and genetic investigation. The patients presented with hepatic dysfunction: fatigue, abdominal pain, jaundice, oedema, ascites, hepatomegaly; elevated aminotransferases, decreased prothrombin time, serum albumin and cholesterol, elevated γ-globulines, (+) antimitochondrial antibodies. Kayser–Flaisher corneal ring was not found in either patient. Specific examinations showed: decreased ceruloplasmin, decreased serum copper and increased 24-h urinary excretion of copper. Testing with 0.5 g D-penicillamine provoked an 8–10-fold elevation of urinary excretion of copper. In these cases a mutation in the ATP 7B gene was proved: both patients were found to be homozygotes for H1070 mutation. Ultrasound images showed hepatomegaly, portal hypertension, ascites. The treatment included: prednisone 2 mg/kg + D-penicillamine 15 mg/kg. Both girls died, with signs of autoimmune cirrhosis, after a period of 2 years. In conclusion, the clinical findings of WD in early childhood are very unusual. Autoimmune hepatitis as a clinical finding of WD is very complicated and has a bad prognosis.

S9
Prevalence of autoimmune hepatitis in Austrian children and adolescents

J. DEUTSCH (GRAZ) and E. PENNER (WIEN)

Arbeitsgruppe für Pädiatrische Gastroenterologie und Ernährung der Österreichischen Gesellschaft für Kinder- und Jugendheilkunde und Mitglieder der Österreichischen Gesellschaft für Gastroenterologie und Hepatologie

---

To estimate the prevalence of autoimmune hepatitis in Austrian children and adolescents a collaboration has been initiated using the laboratory results of index cases and existing Austrian working groups.

Up to date 34 patients have been identified below the age of 19 years, 9 males and 25 females (ratio 1 : 2.77). This is an approximate prevalence of 1 : 40 000 in the Austrian population. Thirteen patients had positive autoimmune antibodies against liver–kidney microsomes (LKM), 13 patients had autoimmune antibodies against ds-nucleic acids (ds-ANA) and/or smooth muscles (SMA), and 7 patients against soluble liver antigen (SLA) with/without ds-ANA.

Three patients developed autoimmune antibodies/hepatitis after viral illnesses, 2 after Epstein–Barr virus and 1 after human herpes virus infections.

The course of the disease is analysed.

S10
Prevalence of autoantibodies and the risk of autoimmune thyroid disease in children with chronic hepatitis C virus (HCV) infection treated with α-interferon

S. GEHRING[1], E. LAUSCH[1], U. KULLMER[1], TH. KOFFLER[1], B. ZABEL[1] and S. WIRTH[2]

[1]Children's Hospital, University of Mainz; [2]Children's Hospital Wuppertal, Germany

---

Introduction: It has been reported that autoimmune activation occurs in patients with chronic hepatitis C and α-interferon treatment. One particular target organ is the thyroid, which may develop autoimmune thyroid disease during therapy. Therefore the aim of the present study was to evaluate the prevalence of autoantibodies (LKM: anti-liver and -kidney microsomal antibody, SMA: anti-smooth muscle antibody, ANA: anti-nuclear antibody, TGA: anti-thyroglobulin antibody) and the risk of developing autoimmune disease in children with chronic hepatitis C undergoing treatment with α-interferon.

Patients and methods: Twenty-eight children with chronic HCV infection received treatment with α-interferon. Twenty-one were treated with interferon alone; 7 children received the combination therapy, interferon and ribavirine.

Results: Before starting treatment, only one patient tested positive for one autoantibody (LKM). During therapy, 12 patients (42%) became positive for the autoantibodies LKM, ANA and TGA. Eight of these children were positive for TGA antibodies and two of them developed signs of an autoimmune thyroiditis with hypothyroidism requiring substitution of thyroid hormones.

Discussion: According to our results, a considerable number of children (12/28) developed signs of autoimmunity during α-interferon treatment. Particularly in terms of thyroid dysfunction, α-interferon therapy in children with chronic HCV requires close monitoring for signs of autoimmunity. This should be considered in future treatment regimens.

S11
Autoimmune markers in children with chronic hepatitis C

J. KUPS, T. WOZNIAKOWSKA-GESICKA and M. WISNIEWSKA-LIGIER

3rd Department of Paediatrics Polish Mother's Memorial Hospital, Research Institute, Lodz, Rzgowska 281/289 Street, 93-338 Lodz, Poland

---

HCV is an immunogenic virus that causes the appearance of autoimmunological markers with different clinical and prognostic implications in cases leading to the development of extrahepatic disease. The purpose of this study was the analysis of autoimmune phenomena in the course of chronic hepatitis C in children with respect to genotype. The study covered 60 children with chronic hepatitis C divided into two groups where one group was treated with IFN-1 and the second was left untreated. HCV genotyping and diagnostic tests for the presence of autoantibodies, ANA, AMA, SMA, LKM1 and Ro, before and after the follow-up period, were carried out in all the patients. At the start of the observation period, autoantibodies (ANA and/or AMA and/or SMA) were present in 22/60 patients, especially in children infected with genotype 1b. After 6 months of observation, there was an increase in children with autoantibodies (38/60), in the group of treated children as well as the group of untreated children and this increase was similar in children infected with genotypes 1a and 1b. One child treated with IFN-1 developed characteristics of autoimmune hepatitis. In summary, this study indicates the role of HCV infection in the processes of autoimmune induction.

S12
Upper gastrointestinal lesions in children with inflammatory bowel disease

M. SLADEK, A. WEDRYCHOWICZ, S. PIECZARKOWSKI, U. JEDYNAK, M. DRABAREK, M. GRUSZKA and K. FYDEREK

Department of Pediatrics, Gastroenterology and Nutrition, Jagiellonian University, Faculty of Medicine, Krakow, Poland

---

Ulcerative colitis and Crohn's disease are usually distinguished by a combination of clinical, histopathological and anatomical findings. Few studies have evaluated upper GI involvement in children with IBD.

Thirty-two children with active IBD (24 with ulcerative colitis, 8 with Crohn's disease) with a mean age 12.1y and 13.8y, respectively, were studied. Upper GI endoscopy was performed and biopsy specimens were taken from duodenum, antrum, gastric body and oesophagus, and any visible mucosal lesions were evaluated by histology including Giemsa staining and urea test.

Fifty-four per cent of patients with UC and 88% with CD were found to have inflammatory infiltration in gastric mucosa. In one UC patient, a polyp of the pylori was found, and another patient was additionally diagnosed with Menetrier disease. Only one patient with CD showed gastric mucosal epithelioid non-caseating granulomas. Microscopic inflammation in duodenal mucosa occurred in 33% of UC and 63% of CD patients. In one patient with CD, a type III duodenal mucosa was diagnosed. All patients were *Helicobacter pylori* negative. Within our study group, only one CD patient (4%) was diagnosed with inflammatory lesions in the oesophagus.

Non-specific inflammatory changes were found in both CD and UC patients, with a higher frequency in the CD group (88% vs. 54%). Gastric mucosal epithelioid non-caseating granulomas occurred less frequently than non-specific inflammation in CD patients. Upper GI endoscopy may be helpful when planning treatment.

S13
Serum interleukin-1β decreased faster than interleukin 1 receptor antagonist during recovery in children with active ulcerative colitis

A. WEDRYCHOWICZ[1], J. STOPYROWA[1], K. FYDEREK[1] and W. MIEZYNSKI[2]

[1]Department of Paediatrics, Gastroenterology and Nutrition, [2]Department of Pathology, Polish–American Children's Hospital, Jagiellonian University, Cracow, Poland

---

Introduction: It is known that there are increased concentrations of interleukin 1β (IL-1β) and interleukin 1 receptor antagonist (IL-1ra) in serum, stools and colonic mucosal specimens in ulcerative colitis (UC) children. The aim of the present study was to estimate IL-1β and IL-1ra in serum during recovery, and evaluate their correlations with clinical, endoscopic and histopathological UC activity.

Methods: Twenty children with active UC, 14 children with non-specific colitis (NC, inflammatory control group) and 14 healthy children (normal control group) were included in the study. The interleukin concentrations were measured in the serum of UC children during admission to the hospital and after 4 and 12 weeks of treatment, using commercial quantitative ELISA immunoassays (R&D Systems, MN, USA). The Truelove–Witts clinical activity index was calculated. The endoscopic and histopathological findings were graded by Roths endoscopic scale and standard histopathological scale.

Results: The serum IL-1β and IL-1ra concentrations reached higher levels in UC patients than normal controls ($p < 0.01$) and ($p < 0.001$), respectively, but showed no differences compared with inflammatory controls and decreased gradually during recovery. The serum IL-1ra/IL-1β ratio increased after 4 weeks of recovery, reaching the normal control group level and decreased after 12 weeks of treatment. The serum IL-1β concentrations correlated statistically significantly with the endoscopic and histopathological scales ($r = 0.38$, $p < 0.05$; and $r = 0.51$, $p < 0.05$, respectively) but did not correlate with UC clinical activity. The serum IL-1ra concentrations correlated statistically significantly both with the Truelove–Witts clinical activity index ($r = 0.43$, $p < 0.05$) and with the endoscopic and histopathological scales ($r = 0.52$, $p < 0.05$; and $r = 0.46$, $p < 0.05$, respectively). Serum IL-1ra/IL-1β ratio did not correlate with clinical, endoscopic and histopathological UC activity.

Conclusions: Serum IL-1β decreased faster than IL-1ra in children with active UC during recovery but serum IL-1ra correlated more closely than IL-1β with UC activity. Serum IL-1β and IL-1ra ratings may be a useful means of assessing UC activity during the treatment of children with active UC.

S14 Sonographic diagnostics of ulcerative colitis in children

S. ABRAMOV and V. KOPEIKIN

Research Institute of Children's Gastroenterology, Nizhny Novgorod, Russia

The aim of this study was to increase the possible uses of the sonographic method for the investigation of children with ulcerative colitis.

Eighteen children aged 3–15 y were studied. The duration of disease was from 1 to 11 years. All the children underwent the complex of clinical and laboratory examination, including irrigography and fibrocolonoscopy with biopsy material taken. Sonographic investigation was performed on "ALOKA 680" and "SCANER 250", using sector and convex pump, frequency, 3.5 MHz and 5 MHz. In 100% of cases, irrespective of the duration of the disease, the wall was thickened from 5 to 7 mm, the internal contour of the bowel wall was changed into a form of erosive or ulcerative defects, and the structure of the layers was also destroyed. The change of the gaustration height depended on the duration of disease: if the disease lasted less than 5 years, in 57% of cases, the gaustration height was decreased, in 29%, it was absent and, in 14%, it was unchanged. If the disease lasted more than 5 years, in 36% of cases, the gaustration height was decreased and, in 64% of cases, there was no gaustration. This corresponded with the endoscopic picture.

Moreover, we noticed a new sonographic criterion: an increase in bowel wall echogenicity. This was found in 100% of cases when the duration of disease was more than 5 years. We could not find the description of this criterion in the available literature.

The sonographic criterion of increased bowel wall echogenicity was characteristic of destructive sclerotic changes. This supposition was confirmed by the morphological study of biopsy material, showing the presence of fibrosis of bowel wall mucosa with tough fibrous connective tissue.

We performed a computer transformation of sonographic images of some large bowel parts to digital values of the grey scale. When normal, the bowel wall had an average echogenicity which corresponded to 41–69% of the grey-scale intensity, and heightened echogenicity was 18–36%.

Thus, sonography of the large bowel may be a prospective method of diagnosis and prognosis of ulcerative colitis in children.

S15
Inhibition of NF-κB and induction of apoptosis by sulphasalazine

S. LIPTAY[1], S. FULDA[1], C. WEBER[2], G. ADLER[2], R. M. SCHMID[2] and K. M. DEBATIN[1]

[1]Department of Paediatrics; [2]Department of Internal Medicine, University of Ulm, Prittwitzstraße 43, D-89075 Ulm

---

Objective: Transcription factors of the NF-κB/Rel family are important regulators of the immune response and apoptosis. Sulphasalazine (SS) and its moiety 5-aminosalicylic acid (5-ASA) have long been known for their beneficial effects in the treatment of IBD. However, their molecular mode of action is not understood.

Aims: The purpose of this study was to investigate whether SS or 5-ASA affect NF-κB/Rel activation or T-cell viability.

Methods and results: SS inhibits NF-κB activation in T-lymphocytes using electrophoretic mobility shift and transfection assays. In immune complex assays, SS inhibits the NF-κB activating kinases (IKKα and IKKβ) directly, most likely by competitive binding to the ATP binding site. Higher doses or prolonged incubation results in apoptosis of T-lymphocytes as determined by DNA fragmentation, annexin V and Apo 2.7 staining. SS-induced apoptosis is triggered by collapse of the mitochondrial transmembrane potential, which leads to cytochrome c release and activation of caspase-3 and downstream substrates. However, the pan-caspase inhibitor Z-VAD.fmk fails to inhibit SS-induced apoptosis. SS stimulates mitochondrio-nuclear translocation of the novel apoptogenic factor AIF (apoptosis inducing factor) and triggers caspase-independent apoptosis.

Conclusion: These results demonstrate that SS prevents NF-κB activation by direct inhibition of IKKα and IKKβ. In addition, SS is a potent inducer of apoptosis in T-lymphocytes, which is mediated by AIF and occurs in a caspase-independent fashion.

S16
Dexamethasone protects enterocytes from TNF-α-induced apoptosis

F. M. RUEMMELE, J. F. BEAULIEU, T. ROTTMANN, E. G. SEIDMAN and M. J. LENTZE

Children's Hospital Medical Center, University of Bonn, Germany; Cell Biology, University of Sherbrooke and Ste. Justine Hospital, University of Montreal, Canada

---

TNF-α, a key inflammatory mediator in Crohn's disease, is known to alter intestinal epithelial cell turnover, resulting in pathological epithelial functions. Previous studies showed that TNF-α in combination with IFNγ markedly inhibited normal intestinal epithelial cell growth and induced a high degree of enterocyte apoptosis.

Aim: To test the hypothesis that the glucocorticosteroid, dexamethasone, protects enterocytes from TNF/IFN-induced apoptosis.

Methods/results: The non-transformed human intestinal epithelial cell line, HIEC, was stimulated with recombinant TNF-α 1–100 ng/ml plus IFNγ 300 U/ml alone or in the presence of dexamethasone 10–1000 nmol/L for up to 48 h. TNF/IFN induced HIEC apoptosis in a dose-dependent manner with a maximum apoptosis rate of 73 ± 8% ($p<0.01$) after 48 h. Typical signs of apoptosis, such as the loss of membrane asymmetry, condensation and fragmentation of the DNA as well as the formation of apoptotic bodies were observed in TNF/IFN-stimulated cells by immunofluorescence, confocal and electron microscopy. In the presence of dexamethasone, no induction of apoptosis occurred after stimulation with TNF/IFN (14 ± 6%) even at the highest cytokine concentrations used. Receptor-expression analysis of the p55 and p75-TNF-R showed no effect of dexamethasone at the receptor level.

Discussion: Glucocorticosteroids rescue enterocytes from TNF-induced apoptosis. These protective mechanisms seem to be at the post-receptor level, since no effect of dexamethasone on TNF-receptor expression was observed.

S17

α-Interferon effectiveness in treating ulcerative colitis (UC) in children

E. A. KORNIENKO

Pediatric Medical Academy, St. Petersburg, Russia

UC treatment is based upon anti-inflammatory therapy. Immunomodulation serves as an alternative to hormone therapy, including α-interferon.

Aim: α-Interferon effectiveness was evaluated combined with mesalazine (Salofalk) in children with UC of various degrees of severity.

Materials and methods: Fifteen patients were examined, aged 9 to 15 y: 7 with light distal UC; 5 with moderate left-side UC; 3 with total severe UC. All received 1.0 g to 2.0 g Salofalk pills daily; after 2 weeks, 12 were additionally prescribed 2 ml α-interferon 3 times weekly im for 1 month. Three with distal UC received Salofalk in suppository form (750 mg daily) instead of α-interferon. Evaluation was based on clinical/endoscopic data after 1 and 3 months.

Results: Mild UC (4 on α-interferon/3 on Salofalk): clinical and endoscopic remission reached, Salofalk rectally produced a faster effect: stool blood disappeared on the 7th day; α-interferon, on the 10th to 14th day. Three months later, remission persisted.

Out of 5 patients with moderate UC, α-interferon was effective in 4: stool blood disappeared on the 15th to 20th day, 1 month afterwards there were no erosions/ulcers. In 1 patient, α-interferon was ineffective; treatment was cancelled and prednisolone prescribed.

In severe UC, clinical improvement was achieved only in 1 patient on α-interferon; the disease process remained active, and contact bleeding/erosions persisted. In 2, no positive dynamics were observed; α-interferon treatment was cancelled and prednisolone prescribed.

Conclusions: α-Interferon was effective only in children with light or moderate UC; in children with light distal UC, Salofalk introduced rectally is preferable. In children with severe UC, α-interferon is ineffective.

S18
Plasma exchange (plasmapheresis) in complex therapy in children with ulcerative colitis

B. ASSONOV, V. KOPEIKIN, E. FEDULOVA and S. SARALOV

Nizhny Novgorod Research Institute of Children Gastroenterology, Russia

The aim was to improve effectiveness of ulcerative colitis complex therapy by means of extracorporeal detoxification methods. The expediency of therapeutic plasma exchange (plasmapheresis) in complex therapy of autoimmune diseases of the large intestine, ulcerative colitis, was analysed in children aged 5–16 years old, 4 girls and 8 boys.

Severe forms of ulcerative colitis require plasma exchange (plasmapheresis). The severity of the disease state was determined according to an activity index, including a five-point scale of the 13 most significant factors: asthenovegetative and dyspeptic syndromes, the degree of trophic disorders, stool frequency, ESR, haemoglobin level, white blood cell count, the degree of stab neutrophil deviation, coprogram character, and $\alpha 2$- and γ-globulin levels.

The total activity index in all the patients requiring plasma exchange (plasmapheresis) exceeded 35, and showed no tendency to decrease with the basic therapeutic background: the average rate of decrease was 0.05 per day.

The operation was performed in immunocorrective inexhaustible plasma exchange (plasmapheresis) mode; i.e. plasma fusion did not exceed 30–40% TPC (total plasma circulation). Plasma substitution was performed with media not containing antigens–crystalloid solutions (0.9% NaCl and 5% glucose).

We observed no large deviations in laboratory values, showing negative protein balance. They were restored within 48–72 h; therefore, the procedure was repeated twice a week. Only in severe cases of hypoproteinaemia (total protein level <60 g/L) and hypoalbuminaemia (albumin level $<50\%$) at the final stage, was transfusion of small amounts of donor albumin and plasma introduced into the infusion programme.

Three plasma exchange (plasmapheresis) procedures were enough to lower circulating immune complexes and mediomolecular peptide levels accompanied by distinct clinic improvement of trophic processes and reduction of inflammatory deviations in peripheral blood.

Thus, plasma exchange (plasmapheresis) operations in inexhaustible immunocorrective mode are shown to arrest severe exacerbations of ulcerative colitis.

S19
Treatment with azathioprine in children with colitis ulcerosa

K. GRZYBOWSKA, I. PLANETA-MALECKA, A. PODCZASKA-SLOWINSKA, A. KISIEL, J. TROJANOWSKA-LIPCZYK and E. PLEWINSKA

I Department of Paediatrics and Gastroenterology, PMMH–Research Institute, Lodz, Poland

---

Non-specific colitis, including colitis ulcerosa, is a heterogeneous group of chronic diseases of the intestine. The aim of the study was to assess the effectiveness of treatment with azathioprine in children with colitis ulcerosa.

Materials: Between 1990 and 2000, ninety-two children with colitis ulcerosa were treated in I Department of Paediatrics and Gastroenterology, PMMH–Research Institute, Lodz, Poland. The diagnosis was established based on history, clinical symptoms and endoscopic examinations as well as histological assessment of large-intestine biopsy specimens. Depending on the gravity of relapse, in addition to treatment with 5-ASA, steroids were administered locally or generally as well as enteral or parenteral nutrition. Azathioprine was administered with a good effect for a period of 2–3 years in a group of 10 steroid-resistant or steroid-dependent children. The youngest child to receive azathioprine was 10 years old when the treatment was started and she received it for 4.5 years. Undesired effects were observed intermittantly during therapy. Nevertheless, attempts to withdraw the drug proved unsuccessful and resulted in relapses. She has now been in remission for 2 years and does not require treatment.

Conclusions: The period of treatment with azathioprine is longer in younger children and harmful effects are observed more frequently.

S20
Intravenous azathioprine in steroid-refractory paediatric IBD

Å. LINDBLAD[1], H. HILDEBRAND[1], C. PETERSON[2] and Y. FINKEL[1]

[1]*Astrid Lindgren Children Hospital, Stockholm;* [2]*Department of Clinical Pharmacology, Linköping University, Sweden*

Introduction: Recent evidence suggests that intravenous administration of azathioprine, both at very high and at low doses, may allow more rapid onset of clinical efficacy in the management of acute colitis complicating both Crohn's disease (CD) and ulcerative colitis (UC).

Patients and methods: Five children with IBD (3 UC, 1 CD and 1 IC), median age 15 years (range 11–17), with acute colitis unresponsive to steroids or nutritional therapy, received intravenous infusion of azathioprine (Aza) 2.3–3 mg/kg during 30 min on five consecutive days during which oral Aza was stopped but 5-ASA and steroid treatment was unchanged. In 2 patients, iv Aza treatment was repeated after 2–4 months.

Results: Thiopurine methyltransferase activity was normal in all patients. Clinical remission with reduction in steroid doses and weaning of oral Aza was acheived in all patients. No clinical side-effects were seen during iv Aza treatment; neutropenia and pancreatitis did not occur.

Two patients relapsed after 2–4 months. Repeated iv Aza was adminstered with subsequent clinical remission.

Conclusions: Intravenous low-dose azathioprine is effective in acute colitis in IBD. In this small study, there were no clinical side-effects.

S21
(Auto)immune enteropathy – a clinical survey of the GPGE

A. BALLAUFF

Universitäts-Kinderklinik, Essen, Germany

In the year 2000, members of the German Society of Paediatric Gastroenterology (GPGE) were asked to report on patients with proven or suspected (auto)immune enteropathy. Data of 11 patients were collected. At diagnosis, 5 patients were older and 6 patients younger than 24 months. One of the older patients probably had autoimmune polyendocrinopathy with enteropathy. Watery diarrhoea, vomiting and weight loss were the main symptoms at diagnosis and during follow-up. Extraintestinal manifestations included hepatopathy and dermatitis in both groups and arthritis, cardiomyopathy and hypoadrenalism in the older group. Protein-losing enteropathy was present in 4 infants and in 1 older child. Gut epithelial cell autoantibodies were measured in 8 and detected in 5 patients.

Duodenal biopsy showed lymphocytic infiltration of the lamina propria, which was severe in 8 and mild in 2 children; and villous atrophy which was total in 7 and mild or moderate in 4 children. Intraepithelial lymphocytes were increased in 6 and normal in 5 children. Four of the infants had gastritis and 5 colitis while only 1 of the older children had atrophic gastritis. Ten patients were initially treated with steroids and only 4 showed a good response. Azathioprine, cyclosporine and tacrolimus were most often used for additional immunosuppression. All 6 infants and 2 of the older children needed parenteral nutrition. Infants initially received hydrolysed or amino acid formulas. Three of the older patients received a gluten-free diet. At the end of follow-up (10 patients, median 8 months, range 2–22 months) 10 patients still received steroids, 3 with azathioprine, 3 with cyclosporine, 3 with tacrolimus. Four children received normal food, 1 gluten-free diet, 1 cows' milk-free diet, 3 amino acid, 1 hydrolysed formula. Two of the infants still needed additional parenteral nutrition.

Conclusion: Autoimmune enteropathy is a rare disease in German children. Proven cases should be collected for follow up to gain more information about the prognosis and course of this disease.

S22
A new concept of inducing remission in Crohn's disease: anti-interleukin-2-receptor antibody and mycophenolate mofetil

M. LYONS, R. GANSCHOW, A. VENZKE and M. BURDELSKI

Department of Pediatrics, University Hospital Hamburg, Germany

---

Interleukin 2 plays an important role in the T-cell activation and proliferation cascade of the immune system. In a pilot study we tested safety and efficacy of a chimeric monoclonal anti-interleukin-2 receptor antibody (IL-2-RA) used in liver and kidney transplantation to reduce organ rejection in combination with mycophenolate mofetil (MMF) in inducing remission in paediatric Crohn patients.

We studied five patients between the ages of 8 and 15 years (3 males, 2 females) with chronic relapse of Crohn's disease despite conventional immunosuppressive therapy. The IL-2-RA, daclizumab, was given on days 0, 14 and 28 (Zenapax 1 mg/kg body weight). To reduce the possibility of gastrointestinal side-effects the starting dose of MMF was 200 mg/m^2, increasing the dosage to 300 mg/m^2, then a final dosage of 400 mg/m^2 at 14-day intervals.

The response criteria were defined as the normalization of stools, appetite and weight gain and improvement of clinical and laboratory findings according to the paediatric Crohn's disease activity index (Harms 1992). All five patients showed an initial response to the therapy without side-effects. The follow-up over several months showed an ongoing remission in 2 and a transient remission in 3 patients.

In conclusion, the use of IL-2-RA and MMF could be an option in patients with chronic relapse and unresponsiveness to conventional immunosuppression in Crohn's disease. Our data show comparable results to the TNF-α-antibody. Only repeated applications seem to show a prolonged effect in the majority of patients.

Section VII
Mini-posters read by title

CASE REPORTS: I: LIVER

P1
Autoimmune hepatitis (AIH) in transplanted liver

I. JANKOWSKA[1], J. PAWLOWSKA[1], M. TEISSEYRE[1], P. KALICINSKI[2], A. KAMINSKI[2], P. CZUBKOWSKI[1], J. KUSZYK[3], P. KLUGE[3], M. WOZNIAK[1] and J. SOCHA[1]

[1]Department of Gastroenterology, Hepatology and Nutrition; [2]Department of Paediatric Surgery and Organ Transplantation; [3]Department of Pathology, The Children's Memorial Health Institute, Warsaw, Poland

---

Liver transplantation (LTx) is considered the most effective treatment of chronic liver insufficiency. The aim of this work is to highlight autoimmune hepatitis as one of the problems in transplanted liver. We would like to introduce 2 patients with AIH after LTx.

1. A 26-year-old female patient with AIH complicated with HBV infection, who first underwent LTx in 1993 (Widen), followed by retransplantation because of primary liver dysfunction. A third LTx (1994) was necessary due to chronic rejection. Cyclosporin, prednisone and monthly anti-HBs immunoglobulin infusions were administered. Between the second and third LTx, no LKM antibodies were found in blood. Because of chronic CMV infection, immunosuppression was kept as low as possible. Four years after the last LTx, a diagnosis of AIH relapse was established based on high LKM serum level (>640) and histopathological changes in liver biopsy. Cyclosporin was maintained, prednisone doses were increased and additional azathioprine was administered with good clinical and biochemical effect.
2. A 17-year-old female patient who underwent LTx in 1998 due to α-1 antitrypsin deficiency and liver cirrhosis, treated with cyclosporin, prednisone and azathioprine. One year after LTx, immunosuppression was modified (prednisone every second day). For the next 6 months, an increase in aminotransferase activity was measured. Histopathological changes in liver biopsy and ASMA antibodies (1 : 40) found in serum were consistent with autoimmune hepatitis. Prednisone and azathioprine were modified to 1 mg/kg and

2 mg/kg, respectively. After prednisone doses had been decreased, aminotranspherase activity increased and the liver biopsy was consistent with AIH again. Cyclosporin was switched to tacrolimus which was beneficial. There has been follow up of 2 months so far.

Conclusions:

1. Patients after LTx due to AIH are susceptible to that disease in transplanted liver.
2. There is a possibility of AIH *de novo* in transplanted liver.

P2
Diabetes mellitus – a complication of the treatment or an associated autoimmune disorder of chronic C hepatitis in children

V. TZANEVA, M. GEORGIEVA-SHAKOLA and E. SHEITANOVA

Department of Pediatrics, Medical University, Varna, Bulgaria

---

Interferon alpha (INF-α) has been widely used to treat chronic hepatitis C virus (HCV) infection. Side-effects are common; they are usually minor but some major adverse events can occur. Tolerance in elderly patients and children is usually similar. We report on a case of diabetes mellitus in the course of treatment of HCV infection with INF-α. In 1997, a haemophiliac boy (14 years) with HCV infection was treated with INF-α, 3 MU/m^2, 3 times a week for 6 months. HCV was diagnosed by clinical, laboratory (elevated aminotransferases) and serological tests (HCV antibody (+)), HCV RNA (+) tests. At 1-week intervals during the treatment, the patient was tested for haemoglobin, leucocytes, granulocytes and platelet cells, and, at 2 weeks intervals, for aminotransferases. There were clinical and laboratory (+serologic, +HCV RNA) controls after the end of the treatment. At the 6th month, the boy developed a diabetes mellitus (insulin related) and the treatment was stopped. The patient only had a biochemical response; he had no antibodies for autoimmune hepatitis or other autoimmune abnormalities: thrombocytopenia, rheumatoid factor, antithyroglobulin. We discussed two possibilities: first, an association of two autoimmune disorders, which is supported by some research and publications in the literature, and second, a side-effect of the treatment which is not very well investigated yet. This case indicates the importance of selecting patients for therapy and optimizing response. Careful assessment is required before treatment, and monitoring is required during treatment. Relatively little is known about the mechanisms of many of the side-effects of INF-α.

P3
Autoimmune or toxic liver injury – a diagnostic dilema

J. PAWLOWSKA, M. TEISSEYRE, M. WOZNIAK and J. KUSZYK

The Children's Memorial Health Institute, Warsaw, Poland

Autoimmune hepatitis (AIH), primarily a paediatric disease, may present as an acute, fulminant or subfulminant hepatitis. The aetiology is still unknown and, in some cases, the toxic liver injury may play a role. In children, idiosyncratic hepatotoxity is an infrequent but well-recognized complication of a variety of therapeutic agents. We present a case of cholestatic liver disease with probable toxic and immune-mediated injury.

A 14-year-old boy, previously healthy, was admitted to the hospital with abdominal pain, jaundice (maximal total bilirubin 19.5 mg/dl, conjugated 17.4) and hepatosplenomegaly. Two weeks earlier, he had received Bactrim for upper respiratory tract infection. Laboratory tests revealed high activity of aminotransferases (max. GPT 2305 U/L, GPT 2405 U/L, GGTP 128 U/L), decreased prothrombin index (INR min. 1.42). Evaluation for known viral and metabolic causes of cholestasis was negative. Ultrasound showed a homogenous enlarged liver with no gallstones or dilatation of the biliary tree. A percutaneous liver biopsy specimen obtained two weeks after the beginning of symptoms revealed acute liver injury, probably of toxic origin. Because no clinical or biochemical improvement was achieved after treatment with UDCA, a second percutaneous liver biopsy was performed one month later. The microscope pattern (lymphocyte infiltration) was suggestive of AIH. Treatment with prednisone and azathioprine was started with quick normalization of laboratory parameters. No elevation of total proteins, γ-globulins or presence of autoantibodies was ever observed. The biopsy taken one year later was normal.

P4
Association between HBV infection and autoimmune hepatitis – case report

M. WOYNAROWSKI, M. WOZNIAK and J. SOCHA

Department of Gastroenterology, Hepatology and Nutrition, Child's Health Memorial Institute, Warsaw, Poland

---

The aetiology of autoimmune hepatitis (AIH) is unknown. There are reports describing the association of AIH with chronic hepatitis C but the role of HBV infection in AIH has not been determined. We describe a patient with HBV infection which probably triggered autoimmune response.

A male patient, born in 1982 of an HBs-positive mother, received a blood transfusion in the neonatal period. The patient was found to be HBsAg positive on a routine blood tests performed in 1988. The patient was asymptomatic and liver function tests were not impaired until June 1995 when the patient presented with signs and symptoms of subacute liver failure with mild encephalopathy, high ALT (4000 U/L), bilirubin (20.0 mg%), IgG (>3000 mg%), increased serum ammonia level (180 μg%) and prolonged prothrombin time. The patient received steroid treatment and rapidly improved with return of ALT activity to normal values. For several weeks, the HBe/antiHBe seroconversion was observed. Liver biopsy performed 5 months later showed mild chronic hepatitis which justified steroid discontinuation. The patient developed a second episode of subacute liver failure, with rises in ALT, γ-globulin and IgG, and steroid treatment was rechallanged in September 1996. Autoimmune aetiology was not confirmed by the presence of serum autoantibodies but liver function tests improved with the return of IgG and γ-globulins to normal values. Steroid treatment was stopped in April 1997. In September 1997 the patient had high ALT (308 U/L), normal IgG and positive HBeAg. Liver biopsy showed progression of inflammatory changes. The patient started on interferon-α treatment (3 MU TIW) and initially normalization of ALT was observed. After 3 months of therapy, ALT and IgG started to rise again. Interferon was stopped and steroid treatment was restarted in March 1998. The patient continued on low doses of steroids, modified according to the actual ALT and IgG levels. A control liver biopsy in March 2000 showed progression of liver damage (grading 3 and staging 3 Sheuer classification) and the patient was positive for HBV-DNA and HBeAg. The patient began combined steroid + lamivudine treatment in April 2000 and steroids were discontinued in June 2000. The patient completed one year of lamivudine treatment with no ALT, IgG or γ-globulin flare. The patient seroconverted to antiHBe but remained HBV-DNA positive.

We did not manage to demonstrate the presence of serum autoantibodies but we believe that liver disease exacerbation with high IgG and γ-globulins, deterioration of the disease during interferon and good response to steroid treatment and advanced liver damage found on biopsy justify a diagnosis of AIH that could have been triggered by HBV infection.

P5
Multiple allergies in a child treated with FK 506 after liver transplantation

T. SAUERWALD[1], D. MÜHLBAUER[1], M. BURDELSKI[2] AND S. KOLETZKO[1]

[1]*Dr. v. Haunersches Kinderspital, University of Munich;*
[2]*Universitätskrankenhaus Eppendorf, Hamburg*

Introduction: Induction of multiple allergies secondary to immunosuppression is uncommon. We present a 3-year-old girl who developed severe food and drug allergies after the initiation of FK 506 therapy.

Case report: A preterm infant (31 weeks of gestation) was diagnosed with biliary atresia at 2 months of age. A Kasai procedure failed and liver transplantation was performed at 10 months of age. Initial nutrition consisted of a preterm formula and human milk; later Heparon junior and a normal diet was well tolerated. Because of two episodes of acute rejection during cyclosporine therapy, she was switched to FK 506. Thereafter, she developed severe allergic reactions against drugs (several classes of antibiotics and anaesthetics) and food. Early and late allergic symptoms occurred including severe eczema, rashes, itching, high fever, diarrhoea and wheezing. Total IgE increased from 2.8 IU/ml before transplantation to >1100 IU/ml after FK 506 was introduced. She only tolerated an amino-acid-based formula (Neocate). Unfortunately, chronic rejection developed and the child is listed for retransplantation.

Discussion: Few cases of multiple allergies after FK 506 therapy have been reported. The severity of some of these unexpected reactions warrants careful observation and close follow-up. Cytokine profiles may help to prove a link between immunosuppressive therapy and development of allergies.

P6
Autoimmune chronic hepatitis combined with coeliac disease and IgA deficiency

G. DOCKTER[1], J. BRUNNER[1], H. BONKHOFF[2] and M. MENGES[3]

[1]Paediatric Gastroenterology; [2]Department of Endoscopy; [3]Department of Pathology, University Hospital of Saarland, D-66424 Homburg

---

A 5-year-old boy (father Irish, mother Hispanic) presented with a history of chronic diarrhoea and vomiting, Hirschsprung-like abdomen, wasted weak muscles, abdominal pain and anorexia. Gluten antibodies (AGA, EMA) were reported as negative, aminotransferases elevated, albumin very low. The first diagnosis was coeliac disease and secondary hepatotoxic injury, complicated by IgA-deficiency.

The initial lab screening was confusing: ASAT 40; ALAT 51; IgG 2956; IgA negative; AGA negative; EMA negative; ANA 640.

Completing lab data:

SMA-antibodies negative; LKM-AG negative; SLA-antibodies negative; AMA-M2-antibodies positive; Reticulin antibodies 1 : 32 000 positive; HLA A3, B35, B47, Cw4, Cw6, DR7, DR17, DQA1*0201

and doing liver and jejunal biopsies:

Jejunum: flat mucosa with a high count of intraepithelial lymphocytes.
Liver: medium-grade inflammation (lymphocytes, histiocytes), beginning of fibrosis but no cirrhosis, focal liver cell damage, no bile duct proliferation but destruction of small bile ducts.

We diagnosed IgA deficiency, chronic autoimmune hepatitis and primary biliary cirrhosis or beginning primary sclerosing cholangitis with secondary immunopathy of intestinal mucosa.

Treatment with prednisolone and gluten-free diet was followed by a slow improvement in intestinal and liver symptoms. Lab parameters and autoimmune antibodies became negative. After stepwise reduction to stop corticoids, antibodies and liver enzymes rose again. Now on 5 mg prednisolone daily and a gluten-free diet, he is in a good clinical condition, liver enzymes are normal, but IgG (1710), IgE (1860) and ANA (1280) are rising again.

P7
Crohn's disease in a 3.5-year-old patient

A. PODCZASKA-SLOWINSKA, K. GRZYBOWSKA, I. PLANETA-MALECKA and E. PLEWINSKA

I Department of Paediatrics and Gastroenterology, Polish Mother's Memorial Hospital Research Institute, Lodz, Poland

Crohn's disease is a chronic non-specific enterocolitis that is characterized by occurrence of lesions in any part of the intestine.

Aim: The aim of the study was to present diagnostic and therapeutic problems in a 3.5-year-old girl treated for chronic bloody and mucous diarrhoea. The disease was first manifested at the age of 2.5 by loose stools and ulcerations in the mouth cavity which were not susceptible to the treatment. The cause was not established and therapy proved ineffective. Results of the diagnostic endoscopic and histopathological examinations performed a year later show Crohn's disease. Steroids proved effective; nevertheless, attempts to finish the therapy were unsuccessful.

Conclusion: The younger the patient is, the more frequently diagnostic and therapeutic problems occur.

P8
Crohn's disease presenting with enterovesical fistula: a case report

J. UTESENY and D. KLUSACEK

IInd Department of Pediatrics, University Childrens Hospital, Brno

Introduction: The course of Crohn's disease is quite variable in children and enterovesical fistula is a relatively rare condition (1.6%).

Results: We report a case of a 15-year-old boy presenting with typical clinical signs of fistulous communication between the intestinal tract and bladder. This caused complications (abdominal abscess with concomitant sepsis), cystoscopic findings, intravenous urography and charcoaluria underlining the importance of respective clinical signs. In this patient we found the combination of clinical symptoms most often described: pneumaturia, fecaluria and haemorrhagic cystitis.

Conclusion: Rare complications of Crohn disease (for example enterovesical fistulas) can be diagnosed in hospitals with limited numbers of patients. Clinical examination and family history should be performed carefully.

P9
Budenofalk® and non-steroidal anti-inflammatory drugs (NSAIDs) for treatment of anal complications of Crohn's disease with peripheral arthritis in a 15-year-old boy

V. SULYMA and O. SULIMA

Medical Academy and Hospital No. 10 of Dniepropetrovsk, Ukraine

---

Thirty-five per cent of patients will have perianal complications of Crohn's disease (fistulas and abscesses) during the course of their disease.

There is significant association between extraintestinal complications and perianal complications (25%), which raises the possibility of a pathogenetic relationship between the two conditions.

Peripheral arthritis as an extraintestinal manifestation can be associated with or complicated by inflammatory bowel diseases (ulcerative colitis and Crohn's disease) in more patients. Some patients with inflammatory bowel diseases have extracolonic problems from the beginning, most of them favorably influenced by treatment and remissions of the disease.

The immune aspects implicated in pathogenesis of inflammatory bowel diseases were clinically evaluated by association with other autoimmune diseases (peripheral arthritis, erythema nodosum, hepatic cirrhosis, conjunctivitis, vasculitis, uveitis, ankylosing spondylitis, Reiter syndrome).

The risk factors have been observed at the beginning and during remission, the patient being, mostly, treated with sulphamide, cortisone or immunosuppressants.

We studied a 15-year-old boy with Crohn's disease with perianal complications (fistulas) and extraintestinal complications (peripheral arthritis).

In the absence of any causal therapy, drugs that relieve symptoms, such as preparations containing or releasing budesonide (Budenofalk®) with non-steroidal anti-inflammatory drugs (NSAIDs), corticosteroids and immunosuppressants, have been used for patients with Crohn's diseases and its perianal complications and extraintestinal manifestations (in particularly, peripheral arthritis).

Thus, therapy with Budenofalk® and NSAIDs is beneficial for perianal complications and extraintestinal manifestations of young patients with Crohn's disease.

P10
Myositis associated with Crohn's disease

M. PERSIC and I. SLAVIC

University of Rijeka, Clinical Hospital Centre Rijeka, Children's Hospital "Kantrida" Istarska 43, HR-51000 Rijeka, Croatia; Tel/fax. +38551659157; E-mail: irena_slavic@yahoo.com

---

A 13-year-old boy was admitted to hospital due to abdominal pain, diarrhoea, mild elevation of body temperature, arthralgia, myalgia and weight loss (10 kg in 3 months). Arthralgia and elevation of body temperature had occasionally been present for two years and some laboratory investigations had been performed previously because two family members had systemic lupus erythematosus. We confirmed Crohn's disease and elevated creatine phosphokinase with abnormal changes in electromyography. Due to the clinical manifestations, family history and skin manifestations (mild macular rash on thorax and extremities, facial erythema), there was a high level of suspicion for juvenile dermatomyositis and polymyositis although specific antibody and muscle biopsy tests were normal. Some symptoms responded to therapy with 5-aminosalicylic acid (intestinal symptoms, normalization of creatine phosphokinase), but myalgia and muscle weakness remain so further clinical and laboratory follow-up is indicated. Although rare, myositis or juvenile dermatomyositis and polymyositis should be included in the differential diagnosis of muscle weakness in patients with inflammatory bowel disease.

P11
Interstitial nephritis in a girl with Crohn's disease: a rare complication of mesalazine therapy

D. MÜHLBAUER, T. SAUERWALD and S. KOLETZKO

Dr. v. Haunersches Kinderspital, University of Munich

Introduction: The use of mesalazine in the treatment of chronic inflammatory bowel disease is well established and, in most cases, tolerated without severe side-effects. However, renal complications have been reported.

Case: A 13-year-old-girl with a 3-year history of long segment ileal Crohn's disease was treated with mesalazine (up to 50 mg/kg per day, depending on the activity of the disease) and budesonide, 3 mg/d. Two years after mesalazine was started, the child presented with malaise, elevated serum creatinine (2.0 mg/dl, normal <1.0), blood urea (53.2 mg/dl, normal <45), and ESR (35 mm/h). Urine analysis revealed the presence of protein (146 mg/dl, normal <15), haemoglobin, granular casts and renal epithelial cells. Sonography showed normal-shaped kidneys with bilateral increased density of the parenchyma, indicating an interstitial nephritis. Mesalazine therapy was discontinued and a daily fluid intake of at least 2.5 L recommended. No immunosuppressive therapy was initiated, but budesonide, 3 mg/d, was continued. After 8 weeks, the girl felt perfectly well, had gained 4 kg body weight, ERS was 6 mm/h, serum creatinine levels had almost normalized (1.1 mg/dl), and urine analysis was normal. Blood pressure was always normal.

Conclusions: Patients with IBD on mesalazine therapy should be closely monitored for serum creatinine levels and urine analysis. When renal impairment is diagnosed, early withdrawal of mesalazine may result in complete recovery. However, long-term impairment leading to renal insufficiency has been reported.

P12
Safety of the *Boswellia serrata* extract H15 – Long-term observation over 6 years

P. G. BUVARI, F. C. SEIFERT and H. GERHARDT

University Hospital Mannheim (Director Prof. Dr. med. D.L. Heene), Faculty for Clinical Medicine Mannheim of the Heidelberg University, Outpatient Clinic for Crohn's disease and Ulcerative Colitis

---

Introduction: Inhibition of 5-lipoxygenase with boswellic acids of the *Boswellia serrata* extract H15 can be shown in *in-vitro* experiments. A large number of single case studies within six years since 1993 have confirmed the assumption of the efficacy of this therapeutic approach in inflammatory bowel diseases. Data indicate that 5-lipoxygenase inhibition can be part of a rational therapy in these diseases.

Patients and methods: Over a period of six years (1993–1999), an investigation was carried out with 2057 patients taking H15 medication. During treatment, blood test results were documented for varying observation periods (median 8 months; range 0.5–60). Nine hundred and eighty-two patients took H15 as their sole therapy with individually adapted daily doses (1–20 tbl/d).

Results: Blood test results before beginning therapy and results at the end of the investigation show no significant differences from normal values that could indicate any toxic or other unwelcome effects. No indications for liver or nephrotoxic effects were found.

Discussion: The approval of safety of this investigation, even in long-term use, underlines the results of the latest 8-week clinical trial that could show the efficacy and safety of H15 therapy compared with mesalazine. The former traditional remedy of the ancient Ayurvedic medicine develops, through this further investigation, to a rational phytotherapeutic treatment.

P13
Anti-TNF-α combined with azathioprine in children with Crohn's disease

V. N. PERISIC

University Children's Hospital, 10 Tirsova Str, YU-11000 Belgrade, Serbia, Yugoslavia

Introduction: The aim of this study was to determine the efficacy of a new modality of treatment of paediatric Crohn's disease (CD) which is composed of a 3-dose course of anti-TNF-α (infliximab) intially combined with parallel continuous Imuran medication.

Methods and results: Two girls aged 11 and 15 years entered this pilot study. The diagnosis of CD was based on ileo-colonoscopy, mucosal histology, and upper GI series. The CD activity index was determined in each case. The first patient had ileo-caecal CD, the second Crohn's colitis of the sidmoid colon. CD was >250 in each case.

Both girls received infliximab 5 mg/kg at the start, then after 12 and 24 weeks. From the beginning, they were receiving Imuran 2 mg/kg daily plus Salofalk tablets 500 mg t.i.d. In both girls, follow-up ileocolonoscopy was performed after 24 weeks.

In both patients, after the first dose of infliximab, resolution of the symptoms occurred between the fifth and fourteen day. CD decreased to <150 in the third week. After the 24th week, ileo-colonoscopy demonstrated CD remission. During the follow-up period of 24 months, the second girl with Crohn's sigmoid colitis experienced a mild relapse on the same site documented by endoscopy. Quick amelioration of the symptoms with normalization of CD activity index was achieved with one Infliximab dose.

Conclusion: This preliminary report indicates that CD immunomodulatory protocol with anti-TNF-α and Imuran is of almost equal efficacy to regimens which include steroids. This protocol seems to be of great importance in teenage CD patients due to steroid unfavourable effects on growth and sexual developments of adolescents.

P14
Gastrointestinal infections in childhood inflammatory bowel disease – diagnostic and therapeutic dilemma

S. BUDERUS, L. BINDL, F.M. RÜMMELE and M.J. LENTZE

University Children's Medical Center, D-53113 Bonn, Germany

Introduction: Gastrointestinal infections are common especially in childhood. We report on two boys with ulcerative colitis in whom diagnosis and treatment of the disease was complicated by Salmonella and CMV.

Patient 1: A 12-year-old boy was referred because of protracted diarrhoea and elevated ESR. Physical examination was normal. Ultrasound revealed thickening of the ileo-caecal wall and mesenteric lymphadenopathy. Stool cultures were positive for Salmonella. Lactulose and Lactobacillus GG decreased stool frequency; cultures remained unchanged. At colonoscopy there was pancolitis with several caecal ulcerations. Biopsies demonstrated features of inflammatory and of infectious bowel disease. Treatment with ciprofloxacin and sulphasalazine resulted in normalization of stool frequency, ESR and elimination of Salmonella. Biopsies of re-colonoscopy were compatible with ulcerative colitis.

Patient 2: A 12-year-old boy had suffered from bloody diarrhoea for 4 weeks. Endoscopically and histologically ulcerative colitis was diagnosed. The patient responded to sulphasalazine and metronidazole. After termination of the antibiotic he developed 5-aminosalicilate intolerance. Therapy was switched to prednisolone but, because of a relapse, cyclosporine was added. After short-term response, the patient deteriorated. Now, CMV was positive on histology, viral culture and PCR from blood. Immunosuppressive therapy was decreased and ganciclovir was initiated. After CMV eradication, the patient was treated successfully with azathioprine and low-dose prednisolone.

Conclusion: These case reports stress the importance of monitoring infectious agents in the diagnosis and long-term treatment of inflammatory bowel disease. Besides stool cultures, endoscopy with histology and culturing of biopsies, and PCR techniques may be needed.

P15
Observation of ulcerative colitis in children under the age of three

E. G. TSIMBALOVA, A. S. POTAPOV, P. L. SCHERBAKOV and B. S. KAGANOV

Department Gastroenterology and Hepatology, Research Center of Children's Health, Moscow, Russia

---

Ulcerative colitis is a rare autoimmune disease, which starts most often at the age of 12–14 years.

Aim: To present the observation of ulcerative colitis in children of early age.

Methods: Three children with ulcerative colitis before the age of 3 were observed for 2 years. Evaluation included clinical and laboratory methods, colonoscopy and histological examination of biopsy specimens of the large intestine.

Results: All the children had diarrhoea from birth. Blood appeared in their stool for the first time at the age of 1.5–1.9 years. The duration of the disease before admittance to the clinic was 6–8 months. The children's condition was moderate; abdominal pains were absent. Observations included paleness of the skin, bulging of the stomach and hepatomegaly. The stool was liquid, mixed with up to 20–30 ml blood. The blood analysis showed: a decrease in haemoglobin, up to 66 g/L, and iron, up to 5.5 μmol/L, leucocytosis, up to 20×10^9/L, an increase in sedimentation rate, up to 20 mm/h, and decrease in proteins, up to 50 g/L. One child had an increase in transaminases, up to 10 quotas, GGT up to 5 quotas. Colonoscopy: all the children had oedema and hyperaemia mucous, 2 children had ulcers and erosions. Inflammation was detected in distal parts and was absent in the rectum. Histological examination of biopsy specimens of the large intestine showed increases in goblet cells, neuthrophilic infiltration and crypt abscesses. All the children received Salofalk, 30 mg/kg per day for 1 month, then a maintenance dose of 10 mg/kg per day for 3 months. In addition, one child received prednisolone 3 mg/kg per day. All the children had complete remission after 1–2 weeks from the start of treatment which remained stable for 2 years.

Conclusion: Infrequency of ulcerative colitis at early age causes difficulties in diagnosis. Salofalk treatment resulted in remission for 2 years.

P16
Cyclosporine-induced coma: rare complication in treatment of autoimmune enteropathy

M. HEIDUK[1], L. CLARA[1], A. FINDEISEN[2] and D. BRETSCHNEIDER[1]

[1]Zentrum für Kinderheilkunde, Otto-von-Guericke-Universität Magdeburg, Wiener Straße, D- 39112 Magdeburg;
[2]Ernst–Moritz–Arndt–Universität Greifswald

The use of cyclosporin A (CsA) is associated with neurotoxic side-effects in up to 40% of patients, including tremor, posterior leukoencephalopathy, seizures and others. There are only a few reports of coma during CsA therapy in patients with primary immune related disorders.

We report the case of a $4\frac{1}{2}$-year-old girl with severe steatorrhoea, flatulence, failure to thrive and signs of malabsorption. Autoimmune enteropathy was diagnosed and initial therapy with azathioprine and prednisolone was ineffective. Therefore, we started with CsA, supported by methylprednisolone pulse therapy for 6 months. After 4 days of intravenous CsA, the girl fell into a coma which required mechanical ventilation. No causes of coma were found on laboratory investigations, EEG, chest X-ray and MRI. The CsA levels in the blood (158.6 ng/ml) and liquor (0 ng/ml) were normal. The CsA level on the day before had been 57.9 ng/ml. After cessation of CsA consciousness returned within a few hours.

Cofactors of coma in our patient may be hypertension (up to 168/100 mmHg) under therapy with methylprednisolone or the rapid increase in CsA level during intravenous therapy. Rechallenge at a lower oral dose of CsA was well tolerated.

Low cholesterol and magnesium blood levels are found in some patients with CsA neurotoxicity. In our patient, we did not measure these parameters during the coma, but, a few days before and after coma, the magnesium level was decreased.

We conclude, after exclusion of other causes, that the coma in our patient was a rare complication of CsA therapy. We assume that hypertension and hypomagnesaemia were cofactors. In CsA therapy, monitoring and correction of blood pressure, magnesium and cholesterol levels may prevent neurotoxicity.

P17
Lymphocytic colitis in a patient with coeliac disease. A case report

J. UTESENY and D. KLUSACEK

IInd Department of Pediatrics, University Childrens Hospital Brno

---

Introduction: It has been shown that the frequency of coeliac disease in patients with lymphocytic colitis is increased. However, clinical symptomatology of these patients remains unclear.

Results: We present a case of a 12-year-old boy with spastic diparesis and chronic watery diarrhoea which was refractory to medication with cholestyramine and a milk-protein-free diet. Because of intercurrent febrile virosis, ibuprofen, 20 mg/kg, was administered resulting in disappearance of the diarrhoea within two days of this therapy. In this patient, we found positive HLA Dq heterodimer, positive EMA and tTG; strongly increased total IgE and positive IgE antibody antigliadin and casein. Coeliac disease was diagnosed using enterobiopsy. Colonic biopsy specimens were consistent with lymphocytic colitis. After administration of mesalazine, diarrhoea disappeared within 3 days.

Conclusion: The question remains: what is the relationship between these two diseases entities.

P18
Hepatobiliary complications of inflammatory bowel diseases in children and adolescents

M. GEORGIEVA-SHAKOLA, V. TZANEVA, I. RUSSEVA, M. POPOVA and D. PAVLOVA

Dept. of Pediatrics, Medical University, Varna, Bulgaria

In a high percentage of cases, other organs produce different symptoms and mask inflammatory bowel disease (IBD). An exact diagnosis reveals hepatobiliary abnormalities. This was a retrospective study and its aim was to reveal hepatobiliary complications in children and adolescents with IBD. In 1987– 2001, we had 15 patients with IBD: 8 ulcerative colitis (UC), 6 Crohn's disease (CD) and 1 indeterminate colitis (IC) (mean age 12.3 years). They were investigated clinically by laboratory and microbiological (stool culture) examinations, barium radiography, lower endoscopy with histology, ultrasonography, spiral scan, flow cytometry or by operation. Ten of them had abnormalities of liver and/or gallbladder: fatty liver – 10/15 (5 UC, 5 CD), gallstone disease – 3/15 (3 CD), pericholangitis – 1/15 (1 CD), biliary cirrhosis – 1/15 (1 CD), autoimmune chronic hepatitis – 1/15 (1/15). Autoimmune abnormalities were treated by prednisone 2 mg/kg per day, gallstone disease by ursodeoxycholic acid (Ursofalk 15 mg/kg per day; 1 case) or stone extraction (2 cases). One of the patients (biliary cirrhosis) died. In conclusion, hepatobiliary complications are common in children and adolescents with IBD. Autoimmune abnormalities are severe, difficult to treat and have a bad prognosis.

P19
Indications for surgery of ulcerative colitis in children

V. KOPEIKIN, E. FEDULOVA, S. ABRAMOV and A. DIKUSHIN

Research Institute of Children Gastroenterology, Nizhny Novgorod, Russia

Nowadays, ulcerative colitis (UC) in children is characterized by early development of extraintestinal manifestations, invalidism and resistance to traditional therapy. UC treatment including (besides 5-ACK preparations) hormonal and cytostatic remedies allows the doctor – according to R. Cohen *et al.* (1999) – to make time for a 'planned' colectomy.

The aim of this study was to reveal clinical parameters of unsuccessful conservative treatment and indications for UC surgery in children.

The course of UC in 24 patients aged 3–15 years was analysed. Twelve children had a continuous progressive course of disease, resistant to 5-ACK and hormonal therapy; that is why subtotal colectomy was performed. Another group of 12 patients treated by 5-ACK had remissions lasting from 3 to 6–12 months.

By factor analysis, we chose 13 parameters: premorbid background, age, character of onset, course of disease, severity, duration, causes of exacerbations, presence of extraintestinal manifestations (EIM), clinical and endoscopic activity indexes (CAI, EAI according to Rachmilevich, 1989 in our modification), and presence of pseudopolyposis. In the first group of patients, we chose 3 main factors pointing to the surgical necessity. The first factor, 'aggressiveness' of the disease course, includes acute onset, high CAI in exacerbation periods and EIM. The second factor, indicating the chronic character of process, includes duration of disease over 5 years, persistent high EAI and pseudopolyposis. The third factor, aetiopathogenetic, indicates the absence of evident reasons for UC and subsequent UC exacerbations.

To compare, we chose 3 determining factors: the first factor: medium degree of severity and absence of EIM; the second factor: moderate degree of process activity ($CAI < 10$, $EAI < 10$); the third factor: short duration (up to 3 years) and gradual character of the disease. In CAI, increasing stool frequency and worsening indexes of general state are the most significant indications for surgery.

In EAI, a large part (in comparison with children treated successfully by 5-ACK) is contact bleeding. To determine the necessity for operation, we should estimate the degree of wall echogenic increase in transabdominal ultrasound examination, and the degree coincides with the depth of destructive sclerotic changes in intestine wall; these changes we observe in biopsy material and then in surgical material.

Thus, the complex of clinical data – acute onset, high CAI, EAI, presence of extraintestinal manifestations, pseudopolyposis and vague causes of disease manifestation and/or its exacerbation, in combination with high level of echogenicity of intestinal wall on ultrasound examination – are the indicators for planned surgery of patients with ulcerative colitis.

P20
How long does it take to diagnose ulcerative colitis in children and adolescents?

M. DICULESCU, M. CIOCIRLAN, M. IONESCU, O. PAPUC, T. ARBANAS and C. CIORA

Fundeni Gastroenterology and Hepatology Center, Bucharest

Background: Ulcerative colitis (UC) is one of the most important chronic diseases afflicting children and adolescents. Many of the characteristics of UC are similar in adults and children. There are, however, a number of aspects that are unique to the paediatric population. The purpose of this study was to identify those features.

Method: A case–control study has been made. The test group consisted of 25 children and adolescents (under 18 years old) diagnosed with UC. The matched control group was 50 adult patients (over 18 years old) with UC.

Results: At the inaugural episode of ulcerative colitis, time to diagnosis – measured from the moment when complaints started until a positive diagnosis had been made – was recorded. Median values were: test group 2 months, control group 1 month. A time to diagnosis of longer than 1 month significantly correlates with children and adolescents with UC (OR = 5.12, p = 0.002). The presence of intestinal parasites (*Giardia lamblia*, *Ascaris lumbricoides*), finding and treating them during this period of time is associated with the UC inaugural episode in children and adolescents (OR = 11.67, p = 0.01).

Conclusions: The time to diagnosis from the beginning of clinical manifestations of ulcerative colitis in the paediatric population tends to be higher than in adults. The presence of intestinal parasites might be responsible for this delay in diagnosis.

P21
Associated parasitic infection delays early diagnosis of Crohn's disease in paediatric population?

M. CIOCIRLAN, M. IONESCU, O. PAPUC, T. ARBANAS, C. CIORA and M. DICULESCU

Fundeni Gastroenterology and Hepatology Center, Bucharest

Background: Sometimes the age of the patient produces considerable particularities regarding presentation and course of the disease. The objective of this study was to find significant differences between the paediatric and adult populations with Crohn's disease (CD).

Method: An investigation (case–control study) has been made. The test group included 19 children and adolescents, less than 18 years old, diagnosed with CD and the control group had 38 adult CD matched patients (over 18 years old).

Results: At the inaugural episode of CD, time to diagnosis – measured from the moment when symptoms started until a positive diagnosis was made – was recorded Median values were: 10 months for the test group, 3 months for the control group. A time to diagnosis longer than 12 months significantly correlates with the children and adolescents group with CD (OR = 4.94, $p = 0.028$). The presence of intestinal parasites (*Giardia lamblia, Ascaris lumbricoides*) diagnosed in this period of time and treatment for these infections are more frequently found associated with the CD inaugural episode in children and adolescents (OR = 13.37, $p = 0.01$).

Conclusions: Time passed from the beginning of clinical manifestations to diagnosis of CD in the paediatric population tends to be higher than in adults. One possible explanation is the presence of intestinal parasites considered responsible for symptoms.

P22
National data on inflammatory bowel disease in children in Lithuania

V. URBONAS

Vilnius University Children's Hospital Centre for Paediatrics

Background: The expectations behind epidemiological studies are that they will be able to provide information on the aetiology and pathogenesis of a disease. Epidemiological studies have shown an increased incidence of paediatric inflammatory bowel diseases (IBD) during recent decades. Crohn's disease (CD) has become more prevalent than ulcerative colitis (UC) in US, Canada, UK, Sweden. There is a lack of such data from the East Europe countries.
Aim: To study the incidence of IBD (UC, CD) over a four-year period in Lithuania.
Methods: During 1997 to 2000, we analysed data to identify newly diagnosed cases of IBD from the Statistical Department of Lithuanian Ministry of Health. Paediatric gastroenterologists, paediatricians and surgeons presented the data. The age of the children was from 0 to 14 years old.

Results:

	Mean	*2000*	*1999*	*1998*	*1997*
CD Number	2	3	2	1	2
Per 100000 children	0.27	0.4	0.27	0.13	0.26
UC Number	15.5	19	14	16	23
Per 100000 children	2.1	2.6	1.9	1.4	2.3
CD/UC ratio	0.13	0.15	0.14	0.09	0.11
Total number of children (0–14 years)	753675	731000	742300	762200	779200

Conclusions: 1. The incidence of UC in Lithuanian children is similar to the northern Stockholm (1) data. 2. The incidence of CD and the ratio between CD and UC is very low.

Reference: 1. Hildebrand H *et al.* Abstract book. 34th Annual Meeting of ESPGHAN, Geneva 2001; p35.

P23
How age influences lesion topography and symptoms in Crohn's disease inaugural episode

M. IONESCU, M. CIOCIRLAN, O. PAPUC, T. ARBANAS, C. CIORA and M. DICULESCU

Fundeni Gastroenterology and Hepatology Center, Bucharest

Background: The objective of this study was to find significant differences between paediatric and adult populations with Crohn's disease (CD).

Method: A case–control study was made. The test group was 19 children and adolescents with CD less than 18 years old, and the control group was 38 adult CD-matched patients (over 18 years old). The severity of the first episode was assessed using the Crohn's Disease Activity Index scale.

Results: At the first episode of CD, a difference between the ideal weight and the actual weight of over 10% is more frequently found in adults (odds ratio (OR) = 6.46, $p = 0.005$). Positive correlations for children and adolescents: rectal involvement (OR = 3.76, $p = 0.03$), fever at first episode with involvement of caecum and ascending colon (OR = 5.22, $p = 0.03$) and also transverse colon involvement (OR = 5.42, $p = 0.003$). No differences were found concerning the number of liquid stools, grade of abdominal pain, general status, and other bowel involvement sites.

Conclusions: Nutritional impact is higher and the rectum is more frequently involved in the paediatric population with CD at the inaugural episode. Some colon involvement sites are associated with fever in adults with CD at first episode. No difference in severity at first episode was found.

P24
Activity index in administering the treatment in ulcerative colitis in children

E. FEDULOVA and V. KOPEIKIN

Research Institute of Children Gastroenterology, Nizhny Novgorod, Russia

---

Aim: To increase the effectiveness of non-specific ulcerative colitis (UC) therapy in children by individual administration of medication on the basis of activity index development.

Methods: We analysed the cases of 32 children aged 3–16 years with UC during their first hospitalization in SRICG (Scientific Research Institute of Children Gastroenterology). Basic therapy (BT) of 5-aminosalicylic acid preparations was administered to all children. Seventeen patients showed a good therapeutic effect. Since 15 children did not show any clinical improvement within 30 days, hormonal therapy (HT) with prednisolone was administered.

We made a factor analysis of 87 clinical and laboratory parameters characterizing the child's condition and chose 13 as the most significant factors. These included: asthenovegetative, dyspeptic syndrome, the degree of trophic disorders, stool frequency, the presence of blood in stool, ESR, haemoglobin, white blood cells, relating to stab neutrophile shift in leukocytic blood count, coprogramme, level L2 and γ-globulin.

The chosen factors were assessed on a scale from 1 to 5; on this basis, we obtained a total activity index (AI), which was calculated when admitting the children, administering HT and on discharging them from the hospital. Moreover, we calculated the AI decrease in groups of patients receiving different therapeutic procedures.

Results: We found that the initial AI in the group of children with BT only (1st group) averaged 30.4 ± 5.6; and, in patients with HT (2nd group), 30 ± 9. So, the initial AI value at initial hospitalization in both groups did not differ significantly. Dynamic observations showed a more essential difference in AI decrease speed. In children of the 1st group, this value was 0.3 per day. Besides, in children taking Salofalk, AI decrease speed was higher than in children taking sulphasalazine. In the 2nd group, before HT was administered, AI decrease speed averaged 0.05 per day, and, after glucocorticoid administration, it increased up to 0.25. Therefore, slow dynamics of improvement of the chosen clinical and laboratory parameters is a convincing criterion for HT administration.

Conclusions: Thus, a quantitative approach to parameters, which were considered particularly qualitative formerly, makes it possible to change in good time the tactics of conservative treatment, reducing the period necessary for eradication of UC exacerbation.

P25
The significance of the assessment of anti-rabbit asialoglycoprotein receptor (ASGPR) antibodies in the diagnosis of autoimmune hepatitis (AIH) in children

P. DEDEK[1], J. HAVLASOVÁ[2] and O. POZLER[1]

[1]Department of Pediatrics, [2]Department of Clinical Immunology and Allergy, Teaching Hospital, Hradec Králové, Czech Republic

---

Introduction: Anti-ASGPR antibodies are considered to be very useful in the diagnosis of AIH.

Aim: To evaluate the significance of anti-rabbit ASGPR antibody determination in the diagnosis of AIH in children.

Patients and methods: Four study groups were selected for analyses:
Group I – 6 children with AIH before the beginning of treatment.
Group II – 22 children with other defined non-autoimmune liver diseases.
Group III – 22 healthy children.
Group IV – 20 healthy adults.
Antibodies were detected by Medizym anti-rabbit ASGPR ELISA (Medipan Diagnostica, Germany). The results were presented by means of the binding index (BI). A BI<0.9 was negative; BI>1.1 was positive. The Mann–Whitney test was used for statistical analysis.

Results: In these groups, statistically significant differences were found between groups I and III ($p < 0.05$), I and IV ($p = 0.003$), II and III ($p = 0.002$), and II and IV ($p < 0.001$). There was no statistically proven significant difference between groups I and II.

Conclusion: We proved stastistically higher levels of anti-rabbit ASGPR antibodies in patients with AIH before treatment in comparison with healthy children and adults. However, we did not manage to prove the significance of the assessment of these antibodies for differential diagnosis of AIH. There was no statistically significant difference between patients with AIH and non-autoimmune liver diseases.

P26
Serological markers of autoimmunity in chronic infections with hepatitis B virus in children

S. BEZNA, M. BEZNA, P. CIUREA and T. CIUREA

University of Medicine and Pharmacology Craiova, Str. Nicolae Balcescu Nr.12 1100 Craiova, Romania

---

Chronic infections with hepatitis viruses are frequently associated with autoimmune diseases or serological markers of autoimmunity.

We are interested in the exact determination of the relationship between chronic viral hepatitis and immune system modifications that lead to viral-induced autoimmunity.

The serological immune manifestations were studied by analysing the serum levels of immunoglobulins, C3 component of complement, and prevalence of antinuclear antibodies, anti-DNA autoantibodies and rheumatoid factor.

In this study, we investigated 21 children with chronic hepatitis B. Their ages were between 3 and 16 years.

Serological markers of autoimmunity were detected in 5 of these 21 patients. In one patient, the presence of antinuclear antibodies was due to the interferon treatment. Interferon is the main treatment for chronic viral hepatitis and the study of serological markers of autoimmunity represents a necessity for immunostimulant treatment.

P27
Aetiological structure of chronic liver disease in children in Moscow

B. KAGANOV, Z. ZAINUDINOV, O. BUKANOVICH, T. STROKOVA and A. POTAPOV

Department of Gastroenterology and Hepatology, Research Center of Children's Health, Moscow, Russia

---

Investigation of the aetiological structure and natural history of chronic liver disease is a very real problem in modern hepatology.

Aim: To determine the aetiological structure and severity of chronic liver disease in patients of the Paediatric Gastroenterology Department in Moscow in 2000.

Methods: All patients were evaluated using blood chemistry, serology, polymerase chain reaction, ultrasonography and liver biopsy.

Results: 172 patients were evaluated: chronic hepatitis B was revealed in 48 (27.9%) (including 1 patient with cirrhosis); chronic hepatitis C in 32 (18.6%) (including 1 with cirrhosis); chronic hepatitis B+C in 5 (2.9%); chronic hepatitis D in 6 (3.5%) (including 4 with cirrhosis); autoimmune hepatitis in 14 (8.1%) (8 with cirrhosis); Wilson disease in 11 (6.4%) (4 with cirrhosis); glycogen-storage disease in 22 (12.8%); drug-induced hepatitis in 2 (1.2%); cryptogenic liver disease in 8 (4.7%); and other hepatobiliary diseases in 24 (14%).

Conclusions: According to data from the Paediatric Gastroenterology Department, viral hepatitis, especially HBV (27.9%), is the leading cause of chronic liver diseases in children. End-stage liver disease is more often revealed in patients with autoimmune hepatitis (in 57.1% revealed cirrhosis of the liver). Drug-induced liver disease is rarely encountered in children (1.2%).

P28
Morphofunctional state of upper gastrointestinal tract in children with chronic autoimmune hepatitis

S. SARALOV, V. KOPEIKIN and B. ASSONOV

Research Institute of Children's Gastroenterology, Nizhni Novgorod, Russia

---

Eleven children (10 girls and a boy) aged 8–16 years with a chronic autoimmune hepatitis were surveyed. During treatment, all children received corticosteroids. The control group included 10 children (4 boys and 6 girls) aged 10–14 years with chronic non-autoimmune hepatitis, who also were given prednisolone.

All children had an endoscopy of the upper gastrointestinal tract (UGIT) and gastric acid was estimated.

Results: In all children with autoimmune hepatitis, there were pathological changes of UGIT mucus: one girl had varicose phlebectasia of the oesophagus distal region (1st degree.). The mucous inflammation revealed in all children of this group was of a widespread character and was localized in the gastroduodenal zone, and 5 children had symptoms of distal oesophagitis. In seven patients (63.6%), flat erosions of the antral part of the stomach were determined.

In the control group, pathological changes of UGIT mucus were revealed in 70% of cases only. Two patients had varicose phlebectasia of the oesophagus. Three children had pangastritis, 40% antral gastritis, 30% gastroduodenitis. Two children (20%) had flat erosions in the antrum.

In 10 children (90.9%) with an autoimmune hepatitis, high acid production of the gastric mucus with a disorder of the alkalizing function of the antral region was revealed. In the control group, only four children (40%) had these disorders.

Conclusions: Children with an autoimmune hepatitis have marked morphofunctional changes of upper gastrointestinal tract mucus. Examination of patients with this disease should include UGIT endoscopy and estimation of acid-production gastric function to correct the revealed disorder.

P29
Indications for liver transplantation in children

Z. ZAINUDINOV[1], S. GAUTIER[2], O. TCHIRULNIKOVA[2], B. KAGANOV[1], O. BUKANOVICH[1], O. GUNDOBINA[1] and A. POTAPOV[1]

[1]Research Center of Children's Health, [2]Research Center of Surgery, Moscow, Russia

---

End-stage liver disease of various origins is a direct indication for liver transplantation. Taking into consideration lack of donor organs and unsettled law problems of paediatric transplantation in Russia (cadaveric organ donation in children is prohibited in Russia), living related liver transplantation has become the therapeutic option for end-stage liver disease in children.

Aim: To determine the need for liver transplantation in patients of the Pediatric Gastroenterology Department in Moscow during 2000.

Methods: All patients were evaluated using blood chemistry, serology, polymerase chain reaction, ultrasonography and liver biopsy.

Results: In 15.7% cases cirrhosis of the liver was revealed (27/172). The aetiological structure of cirrhosis follows: HBV – 1 patient, HCV – 1, HDV – 4, AIH – 8, WD – 4, Budd–Chiari syndrome – 2, α_1-antitripsin deficiency – 1 and cryptogenic liver disease – 6. The mean age of patients with cirrhosis was 12.6 ± 1.1 years. In 6 cases, contraindications for orthotopic living related liver transplantation were revealed – replicative phase of HCV, HBV and HDV. Seven patients (5 – WD, 1 – AIH and 1 – α_1-antitrypsin deficiency) were included on a waiting list. In 3 patients (2 – WD, 1 – α_1-AT) OLT was successfully performed. Eleven patients were not listed due to various medical and social reasons (lack of appropriate donor by ABO system, compensated liver disease etc.). In 1 child, the parents refused liver transplantation for religious reasons. One girl of 13 years old with autoimmune liver cirrhosis died before transplantation from hepatic decompensation.

Conclusions: In our Pediatric Gastroenterology Department during 2000, 15.7% (27/172) cases of chronic liver disease had cirrhosis of the liver, which is an indication for OLT. In 3 cases liver transplantation was performed; 1 patient died before transplantation.

P30
Zinc increases viability of fetal liver cells during oxidative stress

V. BARAN and A. DAVIDOVSKY*

Belarussian State Medical University, Institute of Physiology, National Academy of the Sciences of Belarus, Minsk, Belarus.
**E-mail: biblio@fizio.bas-net.by*

The effects of zinc (Zn^{2+}) concentrations from 10^{-4} to 10^{-12} mol/L were investigated. Zn^{2+} concentrations from 10^{-5} to 10^{-9} mol/L decreased lipid peroxidation (LPO) and increased lipid reserve for peroxidation (LRP) from 15% to 67%. Zn^{2+} in concentrations from 10^{-5} to 10^{-8} mol/L raised the viability of fetal hepatocytes from 1.3 to 4.7 times during oxidative stress induced by Fenton reagent, containing H_2O_2 and Fe^{2+}. Thus Zn^{2+} has hepatoprotective properties. Moreover, Zn^{2+} in a broad concentration range may modify Ursofalk and purine receptor agonists effects on free radical oxidation in cytoplasm membranes of rat and human fetal hepatocytes. Thus, Zn^{2+}-containing drugs may be effective tools to increase the viability of fetal liver cells from oxidative stress in viral and autoimmune hepatitis, hypoxia, xenobiotic action and transplantation of fetal hepatocytes.

P31
Autoimmune hepatitis in the chronic course of HAV infection

T. WOZNIAKOWSKA-GESICKA, J. KUPS and M. WISNIEWSKA-LIGIER

IIIrd Department of Paediatrics Polish Mother's Memorial Hospital, Research Institute, Lodz, Rzgowska 281/289 street, 93-338 Lodz, Poland

---

In this paper, we present the case of a 13-year-old girl with type 1 autoimmune hepatitis in whom biochemical, serological and histopathological parameters of chronic hepatitis caused by virus A in last 2 years were observed. The diagnosis was based on increased γ-globulin levels and IgG levels and the presence of autoantibodies and was confirmed by the presence of anti-HAV IgM in serum. First, the patient was treated by steroids given by the pulse method for 5 months, and next, because improvement was not observed, continuous steroid therapy for next 5 months. After this period, clinical and biochemical remission and loss of HAV antibodies of the class IgM were observed. In the follow-up, when sustained steroid therapy was given, a clinical and biochemical exacerbation of the disease was observed, accompanied by anti-HAV IgM and insignificant intensification of the autoimmune process parameters.

This case suggests that HAV infection may cause chronic hepatitis and autoimmunological reaction.

P32
The role of AKT, a proliferative factor in transforming inflammation to liver fibrosis

R. SHIMON, D. BRENNER and R. RIPPE

Dept of Pediatrics, Tel Aviv Medical Center, Israel, and Department of Digestive Diseases, UNC Chapel Hill, UA

Background: Following an inflammatory stimulus, the hepatic stellate cell (HSC) undergoes a complex activation process. Increased cell proliferation and excess deposition of extracellular matrix (ECM) proteins are characteristic of HSC activation. Our laboratory has shown that PDGF, a potent proliferative cytokine for HSCs, activates and requires focal adhesion kinase and phosphoinositol 3-kinase (PI3-K) for HSC proliferation. AKT, a protein kinase, is activated by phosphorylation following growth factor stimulation in several cell types in a PI3-K-dependent manner. Increased cell proliferation and anti-apoptotic proterties are associated with AKT activation. TNF-α can also lead to AKT phosphorylation leading to NFκB activation.

Aim: The aim of this study was to investigate the role of AKT in HSC proliferation.

Methods: To assess the role of AKT in growth factor-induced HSC proliferation, rat HSCs were isolated and culture activated. Cells were transduced with Ad5myrAKT (a constitutively activated AKT), Ad5dnAKT (a dominant negative AKT), or Ad5LacZ as an adenovirus control. Transduction efficiency was determined by immunochemistry. HSC proliferation was assessed using ^{3}H-thymidine incorporation following treatment with 10% serum or 20 ng/ml PDGF-BB. Total and phosphorylated AKT protein levels were assessed by Western blot analysis. The effects of TNF-α on AKT phosphorylation and TGF-β on PDGF-stimulated AKT phosphorylation were also assessed.

Results: Ad5myrAKT stimulated HSC proliferation approximately 2.5-fold in serum-starved HSCs while Ad5dnAKT inhibited serum-induced proliferation nearly 3-fold. Following serum starvation, both serum and PDGF rapidly induced AKT phosphorylation within 10 min. Serum and PDGF-induced AKT phosphorylation was completely inhibited by pretreating the cells with 25 μmol/L LY294002, an inhibitor of PI3-K, without affecting total AKT protein levels. TGF-β, an inhibitor of HSC proliferation, did not activate AKT, but, more importantly, did not block PDGF-induced AKT phosphorylation suggesting that TGF-β mediates its antiproliferative effect downstream of AKT. Similar to vascular smooth muscle cells, but unlike endothelial cells, treatment of HSCs with 10 ng/ml TNF-α failed to induce AKT phosphorylation.

Conclusion: AKT is important for growth factor-stimulated HSC proliferation and is positioned downstream of PI3-K. Therefore, AKT may represent a potential therapeutic target to inhibit HSC proliferation and subsequent ECM deposition during fibrosis.

P33
Autoantibodies in patients with clinical suspicion of coeliac disease

L. GÜRTLER

St Cyril and Method Hospital, Dept. of Clinical Immunology, Bratislava, Slovakia

---

Objective: To assess results of detected autoantibodies in patients with clinical suspicion of coeliac disease (CD).

Methods: Prospective evaluation and analyses were made in the period of October 1998 to September 2000. Serum samples (895) diluted 1 : 20, were evaluated on monkey oesophagus for IgA endomysial antibody (EmA) by indirect immunofluorescence (IF). Anti-gliadin (AGA) IgA, IgG, anti-transglutaminase (anti-tTG) IgA and anti-endomysium IgA were detected by ELISA.

Results: 64/895 (7.1%) sera were EmA, and 72/895 (8.0%) smooth muscle (SMA) positive; 48 of 879 (5.4%) patients had EmA. Out of 461 sera 80.9% were negative (8.5% positive) against both AGA IgA and EmA. 5.4% of sera were EmA positive but AGA IgA negative, and 5.2% were AGA IgA positive but EmA negative. A comparison between AGA IgG and IgA showed that, out of 84 sera, 64 were negative to both (14 were positive to both). Detection of EmA showed that, out of 46 sera, 6 were negative by ELISA but positive by IF. In the correlation of anti-tTG IgA with EmA, out of 74 sera, 3 were anti-tTG IgA positive but EmA negative, and 5 anti-tTG IgA negative inspite of EmA positivity.

Conclusions: We found EmA in 5.4% of sera. EmA and SMA could have been present at the same time. There were small advantages of IgG AGA over IgA. Anti-gliadin IgA did not correlate with EmA. Some patients had EmA or AGA IgA alone. Anti-tTG IgA correlated with EmA.

P34
The importance of antibodies in the follow-up of coeliac patients

G. JESSERNIGG, U. GORIUP, J. DEUTSCH and G. GRANDITSCH

Aims: To evaluate dietary compliance (DC) and to identify relapses of our coeliac patients in the outpatient department by means of endomysial (EMA) and anti-gliadin (AGA) antibodies.

Patients and methods: 139 coeliac patients were followed for a 2-year period. Patients younger than 1 year were excluded from the study. EMA were assessed by indirect immunofluorescence and AGA by enzyme-linked immunosorbant assay. DC was determined by an accurate dietary history and questioning, and, according to the assessed DC, patients were divided into 7 groups. Jejunal control biopsies were performed in 20 patients.

Results: 32/139 (23%) were positive for EMA, 13/139 (9%) were positive for IgA-AGA, 22/139 (15%) were positive for IgG-AGA. In 96/139 (69%) DC was good, in 16/139 (12%) moderate and in 21/139 (15%) bad; 6/139 (4%) were on gluten challenge. 86% (12/14) of the patients between 0 and 6 years, but only 50% (11/22) of the patients 18 years or older, were on a strict gluten-free diet. DC of 32% (7/22) of the patients 18 years or older was bad.

5/107 of the patients negative for EMA were biopsied because of discordant DC. (One of them showed a flat mucosa.) 15/32 patients positive for EMA were biopsied and the suspected mucosal relapse was confirmed in all of them.

Conclusions: The control of DC requires continuous interdisciplinary medical care, based on accurate dietary history and combined determination of EMA and AGA.

P35
Coeliac disease among children with insulin-dependent diabetes mellitus in the northern coastal part of Croatia

I. SLAVIC, M. PERSIC, K. CVIJOVIC and S. SEVERINSKI

University of Rijeka, Clinical Hospital Centre Rijeka, Children's Hospital "Kantrida" Istarska 43, HR-51000 Rijeka, Croatia; Tel/fax: +38551659157; e-mail: irena_slavic@yahoo.com

---

We investigated the prevalence of coeliac disease among children with insulin-dependent diabetes mellitus (IDDM) in the northern coastal part in Croatia. In our care are 131 children with IDDM; 105 (80%) children were tested for endomysial antibodies (EMA). Seven from them (6.6%) were EMA positive (five boys and two girls) and small bowel biopsy was performed. We have found different degrees of mucosal atrophy. HLA types were characteristic (DR3, DQ2) in four patients. After one year of gluten-free diet, we investigated glycosylated haemoglobin (HbA_{1c}), and percentiles of stature and weight. There was significant difference only in body mass index before and after one year of gluten-free diet ($p = 0.03$). Due to the higher prevalence of coeliac disease among patients with IDDM, these patients should be tested regularly for EMA.

P36

Changes of mucosa of the upper gastrointestinal tract in children with atopic dermatitis

O. NIKANDROVA

Novomoskovsk Children Municipal Hospital, Novomoskovsk, Tula Region, Russia

---

The circulation of autoimmune complexes in blood vessels damages the mucosa of the digestive tube and promotes entering of allergens into the internal environment of the organism. Therefore a state of sensibilization arises and the chronic course of atopic dermatitis appears.

Sixteen children with atopic dermatitis had an endoscopy of the upper gastrointestinal tract (UGIT). In 11 children (68.7%), changes of UGIT mucosa were revealed. These changes were dependent on the age of the patients.

In three of six children of early age examined we found marked distal duodenitis (50%), and, in one child, the change was localized on the antral region of the stomach.

In nine children aged 7–10 years, pathology of gastroduodenal mucus was revealed in 62.5% of cases. In most of these cases (in four patients), marked combined gastric and duodenal lesions were observed; in one boy, only isolated duodenitis.

At endoscopy of two children of senior school age (11–14 years), gastroduodenitis was diagnosed in one girl.

Conclusions:

1. The majority of children with atopic diseases of the skin has changes of the mucosa of the upper gastrointestinal tract
2. In children of early age with allergic skin diseases, isolated mucous lesions of distal regions of duodenum prevail.
3. With increasing age, children suffering from these diseases have excavation and diffusion of pathological process in the upper gastrointestinal tract mucosa.
4. To reveal and treat pathological changes of GUIT mucosa, it is necessary to carry out endoscopy of children with allergic skin manifestations.

P37
Autoimmune components in the damaged mucosa of the stomach of children with yersiniosis

A. V. GORDEETS, S. N. BENIOVA and O. F. SEDULINA

Infections Diseases Clinical Picture, State Medical University, Vladivostok, Russia

---

Morphofunctional differences in the stomach mucosa of children with allergy and chronic HP infection are described.

Structure–functional state of the stomach mucous lining in 86 children with yersiniosis has been studied by us, although they had no dyspeptic complaints previously. Gastrofibroscopy with the special cleansing of the image and morphological valuation of the changes in the bioptates of the stomach mucous lining on the day of hospitalization (the first days of the disease) and after 10 days of the treatment were tested on all patients. The investigations showed an inflammatory character of the changes of the stomach mucous lining. Usually focal superficial, and seldom erosive, gastritis developed in all the patients. Biopsy material was taken from the more changed parts of the stomach mucous lining and was characterized in all yersiniosum patients with neutrophilic emigration in the clear space of the stomach body glands and mononuclear infiltration of the stomach mucous plate. Eosinophilic infiltration was observed, but not often. However, morphofunctional parameters of autoimmunoprocess were revealed in patients with the recurring form of yersiniosis.

Test investigations after 10–12 days of traditional treatment demonstrated minimal clinical yersiniosum manifestations. Epithelization foci were noted visually on the stomach mucous lining; morphologically marked stroma cellular reaction in the proper plate of the mucous membrane.

Opticomorphological changes of the stomach mucous lining, revealed in convalescent patients 12 months after having the illness, but not accompanied with yersiniosum recurrence, are of great interest.

P38

New immunomodulatory treatment of Crohn's disease after surgical intervention in adolescence: case report

M. POLGÁR, I. GALÁNAI and F. FEKETE

Madarász Children's Hospital Budapest, Hungary

INTRODUCTION

Numerous epidemiological studies have reported an increasing incidence of Crohn's disease (CD) in most European countries. Improvements in socioeconomic levels and diffusion of the modern lifestyle influence the rising incidence of CD. In recent years the incidence of CD has increased in children and adolescents. This indicates the importance, for the paediatrician, of considering this illness more often. The early recognition of CD has great importance because short- and long-term prognosis depends on time from appearance of the symptoms to diagnosis. In respect of the course of CD, the location of the disease, the severity of the symptoms, the complications, the response to medical therapy, and the age at onset are also important. In childhood, in prepuberty and in adolescence treatment is difficult because of the risk of side-effects of the drugs used, which retard growth and sexual maturation of patients[1].

We here present two cases from our practice in which surgical intervention preceded the recognition of CD. Severe conditions evolved in the patients which made it necessary to look for a new therapy. In the course of the therapy in one patient cyclosporine was given for closure of fistulas. In the other patient somatostatin has been used, and after the failure of this treatment infliximab (anti-TNF-α antibody) was introduced. We report our clinical experience with various immunomodulatory drugs.

CASE 1

Diagnosis

Morbus Crohn, abscesses regio ileopsoas, fistula stercoral. Sepsis, shock. St. post. resectionem intestini ileocoecalis.

First admission

D.P., a 14-year-old boy, had experienced diarrhoea, weight loss and anaemia over a period of some months. He was admitted to the Children's Hospital. After the 4th day of his hospitalization acute phlegmonous appendicitis developed, and he was operated upon. Histological examination of the biopsy and inflammation of the terminal ileum proved the former suspicion of CD. Inflammatory markers were raised: erythrocyte sedimentation rate: 80 mm/h, C-reactive protein: 253 mg/L, full white blood cell count: 19.7 g/L, band count: 20%, neutrophil granulocyte: 58%, eosinophil: 4%, lymphocyte: 11%, monocyte: 7%, blood cell count: 5.09 T/L, haemoglobin: 8.0 mg/dl, PLT: 600 g/L. Severe iron deficiency and hypoproteinaemia were also detected. He was treated by intravenous steroid, 5-ASA, metronidazole, ciprofloxacin and received total parenteral nutrition (TPN), with vitamin supplementation; after some days an elementary diet was introduced. The condition of the patient improved, activity signs of CD returned to normal, and he was released.

Second admission, 2 months later

The patient was again admitted to hospital because of fever and increasing pain in the right hip. Laboratory data showed signs of sepsis. CT, MRI and selective enterography showed some abscesses and fistulas connected with each other and with the ileo-caecal region and duodenum. The treatment was surgical – drainage of abscesses and antibiotics. For closing the multiplex fistulas it was decided to give cyclosporine intravenously 5 mg/kg per day. Parenteral nutrition with vitamin supplementation was again introduced.

After transient improvement (1 month) the condition of the patient has again worsened. At this time the CT showed no change of size or extent of abscesses and the activity index increased. Extended surgical intervention and permanent drainage were again introduced and antibiotic combinations were given according to the antibiogram. The condition of the patient improved, the abscesses healed, cyclosporine treatment was ended, and the steroid dose was decreased. At this point it was decided to operate, because of entero-enteral fistulas.

The elective operation was made 4 months after the diagnosis of CD. Ablation of the terminal ileum, the caecum and the short part of the ascending colon was performed. Ileocolic anastomosis was also performed.

After surgical intervention a severe postoperative condition developed. The condition of the patient got dramatically worse: fever, hypotension, oligoanuria, and cardiomegaly appeared. He received intensive therapy, a water–electrolyte imbalance was corrected and antibiotic treatment was changed.

The nutrition was all-in-one TPN. After stabilization of the patient's condition, oral nutrition was gradually introduced. The steroid dose was slowly decreased and 5-ASA was maintained.

In the course of the cardiological echographic control thrombus was found on the chords in the heart without clinical symptoms. The cardiological opinion was that the thrombus showed no danger of emboli. No intervention was needed.

1 month later

The patient was released home in good general condition. He had gained about 10 kg in body weight since the operation. He does hygienic gymnastics for rehabilitation. It was proposed to take, for maintenance, mesalazine 2.0 g/day and 6-mercaptopurine 50 mg/day.

Present condition

In the past 3 years the boy has shown no relapse with the above therapy. The laboratory findings were: erythrocyte sedimentation rate: 3 mm/h, C-reactive protein: 7.83 mg/L, full white blood cell count: 7.2 g/L, neutrophil granulocyte: 61.3%, eosinophil: 2.64%, lymphocyte: 28.5%, monocyte: 7.1%, blood cell count: 5.09 T/L, haemoglobin: 14.5 mg/dl, PLT: 244 g/L. The iron deficiency is very moderate, and hypoproteinaemia is no longer. He has gained body weight, and his height and sexual maturation are normal.

CASE 2

Diagnosis

Morbus Crohn. St. post-appendectomy. Ileo-caecal resection. Fistula enterocutan. Suppuration of the sutures.

First admission

B.M., a 15-year-old boy, had CD at the time of diagnosis. In the anamnese of the young boy abdominal discomfort had been felt for 1 month.

The patient was admitted to surgery with fever and acute abdominal pain. The localization and symptoms corresponded to phlegmonous appendicitis. Ultrasonography showed periumbilical thickened small bowel with extraluminal fluid. Appendectomy was performed. During the course of the operation conglomeratum of the ileum was found with intramesenterial abscess, then the operation was broadened and ileocaecal resection was carried out. The *in-situ* findings and histology proved the diagnosis of CD. In the postoperative period the patient had lost weight and suffered from enteritis.

At 20 days after the operation

The patient was admitted to the department of gastroenterology. At physical examination a palpable abdominal mass was detected in the ileocaecal region.

Ultrasonography, CT and selective enterography showed more abscesses in the cicatrice of the operation, and an enterocutaneous fistula soon developed. Laboratory data also proved the activity of CD. The findings were: erythrocyte sedimentation rate: 40 mm/h, C-reactive protein: 62.6 mg/L, full white blood cell: 16.0 g/L, band count: 7%, neutrophil granulocyte: 69%, lymphocyte: 19%, monocyte: 3%, plasma cell: 2.0%, blood cell count: 4.89 T/L, haemoglobin: 11.0 mg/dl, PLT: 550 g/L. Severe iron deficiency (2.2 μmol/L) was also shown. The suppuration was drained, antibiotics (metronidazole, ciprofloxacin, cefotaxim, netromycin, meropenem) were applied and, as basic therapy, 5-ASA 3.0 g/day steroid was given. Azathioprine 50 mg/day was also introduced. After temporary improvement a large quantity of intestinal fluid again drained through the fistula.

We attempted to close the fistula by using intravenous somatostatin. Therapy was completed by TPN for 3 days in 6 mg/day doses, and for a further 4 days at 3 mg/day. The loss of small bowel fluid decreased but did not cease completely. The activity of the CD was low, but suppuration in the suture was permanent and the fistula was again opened to a great extent. The patient had to use a colostomy bag, which significantly worsened his quality of life.

At 3 months after the appendectomy infliximab was introduced (anti-TNF-α antibody treatment). This was given 5 mg/kg per dose, three times. The second treatment was given 2 weeks after the first one, and the third one at 6 weeks after the start of treatment. After the first administration of the drug the fistula had already healed. No side-effects were observed.

Present condition

The patient is in good general condition, he has gained body weight and laboratory findings were normal except for iron deficiency. The data are: erythrocyte sedimentation rate: 5 mm/h, C-reactive protein: 12 mg/L, full white blood cell 8.2g/L, neutrophil granulocyte: 56.%, lymphocyte: 34%, monocyte: 6%, eosinophil: 2.0%, blood cell count: 4.75 T/L, haemoglobin: 14.3 mg/dl, PLT: 251 g/L. Iron concentration normalized at 10.8 μmol/L. The present medication for admittance is 5-ASA, azathioprine, vitamins and trace element supplementation.

DISCUSSION

In this report our two presented cases were misdiagnosed at an early phase of the illness. On the basis of symptoms, such as fever and right-side abdominal pain, appendicitis was diagnosed and both patients were operated upon. It is observed that surgical intervention increases the risk of early and severe complications and a second operation often follows the first one[2,3]. Both cases had a number of risk factors of clinical recurrence. Both children were operated by CD with perforation. They showed some ileal involvement and an end-to-end anastomosis was performed. In both cases the operation worsened the course of the illness. A short time after the operation abscesses and fistulas appeared. On the basis of our experience our aim was to draw attention to the importance of early recognition of CD, and to the risk of unsuitable surgical intervention. On the other hand, we wanted to demonstrate the effect of the immunomodulatory treatment, especially the experience with applied anti-cytokine treatment in fistulizing CD.

In our first case the conventional treatment was not successful; therefore intravenous cyclosporine was applied for the closure of entero-entero and entero-ileal fistula[4,5]. Closure of the fistula had not been successful, so surgical intervention was needed. For admittance to prevent the risk of relapse immunomodulatory 6-mercaptopurine treatment was proposed[6–10].

The second patient had already been admitted with fistulas after the perioperative period. For this reason the treatment had to focus on both closure of the fistula and basic treatment of the active CD. For basic medication 5-ASA, steroids, and initiating azathioprine were given as prophylaxis[6,11]. For the closure of the fistula somatostatin was tried without success. However, there are reports that somatostatin with antisecretory properties and TPN can be potentially useful in reducing fistula output[12,13]. Spontaneously enterocutaneous stoma appeared, and through the stoma a very large quantity (800–900 ml/day) of intestinal fluid was lost. In this very severe condition it was decided to try new anticytokine treatment. In recent years several proinflammatory cytokines have been involved in the pathogenesis of inflammatory bowel diseases. A significant role has been given to tumour necrosis factor alpha (TNF-α) in CD. This has a fundamental role in formation of granuloma in CD, and there is a high level of TNF-α in the intestinal mucosa and stools of IBD patients[14,15]. Controlled trials have shown the effectiveness of anti-TNF-α antibody treatment in CD[16]. Based on the published data it was decided to use anti-TNF-α antibody (infliximab) for closure of the enterocutaneous fistula in the second case. A positive result was achieved. Disappearance of the fistula promoted a better quality of life for the adolescent patient, and improved his chances for the course of the illness.

There were some difficulties with the paediatric use of infliximab, such as the high price and lack of official permission for use in this age group. Consequently we had to obtain Ethical Committee and parental consent, and agreement regarding social insurance to use the drug in our clinical practice.

In the treatment of CD childhood and adolescence are very delicate ages. It is considered that the treatment of CD by infliximab (Remicade) was effective for the closure of fistulas. The new drug is quite promising, but it needs more experience to know whether it fulfils expectations.

An additional aim was to avoid relapses of CD. Some studies have reported that administration of 6-mercaptopurine and azathioprine is effective in a large majority of patients to prevent relapses without steroids, promising better growth, somatic development and better quality of life[6–8]. Especially favourable effects were found with application of 6-mercaptopurine in the perioperative state[17]. On this basis both patients were treated with immunomodulatory drugs (azathioprine, 6-mercaptopurine) for maintenance. The administration of immunomodulatory drugs has not shown any side-effects over 3 years. Patients do not need steroids. Pancreatic disorders have not appeared, and the number of infectious diseases has not increased. Growth, general condition, and sexual development of both patients are normal.

References

1. Kirschner BS. Ulcerative colitis and Crohn's disease in children. Diagnosis and management Gastroenterol Clin N Am. 1995;24:99–117.

2. Whelan G, Farmer RG, Fazio VW. Recurrence after surgery in Crohn disease. Gastroenterology. 1985;88:1826–33.
3. Williams JG, Wong WD, Rothenberger D, Goldberg A. Recurrence of Crohn's disease after resection. Br J Surg. 1991;78:10–19.
4. Grand RJ, Ramakrishna J, Calneda KA. Therapeutic strategies for pediatric Crohn disease. Clin Ivest Med. 1996;19:373–80.
5. Hanauer ST, Smith MB. Rapid closure of Crohn's disease fistulas with continuous intravenous cyclosporin A. Am J Gastroenterol. 1993;88:646–9.
6. Kader HA, Raynor SC, Young R *et al.* Introduction of 6-mercaptopurine in Crohn's disease patients during the perioperative period: a preliminary evaluation of recurrence of disease. J Pediatr Gastroenterol Nutr. 1997;25:93–7.
7. Bousvaros A. Preventing relapse after surgery for Crohn's disease: Where do we go from here? J Pediatr Gastroenterol Nutr. 1997;25:114–15.
8. Kirschner BS. Safety of azathioprine and 6-mercaptopurine in paediatric patients with inflammatory bowel disease. Gastroenterology. 1998;115:813–21.
9. Markowitz J, Rosa J, Grancher K *et al.* Long-term 6-mercaptopurine treatment in adolescents with Crohn's diasease. Gastroenterology. 1990;99:1347.
10. Verhave M, Winter HS, Grand RJ. Azathioprine in the treatment of children with inflammatory bowel disease. J Pediatr. 1990;117:809–14.
11. Chehake M, Benkov K. A multicenter trial of 6-mercaptopurine and prednisone in children with newly diagnosed Crohn disease. J Pediatr Gastroenterol Nutr. 2001;32:120–1.
12. Ysebaert D, Van Hee R, Hubens G *et al.* Management of digestive fistulas. Scand J Gastroenterol. 1994;29:42–4.
13. Ysebaert D *et al.* Treatment of postoperative pancreatic and enterocutaneous fistulae with total parenteral nutrition and somatostatin. Br J Surg. 1992;79(Suppl.).
14. Targan SR, Rutgeerts P, Hanauer SB *et al.* A multicenter trial of anti-tumor necrosis factor antibody (cA2) for treatment of patients with active Crohn disease. Gastroenterology. 1996;110:A1026.
15. Stack WA, Mann SD, Roy AJ *et al.* Randomly controlled trial of CDP571 antibody to tumor necrosis factor in Crohn disease. Lancet. 1997;340:521–4.
16. Kohen RD, Tsang JF, Hanauer SB. Infliximab in Crohn's disease. First anniversery clinical experience. Am J Gastroenterol. 2000;95:3469–77.
17. Mc Lain BI, Davidson PM, Stokes KB *et al.* Growth after gut resection for Crohn's disease. Arch Dis Child. 1990;65:760.

Index

Falk Symposium Series

43. Reutter W, Popper H, Arias IM, Heinrich PC, Keppler D, Landmann L, eds.: *Modulation of Liver Cell Expression*. Falk Symposium No. 43. 1987 ISBN: 0-85200-677-2*
44. Boyer JL, Bianchi L, eds.: *Liver Cirrhosis*. Falk Symposium No. 44. 1987 ISBN: 0-85200-993-3*
45. Paumgartner G, Stiehl A, Gerok W, eds.: *Bile Acids and the Liver*. Falk Symposium No. 45. 1987 ISBN: 0-85200-675-6*
46. Goebell H, Peskar BM, Malchow H, eds.: *Inflammatory Bowel Diseases – Basic Research & Clinical Implications*. Falk Symposium No. 46. 1988 ISBN: 0-7462-0067-6*
47. Bianchi L, Holt P, James OFW, Butler RN, eds.: *Aging in Liver and Gastrointestinal Tract*. Falk Symposium No. 47. 1988 ISBN: 0-7462-0066-8*
48. Heilmann C, ed.: *Calcium-Dependent Processes in the Liver*. Falk Symposium No. 48. 1988 ISBN: 0-7462-0075-7*
50. Singer MV, Goebell H, eds.: *Nerves and the Gastrointestinal Tract*. Falk Symposium No. 50. 1989 ISBN: 0-7462-0114-1
51. Bannasch P, Keppler D, Weber G, eds.: *Liver Cell Carcinoma*. Falk Symposium No. 51. 1989 ISBN: 0-7462-0111-7
52. Paumgartner G, Stiehl A, Gerok W, eds.: *Trends in Bile Acid Research*. Falk Symposium No. 52. 1989 ISBN: 0-7462-0112-5
53. Paumgartner G, Stiehl A, Barbara L, Roda E, eds.: *Strategies for the Treatment of Hepatobiliary Diseases*. Falk Symposium No. 53. 1990 ISBN: 0-7923-8903-4
54. Bianchi L, Gerok W, Maier K-P, Deinhardt F, eds.: *Infectious Diseases of the Liver*. Falk Symposium No. 54. 1990 ISBN: 0-7923-8902-6
55. Falk Symposium No. 55 not published

55B. Hadziselimovic F, Herzog B, Bürgin-Wolff A, eds.: *Inflammatory Bowel Disease and Coeliac Disease in Children*. International Falk Symposium. 1990 ISBN 0-7462-0125-7

56. Williams CN, eds.: *Trends in Inflammatory Bowel Disease Therapy*. Falk Symposium No. 56. 1990 ISBN: 0-7923-8952-2
57. Bock KW, Gerok W, Matern S, Schmid R, eds.: *Hepatic Metabolism and Disposition of Endo- and Xenobiotics*. Falk Symposium No. 57. 1991 ISBN: 0-7923-8953-0
58. Paumgartner G, Stiehl A, Gerok W, eds.: *Bile Acids as Therapeutic Agents: From Basic Science to Clinical Practice*. Falk Symposium No. 58. 1991 ISBN: 0-7923-8954-9
59. Halter F, Garner A, Tytgat GNJ, eds.: *Mechanisms of Peptic Ulcer Healing*. Falk Symposium No. 59. 1991 ISBN: 0-7923-8955-7
60. Goebell H, Ewe K, Malchow H, Koelbel Ch, eds.: *Inflammatory Bowel Diseases – Progress in Basic Research and Clinical Implications*. Falk Symposium No. 60. 1991 ISBN: 0-7923-8956-5
61. Falk Symposium No. 61 not published
62. Dowling RH, Folsch UR, Löser Ch, eds.: *Polyamines in the Gastrointestinal Tract*. Falk Symposium No. 62. 1992 ISBN: 0-7923-8976-X
63. Lentze MJ, Reichen J, eds.: *Paediatric Cholestasis: Novel Approaches to Treatment*. Falk Symposium No. 63. 1992 ISBN: 0-7923-8977-8
64. Demling L, Frühmorgen P, eds.: *Non-Neoplastic Diseases of the Anorectum*. Falk Symposium No. 64. 1992 ISBN: 0-7923-8979-4

64B. Gressner AM, Ramadori G, eds.: *Molecular and Cell Biology of Liver Fibrogenesis*. International Falk Symposium. 1992 ISBN: 0-7923-8980-8

*These titles were published under the MTP Press imprint.

Falk Symposium Series

65. Hadziselimovic F, Herzog B, eds.: *Inflammatory Bowel Diseases and Morbus Hirschprung*. Falk Symposium No. 65. 1992 ISBN: 0-7923-8995-6
66. Martin F, McLeod RS, Sutherland LR, Williams CN, eds.: *Trends in Inflammatory Bowel Disease Therapy*. Falk Symposium No. 66. 1993 ISBN: 0-7923-8827-5
67. Schölmerich J, Kruis W, Goebell H, Hohenberger W, Gross V, eds.: *Inflammatory Bowel Diseases – Pathophysiology as Basis of Treatment*. Falk Symposium No. 67. 1993 ISBN: 0-7923-8996-4
68. Paumgartner G, Stiehl A, Gerok W, eds.: *Bile Acids and The Hepatobiliary System: From Basic Science to Clinical Practice*. Falk Symposium No. 68. 1993 ISBN: 0-7923-8829-1
69. Schmid R, Bianchi L, Gerok W, Maier K-P, eds.: *Extrahepatic Manifestations in Liver Diseases*. Falk Symposium No. 69. 1993 ISBN: 0-7923-8821-6
70. Meyer zum Büschenfelde K-H, Hoofnagle J, Manns M, eds.: *Immunology and Liver*. Falk Symposium No. 70. 1993 ISBN: 0-7923-8830-5
71. Surrenti C, Casini A, Milani S, Pinzani M , eds.: *Fat-Storing Cells and Liver Fibrosis*. Falk Symposium No. 71. 1994 ISBN: 0-7923-8842-9
72. Rachmilewitz D, ed.: *Inflammatory Bowel Diseases – 1994*. Falk Symposium No. 72. 1994 ISBN: 0-7923-8845-3
73. Binder HJ, Cummings J, Soergel KH, eds.: *Short Chain Fatty Acids*. Falk Symposium No. 73. 1994 ISBN: 0-7923-8849-6

73B. Möllmann HW, May B, eds.: *Glucocorticoid Therapy in Chronic Inflammatory Bowel Disease: from basic principles to rational therapy*. International Falk Workshop. 1996 ISBN 0-7923-8708-2

74. Keppler D, Jungermann K, eds.: *Transport in the Liver*. Falk Symposium No. 74. 1994 ISBN: 0-7923-8858-5

74B. Stange EF, ed.: *Chronic Inflammatory Bowel Disease*. Falk Symposium. 1995 ISBN: 0-7923-8876-3

75. van Berge Henegouwen GP, van Hoek B, De Groote J, Matern S, Stockbrügger RW, eds.: *Cholestatic Liver Diseases: New Strategies for Prevention and Treatment of Hepatobiliary and Cholestatic Liver Diseases*. Falk Symposium 75. 1994. ISBN: 0-7923-8867-4
76. Monteiro E, Tavarela Veloso F, eds.: *Inflammatory Bowel Diseases: New Insights into Mechanisms of Inflammation and Challenges in Diagnosis and Treatment*. Falk Symposium 76. 1995. ISBN 0-7923-8884-4
77. Singer MV, Ziegler R, Rohr G, eds.: *Gastrointestinal Tract and Endocrine System*. Falk Symposium 77. 1995. ISBN 0-7923-8877-1
78. Decker K, Gerok W, Andus T, Gross V, eds.: *Cytokines and the Liver*. Falk Symposium 78. 1995. ISBN 0-7923-8878-X
79. Holstege A, Schölmerich J, Hahn EG, eds.: *Portal Hypertension*. Falk Symposium 79. 1995. ISBN 0-7923-8879-8
80. Hofmann AF, Paumgartner G, Stiehl A, eds.: *Bile Acids in Gastroenterology: Basic and Clinical Aspects*. Falk Symposium 80. 1995 ISBN 0-7923-8880-1
81. Riecken EO, Stallmach A, Zeitz M, Heise W, eds.: *Malignancy and Chronic Inflammation in the Gastrointestinal Tract – New Concepts*. Falk Symposium 81. 1995 ISBN 0-7923-8889-5
82. Fleig WE, ed.: *Inflammatory Bowel Diseases: New Developments and Standards*. Falk Symposium 82. 1995 ISBN 0-7923-8890-6

82B. Paumgartner G, Beuers U, eds.: *Bile Acids in Liver Diseases.* International Falk Workshop. 1995 ISBN 0-7923-8891-7

83. Dobrilla G, Felder M, de Pretis G, eds.: *Advances in Hepatobiliary and Pancreatic Diseases: Special Clinical Topics.* Falk Symposium 83. 1995. ISBN 0-7923-8892-5

84. Fromm H, Leuschner U, eds.: *Bile Acids – Cholestasis – Gallstones: Advances in Basic and Clinical Bile Acid Research.* Falk Symposium 84. 1995 ISBN 0-7923-8893-3

85. Tytgat GNJ, Bartelsman JFWM, van Deventer SJH, eds.: *Inflammatory Bowel Diseases.* Falk Symposium 85. 1995 ISBN 0-7923-8894-1

86. Berg PA, Leuschner U, eds.: *Bile Acids and Immunology.* Falk Symposium 86. 1996 ISBN 0-7923-8700-7

87. Schmid R, Bianchi L, Blum HE, Gerok W, Maier KP, Stalder GA, eds.: *Acute and Chronic Liver Diseases: Molecular Biology and Clinics.* Falk Symposium 87. 1996 ISBN 0-7923-8701-5

88. Blum HE, Wu GY, Wu CH, eds.: *Molecular Diagnosis and Gene Therapy.* Falk Symposium 88. 1996 ISBN 0-7923-8702-3

88B. Poupon RE, Reichen J, eds.: *Surrogate Markers to Assess Efficacy of TReatment in Chronic Liver Diseases.* International Falk Workshop. 1996 ISBN 0-7923-8705-8

89. Reyes HB, Leuschner U, Arias IM, eds.: *Pregnancy, Sex Hormones and the Liver.* Falk Symposium 89. 1996 ISBN 0-7923-8704-X

89B. Broelsch CE, Burdelski M, Rogiers X, eds.: *Cholestatic Liver Diseases in Children and Adults.* International Falk Workshop. 1996 ISBN 0-7923-8710-4

90. Lam S-K, Paumgartner P, Wang B, eds.: *Update on Hepatobiliary Diseases 1996.* Falk Symposium 90. 1996 ISBN 0-7923-8715-5

91. Hadziselimovic F, Herzog B, eds.: *Inflammatory Bowel Diseases and Chronic Recurrent Abdominal Pain.* Falk Symposium 91. 1996 ISBN 0-7923-8722-8

91B. Alvaro D, Benedetti A, Strazzabosco M, eds.: *Vanishing Bile Duct Syndrome – Pathophysiology and Treatment.* International Falk Workshop. 1996 ISBN 0-7923-8721-X

92. Gerok W, Loginov AS, Pokrowskij VI, eds.: *New Trends in Hepatology 1996.* Falk Symposium 92. 1997 ISBN 0-7923-8723-6

93. Paumgartner G, Stiehl A, Gerok W, eds.: *Bile Acids in Hepatobiliary Diseases – Basic Research and Clinical Application.* Falk Symposium 93. 1997 ISBN 0-7923-8725-2

94. Halter F, Winton D, Wright NA, eds.: *The Gut as a Model in Cell and Molecular Biology.* Falk Symposium 94. 1997 ISBN 0-7923-8726-0

94B. Kruse-Jarres JD, Schölmerich J, eds.: *Zinc and Diseases of the Digestive Tract.* International Falk Workshop. 1997 ISBN 0-7923-8724-4

95. Ewe K, Eckardt VF, Enck P, eds.: *Constipation and Anorectal Insufficiency.* Falk Symposium 95. 1997 ISBN 0-7923-8727-9

96. Andus T, Goebell H, Layer P, Schölmerich J, eds.: *Inflammatory Bowel Disease – from Bench to Bedside.* Falk Symposium 96. 1997 ISBN 0-7923-8728-7

97. Campieri M, Bianchi-Porro G, Fiocchi C, Schölmerich J, eds. *Clinical Challenges in Inflammatory Bowel Diseases: Diagnosis, Prognosis and Treatment.* Falk Symposium 97. 1998 ISBN 0-7923-8733-3

98. Lembcke B, Kruis W, Sartor RB, eds. *Systemic Manifestations of IBD: The Pending Challenge for Subtle Diagnosis and Treatment.* Falk Symposium 98. 1998 ISBN 0-7923-8734-1

99. Goebell H, Holtmann G, Talley NJ, eds. *Functional Dyspepsia and Irritable Bowel Syndrome: Concepts and Controversies.* Falk Symposium 99. 1998 ISBN 0-7923-8735-X
100. Blum HE, Bode Ch, Bode JCh, Sartor RB, eds. *Gut and the Liver.* Falk Symposium 100. 1998 ISBN 0-7923-8736-8
101. Rachmilewitz D, ed. *V International Symposium on Inflammatory Bowel Diseases.* Falk Symposium 101. 1998 ISBN 0-7923-8743-0
102. Manns MP, Boyer JL, Jansen PLM, Reichen J, eds. *Cholestatic Liver Diseases.* Falk Symposium 102. 1998 ISBN 0-7923-8746-5
102B. Manns MP, Chapman RW, Stiehl A, Wiesner R, eds. *Primary Sclerosing Cholangitis.* International Falk Workshop. 1998. ISBN 0-7923-8745-7
103. Häussinger D, Jungermann K, eds. *Liver and Nervous System.* Falk Symposium 102. 1998 ISBN 0-7924-8742-2
103B. Häussinger D, Heinrich PC, eds. *Signalling in the Liver.* International Falk Workshop. 1998 ISBN 0-7923-8744-9
103C. Fleig W, ed. *Normal and Malignant Liver Cell Growth.* International Falk Workshop. 1998 ISBN 0-7923-8748-1
104. Stallmach A, Zeitz M, Strober W, MacDonald TT, Lochs H, eds. *Induction and Modulation of Gastrointestinal Inflammation.* Falk Symposium 104. 1998 ISBN 0-7923-8747-3
105. Emmrich J, Liebe S, Stange EF, eds. *Innovative Concepts in Inflammatory Bowel Diseases.* Falk Symposium 105. 1999 ISBN 0-7923-8749-X
106. Rutgeerts P, Colombel J-F, Hanauer SB, Schölmerich J, Tytgat GNJ, van Gossum A, eds. *Advances in Inflammatory Bowel Diseases.* Falk Symposium 106. 1999 ISBN 0-7923-8750-3
107. Špičák J, Boyer J, Gilat T, Kotrlik K, Mareček Z, Paumgartner G, eds. *Diseases of the Liver and the Bile Ducts – New Aspects and Clinical Implications.* Falk Symposium 107. 1999 ISBN 0-7923-8751-1
108. Paumgartner G, Stiehl A, Gerok W, Keppler D, Leuschner U, eds. *Bile Acids and Cholestasis.* Falk Symposium 108. 1999 ISBN 0-7923-8752-X
109. Schmiegel W, Schölmerich J, eds. *Colorectal Cancer – Molecular Mechanisms, Premalignant State and its Prevention.* Falk Symposium 109. 1999 ISBN 0-7923-8753-8
110. Domschke W, Stoll R, Brasitus TA, Kagnoff MF, eds. *Intestinal Mucosa and its Diseases – Pathophysiology and Clinics.* Falk Symposium 110. 1999 ISBN 0-7923-8754-6
110B. Northfield TC, Ahmed HA, Jazwari RP, Zentler-Munro PL, eds. *Bile Acids in Hepatobiliary Disease.* Falk Workshop. 2000 ISBN 0-7923-8755-4
111. Rogler G, Kullmann F, Rutgeerts P, Sartor RB, Schölmerich J, eds. *IBD at the End of its First Century.* Falk Symposium 111. 2000 ISBN 0-7923-8756-2
112. Krammer HJ, Singer MV, eds. *Neurogastroenterology: From the Basics to the Clinics.* Falk Symposium 112. 2000 ISBN 0-7923-8757-0
113. Andus T, Rogler G, Schlottmann K, Frick E, Adler G, Schmiegel W, Zeitz M, Schölmerich J, eds. *Cytokines and Cell Homeostasis in the Gastrointestinal Tract.* Falk Symposium 113. 2000 ISBN 0-7923-8758-9
114. Manns MP, Paumgartner G, Leuschner U, eds. *Immunology and Liver.* Falk Symposium 114. 2000 ISBN 0-7923-8759-7

Falk Symposium Series

115. Boyer JL, Blum HE, Maier K-P, Sauerbruch T, Stalder GA, eds. *Liver Cirrhosis and its Development.* Falk Symposium 115. 2000 ISBN 0-7923-8760-0
116. Riemann JF, Neuhaus H, eds. *Interventional Endoscopy in Hepatology.* Falk Symposium 116. 2000 ISBN 0-7923-8761-9
116A. Dienes HP, Schirmacher P, Brechot C, Okuda K, eds. *Chronic Hepatitis: New Concepts of Pathogenesis, Diagnosis and Treatment.* Falk Workshop. 2000 ISBN 0-7923-8763-5
117. Gerbes AL, Beuers U, Jüngst D, Pape GR, Sackmann M, Sauerbruch T, eds. *Hepatology 2000 – Symposium in Honour of Gustav Paumgartner.* Falk Symposium 117. 2000 ISBN 0-7923-8765-1
117A. Acalovschi M, Paumgartner G, eds. *Hepatobiliary Diseases: Cholestasis and Gallstones.* Falk Workshop. 2000 ISBN 0-7923-8770-8
118. Frühmorgen P, Bruch H-P, eds. *Non-Neoplastic Diseases of the Anorectum.* Falk Symposium 118. 2001 ISBN 0-7923-8766-X
119. Fellermann K, Jewell DP, Sandborn WJ, Schölmerich J, Stange EF, eds. *Immunosuppression in Inflammatory Bowel Diseases – Standards, New Developments, Future Trends.* Falk Symposium 119. 2001 ISBN 0-7923-8767-8
120. van Berge Henegouwen GP, Keppler D, Leuschner U, Paumgartner G, Stiehl A, eds. *Biology of Bile Acids in Health and Disease.* Falk Symposium 120. 2001 ISBN 0-7923-8768-6
121. Leuschner U, James OFW, Dancygier H, eds. *Steatohepatitis (NASH and ASH).* Falk Symposium 121. 2001 ISBN 0-7923-8769-4
121A. Matern S, Boyer JL, Keppler D, Meier-Abt PJ, eds. *Hepatobiliary Transport: From Bench to Bedside.* Falk Workshop. 2001 ISBN 0-7923-8771-6
122. Campieri M, Fiocchi C, Hanauer SB, Jewell DP, Rachmilewitz R, Schölmerich J, eds. *Inflammatory Bowel Disease – A Clinical Case Approach to Pathophysiology, Diagnosis, and Treatment.* Falk Symposium 122. 2002 ISBN 0-7923-8772-4
123. Rachmilewitz D, Modigliani R, Podolsky DK, Sachar DB, Tozun N, eds. *VI International Symposium on Inflammatory Bowel Diseases.* Falk Symposium 123. 2002 ISBN 0-7923-8773-2
124. Hagenmüller F, Manns MP, Musmann H-G, Riemann JF, eds. *Medical Imaging in Gastroenterology and Hepatology.* Falk Symposium 124. 2002 ISBN 0-7923-8774-0
125. Gressner AM, Heinrich PC, Matern S, eds. *Cytokines in Liver Injury and Repair.* Falk Symposium 125. 2002 ISBN 0-7923-8775-9
126. Gupta S, Jansen PLM, Klempnauer J, Manns MP, eds. *Hepatocyte Transplantation.* Falk Symposium 126. 2002 ISBN 0-7923-8776-7
127. Hadziselimovic F, ed. *Autoimmune Diseases in Paediatric Gastroenterology.* Falk Symposium 127. 2002 ISBN 0-7923-8778-3

www.ingramcontent.com/pod-product-compliance
Lightning Source LLC
Chambersburg PA
CBHW060743150926
51501CB00003B/76
* 9 7 8 0 7 9 2 3 8 7 7 8 7 *